UNCOVERING
THE SCIENCE OF
COVID-19

UNCOVERING
THE SCIENCE OF
COVID-19

Vincent T K Chow
National University of Singapore, Singapore

Sunil K Lal
Monash University Malaysia, Malaysia

World Scientific

NEW JERSEY · LONDON · SINGAPORE · BEIJING · SHANGHAI · HONG KONG · TAIPEI · CHENNAI · TOKYO

Published by

World Scientific Publishing Co. Pte. Ltd.
5 Toh Tuck Link, Singapore 596224
USA office: 27 Warren Street, Suite 401-402, Hackensack, NJ 07601
UK office: 57 Shelton Street, Covent Garden, London WC2H 9HE

Library of Congress Cataloging-in-Publication Data
Names: Chow, Vincent T. K. (Vincent Tak-Kwong), 1958–   editor. | Lal, Sunil K., editor.
Title: Uncovering the science of COVID-19 / [edited by] Vincent T K Chow,
    National University of Singapore, Singapore; Sunil K Lal, Monash University Malaysia, Malaysia.
Description: New Jersey : World Scientific, [2023] | Includes bibliographical references and index.
Identifiers: LCCN 2022006825 | ISBN 9789811254321 (hardcover) |
    ISBN 9789811254338 (ebook for institutions) | ISBN 9789811254345 (ebook for individuals)
Subjects: MESH: SARS-CoV-2 | COVID-19
Classification: LCC RA644.C67 | NLM QW 168.5.C8 | DDC 616.2/414--dc23/eng/20220412
LC record available at https://lccn.loc.gov/2022006825

British Library Cataloguing-in-Publication Data
A catalogue record for this book is available from the British Library.

For any available supplementary material, please visit
https://www.worldscientific.com/worldscibooks/10.1142/12779#t=suppl

Desk Editors: Soundararajan Raghuraman/Joy Quek

Typeset by Stallion Press
Email: enquiries@stallionpress.com

Dedicated To Our

Loving Families
Talented Colleagues
Persevering Patients
Enthusiastic Students
Steadfast Friends

Foreword

The world has never been more united than it is now. COVID-19 has succeeded where many other multilateral agencies have failed. The SARS-CoV-2 virus has bonded humanity and aligned national interests in a way not seen since the last Great War. As the COVID-19 virus continues to evolve, we are on a global mission to uncover everything about SARS-CoV-2 to strengthen our pandemic responses for future pandemics. This book addresses the molecular biology and evolution of SARS-CoV-2 and the virus–host interactions, and discusses the clinical management, detection technologies, transmission dynamics, and public health efforts to stem the onslaught of COVID-19. The chapters in *Uncovering the Science of COVID-19* have been contributed by health experts and scientists from around the world, who have contributed their experiences and expertise freely to tackle the challenges of this unprecedented pandemic, and to ameliorate the impact of the ones to come.

Since the COVID-19 pandemic struck in early 2020, it has become clear that we are never going back to our pre-pandemic lives. Everything that we have been accustomed to has changed for better or worse. As we pick ourselves up from the ravages of this catastrophe and move into a phase of recovery, it is clear that the COVID-19 pandemic and its aftermath will continue to cause disruptions to our lives, livelihoods, and ways of life. COVID-19 will continue to be a constant companion as we move on, lurking in the recesses of our memories. To be caught unaware and unprepared again would be unforgiveable. It is imperative that we analyze our mistakes and come up with strategies that will better prepare us to cope with future outbreaks. This book also seeks to examine our pandemic responses and derive lessons for future psychological preparedness, crisis management, and adaptability.

I hope this book will be a useful resource for understanding the scientific basis of COVID-19 and the quick decisions that had to be implemented at the peak of the pandemic. Most importantly, I hope readers will use this book as a tool for self-reflection, and as an avenue for more internal and public discussions to take place to influence collective and constructive efforts that would allow us to emerge stronger in anticipation of future public health crises. Let's not be caught out again.

Stay safe and healthy,

Chong Yap Seng
Lien Ying Chow Professor in Medicine
Dean, Yong Loo Lin School of Medicine
National University of Singapore

About the Editors

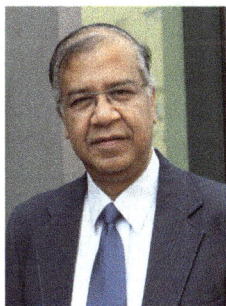

Sunil K. Lal has been at the School of Science, Monash University, Malaysia since 2014. By training, Prof. Sunil is a product of the Georgia Institute of Technology, Atlanta GA (USA) where he earned his PhD in Molecular Virology in 1989. Following this, he was appointed Faculty at the California Institute of Technology, Pasadena (USA). In 1994, Prof. Sunil joined the International Centre for Genetic Engineering & Biotechnology (ICGEB), New Delhi, as a Research Scientist where he worked for 22 years. Professor Sunil is internationally well-known for his research work in the field of RNA viruses including SARS Coronaviruses, Influenza A virus and Hepatitis E virus. Since his primary interests have been focused on emerging viruses in Southeast Asia, he has been a visiting scientist to Universiti Malaysia Sarawak, National University of Singapore, Karolinska Institute, and the Centers for Disease Control (CDC) Atlanta. Professor Sunil has won many prestigious international awards including the Hind Rattan (highest civilian honor from Government of India), and has been the regional representative for the American Society for Microbiology for 9 years, besides being an Elected Fellow of the National Academy of Sciences (India). Professor Sunil is on the editorial board of international journals and is actively involved in peer-reviewing for some of the top-tier scientific journals. He has over 170 publications in international scientific journals, and has published three international books on emerging viral diseases. Currently, Prof. Sunil leads an active research group on Systems Virology of Influenza and Coronaviruses at Monash University, Malaysia.

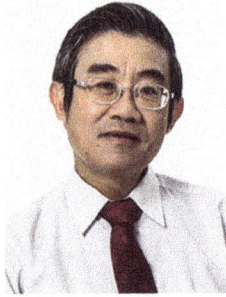

Vincent T. K. Chow is a medical virologist and molecular biologist with the qualifications of MBBS, MD, PhD (Singapore), FRCPath (UK), and MSc (University College London). Dr. Chow has been a faculty member of the National University of Singapore (NUS) since 1984. Currently, he serves as Associate Professor, Education Director of Microbiology and Principal Investigator of the Host and Pathogen Interactivity Laboratory at the Yong Loo Lin School of Medicine, NUS. In 1996, he established the Human Genome Laboratory at NUS that has characterized several novel human genes and proteins of medical significance. He was also a Principal Investigator of the Infectious Diseases Research Program under the Singapore-MIT Alliance for ten years. Dr. Chow previously served as President of the Asia-Pacific Society for Medical Virology, as well as Chair of the Virology Section and Fellow of the International Society of Antimicrobial Chemotherapy. His laboratory has published over 270 articles in international refereed journals, and contributed over 10 book chapters. He has received several awards (including Murex Virologist Award, NUS Special Commendation Award, Faculty Research Excellence Award, Singapore Society of Pathology — Becton Dickinson Award). His research interests have focused on the cellular, molecular and viral pathogenesis of influenza-related pneumonia and enterovirus infections.

Contents

Chapter 1

The Novel SARS-CoV-2: An Overview on its Detection, Prevention and Control

**Anshika Sharma*, Zheng Yao Low*, Sunil K. Lal*,
and Vincent T. K. Chow[†,‡]**

**School of Science, Tropical Medicine and Biology Platform,
Monash University, Bandar Sunway, Selangor, Malaysia*

*†Infectious Diseases Translational Research Program,
Department of Microbiology and Immunology,
Yong Loo Lin School of Medicine, National University Health System,
National University of Singapore, Singapore*

‡micctk@nus.edu.sg

Abstract

On 30 January 2020, the World Health Organization (WHO) character-ized the novel severe acute respiratory syndrome Coronavirus 2 (SARS-CoV-2) outbreak as a Public Health Emergency of International Concern. Subsequently, on 11 March 2020, WHO declared the global spread of Coronavirus disease 2019 (COVID-19) as a pandemic triggered by this causative virus. This COVID-19 pandemic has impacted lives and live-lihoods worldwide, resulting in unprecedented social disruption and economic losses. In order to design and develop effective diagnostics, vaccines and therapeutic interventions against SARS-CoV-2, it is imper-ative to understand the molecular and cellular mechanisms underpinning the complex interactions between this virus, its variants, and its infected hosts. This chapter provides an overview on the classification, genomic organization and evolution of SARS-CoV-2 (including the emergence of variants from Alpha to Omicron), and summarizes existing and emerging testing strategies. With unprecedented speed, an array of conventional and new COVID-19 vaccines has been developed, evaluated in clinical trials, and administered to billions worldwide. Current and novel antiviral drugs and immunomodulatory approaches are discussed for the therapeutic and prophylactic management of SARS-CoV-2 infections. Finally, much remains for humanity to discover and learn as the world must continue to adapt and live with endemic COVID-19 and SARS-CoV-2 evolution.

Keywords: Coronavirus; *Coronaviridae*; bats; SARS-CoV-2; COVID-19; viral evolution; viral variants; diagnostics; RT-PCR; antigen rapid tests; vaccines; spike protein; antiviral drugs; drug repurposing; immunomodulatory agents

1.1. The SARS-CoV-2 Genome Organization and Evolution

The SARS-CoV-2 belongs to the *Coronavirinae* sub-family of the *Coronaviridae* family of viruses (Liu *et al.*, 2020). The *Coronavirinae* sub-family can be further sub-divided into alpha-, beta-, gamma- and delta-Coronaviruses. SARS-CoV-2, along with severe acute Coronavirus syndrome Coronavirus (SARS-CoV) and Middle East respiratory syndrome Coronavirus (MERS-CoV), are classified as beta-Coronaviruses. In recent decades, beta-Coronaviruses have been notorious for causing epidemics of respiratory illness (Pal *et al.*, 2020). The SARS-CoV outbreak occurred in 2002, followed by the MERS-CoV outbreak in 2012. The Coronavirus disease 2019 (COVID-19) pandemic caused by SARS-CoV-2 has resulted in ~280 million confirmed cases, and claimed ~5.5 million lives as of 31 December 2021 (GitHub, 2021).

The SARS-CoV-2 virion is enveloped, with a diameter of about 120–140 nm. The genome organization of SARS-CoV-2 follows the typical structural characteristics of known Coronaviruses, comprising a monopartite, single-stranded, positive-sense RNA of approximately 29.9 kb (Khailany *et al.*, 2020; Lu *et al.*, 2020; Naqvi *et al.*, 2020; Sharma *et al.*, 2021a, 2021b; Zhu *et al.*, 2020). Two-thirds of the genome,

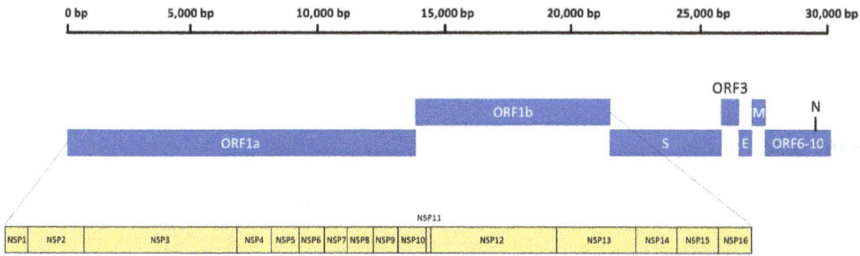

Figure 1.1. Genome organization of SARS-CoV-2.

starting at the 5′ UTR, incorporates the ORF1ab genetic sequence that encodes the polyproteins pp1a and pp1ab. The remaining 3′ one-third region of the SARS-CoV-2 genome encodes the spike (S), envelope (E), membrane (M) and nucleocapsid (N) structural proteins, as well as 9 predicted accessory protein ORFs 3a, 3b, 6, 7a, 7b, 8, 9b, 9c, 10 (Figure 1.1). One study suggested that SARS-CoV-2 expresses only five canonical accessory ORFs 3a, 6, 7a, 7b, 8 (Kim *et al.*, 2020).

High-throughput sequencing of the SARS-CoV-2 genome has facilitated detailed phylogenetic analyses, revealing ~96% identity to the SARS-like bat Coronavirus RaTG13 isolated from Yunnan, China (Zhou *et al.*, 2020). In addition, SARS-CoV-2 shares 88% sequence identity with the bat-SL-CoVZC45, and 87% sequence identity with the bat-SL-CoVZXC21 — thus indicating high genomic close-relatedness to SARS-like bat Coronaviruses. The SARS-CoV-2 whole genome sequence is less genetically similar to SARS-CoV and MERS-CoV, sharing only approximately 79% and 50% identity, respectively (Wang *et al.*, 2020b) (Figure 1.2). At the amino acid level, SARS-CoV-2 proteins share high similarity to SARS-like bat Coronavirus RaTG13, with approximately 95–100% identity. However, it is noteworthy that SARS-CoV-2 encodes for ORF10 which is not documented to be encoded by RaTG13. Moreover, the ORF8 and ORF10 encoded by SARS-CoV-2 are not found to be encoded by SARS-CoV. Although genetically less similar to SARS-CoV compared to SARS-like bat Coronaviruses, SARS-CoV-2 uses the same angiotensin-converting enzyme 2 (ACE2) cell entry receptor as SARS-CoV (Zhou *et al.*, 2020).

Since its initial emergence in late 2019, SARS-CoV-2 has continued to acquire significant mutations (especially within its spike glycoprotein), and has evolved into numerous variants. Indeed, recent virus isolates exhibit

SARS-like coronaviruses: 96.2% identity
to bat RaTG13 collected in Yunnan

SARS-like coronaviruses: 88% identity to
bat-SL-CoVZC45 and bat-SL-CoVZXC21
collected in Zhoushan in 2018

SARS-CoV-2 genomic sequence identity

SARS-CoV (79%)

MERS-CoV (51.8%)

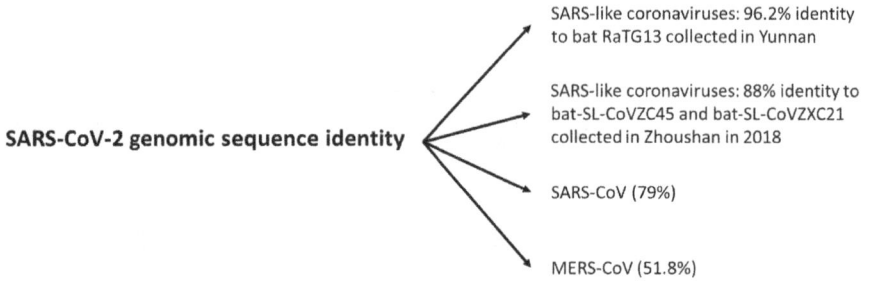

Figure 1.2.   SARS-CoV-2 genomic sequence identity to SARS-like bat Coronaviruses, SARS-CoV, and MERS-CoV.

greater replication efficiency and spread more rapidly among humans, such as the highly transmissible Delta and Omicron variants of concern (VOCs) (Low *et al.*, 2021; Mahase, 2021a; Reardon, 2021).

On 26 November 2021, WHO announced Omicron as the fifth VOC, after the Alpha, Beta, Gamma and Delta VOCs. Omicron is significantly more transmissible than Delta, with a doubling time between 1.5 and 3 days in countries with documented community transmission (Nishiura *et al.*, 2022; WHO, 2021c). Omicron has about 50 mutations, of which 36 are in the spike protein and its receptor-binding domain (RBD) — which confer stronger binding affinity for ACE2 than Delta (Hagen, 2021; Kumar *et al.*, 2022). Experiments using *ex vivo* cultures of human respiratory tract tissues reveal that Omicron replicates about 70-fold more rapidly than Delta and the original SARS-CoV-2 strain in bronchial cells — which may account for Omicron's faster spread. However, the replicative efficiency of Omicron in lung cells is over 10 times less than the other strains, which may suggest lower disease severity (Hui *et al.*, 2022). Modelling studies estimate that the risk of reinfection with Omicron is more than 5-fold greater than that of Delta (Ferguson *et al.*, 2021). Moreover, Omicron can evade prior immunity afforded by both previous infection or immunization with two vaccine doses (Ai *et al.*, 2021; Lu *et al.*, 2021).

1.2. Approach to the Diagnosis and Analysis of SARS-CoV-2 Infection

The approach to the diagnosis of SARS-CoV-2 infection comprises clinical, radiological and laboratory assessments. Clinical assessment entails the evaluation of clinical features such as fever, cough, dyspnea, head-ache, anosmia, and dysgeusia (WHO, 2021a; Wang *et al.*, 2020a; Zanin *et al.*, 2020). In SARS-CoV-2 infection, symptoms may vary between individuals — they may be largely asymptomatic or exhibit mild symptoms upon initial contact. Individuals may have close contact with infected cases, or they may reside within COVID-19 "red zones". Hence, it is important to further evaluate and confirm suspected cases and contacts by diagnostic modalities — which often include lung computerized tomography (CT) imaging as well as various biochemical and specific tests such as nucleic acid amplification tests. It is imperative that individuals seek urgent medical attention if they display the above-mentioned symptoms or in the event of close contact with known COVID-19 cases. The absence or delay in prompt detection and treatment may lead to rapid deterioration, resulting in respiratory distress, loss of movement and speech, and ultimately death (WHO, 2021a).

1.2.1. *Radiological assessment for COVID-19*

The radiological assessment of SARS-CoV-2 infection may involve a series of lung imaging tests. Chest X-ray examination may initially demonstrate small abnormal patchy shadows and interstitial changes, but may exhibit infiltrating shadows and pulmonary consolidation with occasional pleural effusion in severe cases (Huang *et al.*, 2020). Additionally, chest CT scan may reveal clearcut pulmonary lesions, including bilateral ground-glass opacities and segmental consolidation in the lungs — a distinct presentation for SARS-CoV-2 infection that may differentiate it from other pneumonias (Rothan and Byrareddy, 2020).

1.2.2. *SARS-CoV-2 diagnostic tests*

Apart from the lung/chest imaging for suspected lower respiratory tract infection, the gold standard for SARS-CoV-2 detection remains the reverse transcription-polymerase chain reaction (RT-PCR) assay, which entails collection of swab specimens. Clinical specimens can range from nasopharyngeal swabs, anterior nasal swabs, oropharyngeal swabs, saliva, or combinations (CDC, 2021a). Being a well-established molecular biology technique, RT-PCR confers many advantages — it is highly sensitive, rapid, and requires only a minimal amount of sample compared to other detection assays (Peeri *et al.*, 2020). RT-PCR for SARS-CoV-2 detection works well in many successful and widely used assays, such as real-time RT-PCR to identify the consensus pan beta-Coronavirus region of RNA-dependent RNA polymerase or RdRp (Huang *et al.*, 2020; Peeri *et al.*, 2020).

RT-PCR assays have facilitated widespread and large-scale testing for SARS-CoV-2 infections amidst the rapidly growing pandemic, including via "drive-through". Some countries adopted drive-through screening, with the entire service taking only approximately 10 minutes per person including registration, examination, swab specimen collection, and instructions for obtaining test results (Kwon *et al.*, 2020). Similarly, certain hospitals organized appointments via instant messaging applications, followed by a screening process taking only 5–8 minutes (Lee *et al.*, 2021). Coupling RT-PCR tests with popular social media applications achieved major improvements in testing capacity, accompanied by greatly reduced risk of airborne and fomite-mediated transmission — resulting in significant reductions in close contacts and concentrated gatherings at screening locations.

Antigen rapid tests (ARTs) are mainly based on lateral flow immuno-chromatographic assays which can be easily performed on nasal swab specimens. ARTs serve as useful adjunct tests, with their major advantages being their ease of operation and quick turnaround time that yields results in about 15–30 minutes. ARTs are deployed extensively as point-of-care and self tests: for rapid mass screening of infected individuals in large social, religious and other gatherings; and in settings such as institutions, nursing homes, quarantine facilities, etc. Although faster and cheaper, ARTs are generally less sensitive than RT-PCR (Dinnes *et al.*, 2021).

1.2.3. *Serologic tests for SARS-CoV-2 infection*

Apart from RT-PCR and ARTs, serologic testing represents another suitable option for detection of SARS-CoV-2 infection. There are a number of standardized serologic methods for detecting SARS-CoV-2 antibodies, including the enzyme-linked immunosorbent assay (ELISA), colloidal gold immunochromatographic assay, and chemiluminescence immunoassay. For example, Cai *et al.* (2020) developed a chemiluminescent immunoassay that utilizes 20 synthetic peptides based on the SARS-CoV-2 ORF1a/b, spike (S) and nucleocapsid (N) proteins for the detection of IgG and IgM antibodies. Similar approaches to detect SARS-CoV-2 IgG and IgM antibodies have also been reported using ELISA and colloidal gold immunochromatographic assay (Lou *et al.*, 2020; Pan *et al.*, 2020).

Besides aiding the diagnosis of SARS-CoV-2 infection, serologic tests also contribute towards studying the host immunological profile (IgM antibody onset after 3–6 days, IgG antibody onset after 8 days) — thus pinpointing current and past infections based on the antibody levels (Amanat *et al.*, 2020; Shi *et al.*, 2003). However, the disadvantage of this method is the inconsistent detection results, especially during early onset of illness (1–3 days) when antibody levels are low. Hence, serology-based techniques should complement established assays such as RT-PCR. Despite the limitations, the serologic detection approach can provide helpful information to evaluate the immunity status of individuals, e.g. the stage of SARS-CoV-2 infection, and efficacy of vaccination (Pang *et al.*, 2021).

1.2.4. *Alternative approaches to PCR-based assays*

The PCR-based assay remains the preferred detection methodology for SARS-CoV-2 as it is rapid, and has high detection sensitivity and specificity. However, PCR-based assays are generally more costly, require expensive equipment (such as thermocyclers), trained professionals to operate and interpret results, ultraclean settings, and relatively longer waiting times for results (Kashir and Yaqinuddin, 2020). Hence, alternative methods have been explored and considered for SARS-CoV-2 detection, such as loop-mediated isothermal amplification (LAMP), CRISPR-based detection, and DNA sequencing. Some of these newer techniques and their advantages are summarized in Table 1.1.

Table 1.1. Some alternative approaches to PCR-based assays for SARS-CoV-2 detection.

Technique	Efficiency and Significance
Loop-mediated isothermal amplification (LAMP)	Reverse transcription reaction needed to carry out amplification at 60–65°C. Entails the use of 4–6 primers, amplifying up to 8 distinct target sequence sites (Shirato *et al.*, 2018).
	Photometric detection via LAMP within an hour or less (Kashir and Yaqinuddin, 2020).
	Increased sensitivity of detecting only 7–10 initial viral RNA copies per reaction by two-stage LAMP (Hong *et al.*, 2004; Kashir and Yaqinuddin, 2020).

(Continued)

Table 1.1. (*Continued*)

Technique	Efficiency and Significance
	Lower cost as it is isothermal, obviating the need for thermocyclers for PCR assays.
	Shows good agreement with RT-PCR results (Zhang *et al.*, 2020a).
CRISPR-based detection	*DNA Endonuclease-Targeted CRISPR Trans Reporter (DETECTR)*
	Uses RT-LAMP of RNA extracted from nasopharyngeal or oropharyngeal swabs, followed by Cas12a detection (Broughton *et al.*, 2020).
	Cas12a detection with a guide RNA (gRNA) designed to recognize a specific sequence within SARS-CoV-2 N gene or E gene.
	Uses single-strand (ss) DNA fluorescein amidate biotinylated reporter molecule (FAM) for lateral flow detection.
	Simple, efficient, and rapid detection under an hour, without the need for expensive reagents and equipment.
	Promising clinical trial outcomes of 95% positive predictive agreement and 100% negative predictive agreement in patients with COVID-19 and other respiratory viral infections.
	Granted emergency use authorization (EUA) by FDA on 9 July 2020 (Broughton *et al.*, 2020).
	Specific High Sensitivity Enzymatic Reporter Unlocking (SHERLOCK)
	Uses CRISPR Cas13a instead. The targeted DNA or RNA from the sample is first amplified via recombinase polymerase amplification (RPA), or reverse transcriptase RPA coupled with T7 transcription (Gootenberg *et al.*, 2017; Kellner *et al.*, 2019).
	Cas13a-gRNA complex binds to the specific sequence in the SARS-CoV-2 S gene and ORF1ab (Kellner *et al.*, 2019).
	Entails the use of ssDNA FAM for lateral flow detection.
	Fast and efficient detection under an hour, without the need for expensive reagents and equipment.
	Granted EUA by FDA for SARS-CoV-2 detection on 7 May 2020 (Sherlock Biosciences, 2020).
	Testing a cohort of nasopharyngeal and throat swabs showed very high specificity and sensitivity, with fluorescence readout and detection limit of 42 RNA copies per reaction.
	Complete agreement with quantitative RT-PCR in SARS-CoV-2-negative samples (Patchsung *et al.*, 2020).

(*Continued*)

Table 1.1.   (*Continued*)

Technique	Efficiency and Significance
DNA/RNA sequencing-based detection	*Metagenomic RNA Enrichment Viral sequencing (MINERVA)* Based on Sequencing Hetero RNA-DNA-hybrid (SHERRY) system (Chen *et al.*, 2020).
	Uses Tn5 transposase to construct the library which directly tags RNA/DNA heteroduplexes, subsequently adding sequencing adaptor after reverse transcription (Chen *et al.*, 2020; Di *et al.*, 2020).
	Better coverage of SARS-CoV-2 genome accompanied by rapid library construction as compared to conventional double-strand DNA ligation (Chen *et al.*, 2020).
	Detects mutational profiles between SARS-CoV-2 lineages — strong linkages between positions 8,782 and 28,144 in two major S and L lineages (Tang *et al.*, 2020).
	Versatile, highly sensitive, cost-effective, and rapid detection.

1.3. Prevention and Control Strategies

SARS-CoV-2 is known to spread mainly through person-to-person contact via transmission of respiratory aerosols (Coleman *et al.*, 2021). Public health authorities recommend avoiding exposure to the virus through wearing of masks, social distancing, and maintaining proper personal hygiene as effective ways to prevent against COVID-19 (CDC, 2021b). Furthermore, numerous global efforts focus on the development and deployment of safe and effective vaccines and therapeutic agents against COVID-19.

1.4. Vaccine Development Against COVID-19

A range of molecular platforms have been harnessed in the development of COVID-19 vaccines (Shin *et al.*, 2020), including RNA- and DNA-based formulations, purified inactivated vaccines, virus-like particles, and peptide-based formulations (Table 1.2). The process of vaccine development and efficacy evaluation is a lengthy and expensive process, often taking up to 5–10 years before a vaccine is successfully licensed and manufactured for global distribution. The traditional vaccine development

Table 1.2. List of some major COVID-19 vaccines in clinical use (Regulatory Affairs Professionals Society, 2021).

Candidate	Country of Origin	Institution	Funding	Vaccine Technology	Mode of Action
BNT162	Multinational	Multiple study sites in Europe and North America	Pfizer; BioNTech; CEPI; US government	mRNA vaccine delivered via lipid nanoparticles	mRNA encodes for SARS-CoV-2 spike protein and RBD which activates the host immune response
mRNA-1273	Multinational	Kaiser Permanente Washington Health Research Institute	Moderna; CEPI; US government	mRNA vaccine delivered via lipid nanoparticles	mRNA encodes for full-length SARS-CoV-2 spike protein which activates the host immune response
AZD1222	UK	University of Oxford, Jenner Institute	University of Oxford; AstraZeneca; IQVIA; Serum Institute of India; CEPI; US government	Chimpanzee adenovirus vector encoding spike protein of SARS-CoV-2	Expression of SARS-CoV-2 spike protein in the host cell elicits immune response
Sputnik V	Russia	Gamaleya Research Institute; Acellena Contract Drug Research and Development	Russian Direct Investment Fund; Health Ministry of Russian Federation	Recombinant adenovirus vaccine (rAd26 and rAd5) encoding spike protein of SARS-CoV-2	Two-vector vaccine encodes for expression of full-length SARS-CoV-2 spike protein, stimulating an immune response

Janssen (JNJ-78436735; Ad26.COV2.S)	Netherlands; US	Janssen Vaccines, Johnson & Johnson	Janssen; BARDA; NIAID; Operation Warp Speed	Non-replicating adenovirus viral vector	Expression of SARS-CoV-2 spike protein in the host cell elicits immune response
CoronaVac	China	Sinovac	Advantech Capital; Vivo Capital; Sinovac	Deactivation of SARS-CoV-2 cultured in Vero cells using beta-propiolactone (Inactivated virus is mixed with aluminium-based adjuvant)	Inactivated SARS-CoV-2 elicits host immune response
BBIBP-CorV	China	Beijing Institute of Biological Products; China National Pharmaceutical Group (Sinopharm)	Ministry of Science and Technology, China	Deactivation of SARS-CoV-2 cultured in Vero cells using beta-propiolactone (Inactivated virus is mixed with aluminium-based adjuvant)	Inactivated SARS-CoV-2 elicits host immune response

process includes pre-clinical trials of selected targets, Phase 1–3 clinical trials, and licensure followed by large-scale manufacturing.

During a pandemic, urgent control measures are required, and the vaccine development process follows a pandemic paradigm in which multiple steps may be executed in parallel before evaluating the success of the preceding development steps (Lurie *et al.*, 2020). Therefore, although the development of vaccines under this paradigm shift reduces the time it takes to mass-produce effective vaccines, the associated financial risks are also immensely increased. The Coalition for Epidemic Preparedness and Innovations (CEPI) is a global foundation that sources for donations from private, public, philanthropic and civil society organizations to finance research projects aimed at developing vaccines against the WHO list of blueprint priority diseases, including COVID-19. Hence, this partnership aims to reduce the level of financial risks associated with vaccine development (CEPI, 2021). Several hundred candidate vaccines formulated against COVID-19 have been reported, with many candidates in clinical trials or granted approval for clinical use (Regulatory Affairs Professionals Society, 2021). Some examples of COVID-19 vaccines administered worldwide include Pfizer and BioNTech BNT162, Moderna mRNA-1273, University of Oxford and AstraZeneca AZD1222, Sinovac CoronaVac, and Sinopharm BBIBP-CorV (Table 1.2).

Numerous studies have reinforced the life-saving and beneficial impact of COVID-19 vaccines (Scobie *et al.*, 2021; Shoukat *et al.*, 2022). For example, one large study involving 13 US states (representing one quarter of the US population) found that not fully vaccinated persons had about 10 times higher COVID-19 mortality and hospitalization risk, and were over 4 times more likely to be infected compared with fully vaccinated persons (Scobie *et al.*, 2021).

1.4.1. *SARS-CoV-2 spike protein as target for vaccine development*

Most COVID-19 vaccines are designed to target the SARS-CoV-2 spike (S) protein. Depending on the CoV species, the S protein is about 1,100–1,600 amino acids in length with a molecular mass of approximately 220 kDa. This protein adopts a club-shaped trimeric conformation, and is localized at the surface of the virion. The SARS-CoV-2 S protein is of particular interest for vaccine development due to its significant role in facilitating viral entry into the host cell, and it constitutes a crucial target for neutralizing antibodies (Samrat *et al.*, 2020). The SARS-CoV-2 S protein also undergoes extensive glycosylation, suggesting that the S protein has a more organized conformation compared to other non-glycosylated viral counterparts — this lends further support to the S protein as an excellent target for vaccine development (Shin *et al.*, 2020).

Notwithstanding this, the alarming emergence of multiple VOCs with many mutations in the S protein has raised concerns on the efficacy of vaccines based solely on inducing immune responses to the S antigen. Furthermore, the unrelenting circulation and evolution of SARS-CoV-2 and other potentially virulent Coronaviruses in bats and other animal reservoirs continue to pose a pandemic threat to humanity. To counter future CoV epidemics, there must be concerted international research efforts to focus on developing "universal" Coronavirus vaccines that can confer durable and broadly protective immunity (Morens *et al.*, 2022).

1.5. Anti-SARS-CoV-2 Therapeutic Drugs

1.5.1. *Drug repurposing*

Drug repurposing involves the identification of currently existing drugs for new therapeutic purposes. Due to the urgent need for therapeutics against COVID-19, drug repurposing represents an attractive approach to identify potential drugs that may be exploited to treat COVID-19 (Singh *et al.*, 2020b). The development of a novel therapeutic drug is time-consuming, costly, and requires extensive research on safety and efficacy before it can be approved for clinical use (Kraljevic *et al.*, 2004). During a pandemic which requires urgent control measures, repurposing existing drugs (those already in clinical trials or FDA (Food and Drug Administration)-approved) significantly shortens the time and cost to deploy effective therapeutics against the novel pathogen. Hence, a wide array of drugs (and their combinations) have been investigated for their efficacy against COVID-19 and other Coronavirus infections (Drozdzal *et al.*, 2020; Tan *et al.*, 2021; Wu *et al.*, 2020).

1.5.1.1. *Remdesivir*

Remdesivir is a nucleoside analog with broad-spectrum antiviral activity, and was initially designed for treating Ebola virus infection. This agent has antiviral activity against several viruses, including Ebola virus, SARS-CoV, MERS-CoV, Nipah virus, and respiratory syncytial virus (Eastman *et al.*, 2020; Tan *et al.*, 2021). Upon diffusion into the host cell, remdesivir acts as a prodrug which is converted into its active adenosine nucleoside triphosphate form via the activity of esterases and nucleoside-phosphate kinases. The mode of action of the activated remdesivir is by disrupting viral RNA-dependent RNA polymerase activity via "chain termination", thus reducing the rate of viral replication (Ferner and Aronson, 2020; Scavone *et al.*, 2020).

One study found that 68% of patients with severe COVID-19 showed improvement in COVID-19-related symptoms after intravenous administration of remdesivir on day 1, followed by 100 mg daily for the next 9 days of treatment (Grein *et al.*, 2020). On 1 March 2020, the US Food and Drug Administration announced the emergency use authorization of remdesivir for the treatment of COVID-19 (FDA, 2020). The observed side-effects of remdesivir include rash, hypotension, abnormal liver function, and renal impairment — therefore, this drug is not advised for patients with liver and/or kidney dysfunction (Singh *et al.*, 2020a). NIH (National Institutes of Health) guidelines recommend use of remdesivir in hospitalized COVID-19 patients requiring supplemental oxygen through nasal cannula (NIH, 2021a).

1.5.1.2. *Lopinavir-ritonavir*

The combination of lopinavir and ritonavir for the treatment and prevention of human immunodeficiency virus (HIV) infection was approved by the FDA in 2000. The antiviral action of lopinavir is attributed to its ability to inhibit HIV protease activity. Ritonavir slows down the breakdown of lopinavir, and enhances the drug effect via inhibition of cytochrome P450 (Lv *et al.*, 2015; Su *et al.*, 2019). This drug combination has been investigated for its efficacy in treating COVID-19 through randomized controlled open-label clinical trials. However, the administration of lopinavir-ritonavir had no significant effect on the treatment of severe COVID-19 (Cao *et al.*, 2020). On 4 July 2020, WHO announced the discontinuation of these clinical trials due to insufficient evidence of reduction in patient mortality compared to standard care provided in hospitals (WHO, 2020). In addition, reported adverse effects of lopinavir-ritonavir included gastrointestinal discomfort, muscle pains, pancreatitis, abnormal liver function, and high blood pressure (Neuman *et al.*, 2012). WHO strongly recommends against lopinavir and ritonavir in COVID-19 patients of any severity (WHO, 2021b).

1.5.1.3. *Favipiravir and oseltamivir*

Favipiravir is a nucleoside analog used for the treatment of influenza infection in Japan (Du and Chen, 2020). Similar to remdesivir, the mechanism of action of favipiravir is associated with its ability to suppress viral replication by selectively inhibiting the RNA-dependent RNA polymerase activity. Favipiravir has also been reported to have antiviral activity against chikungunya, Ebola, yellow fever, norovirus and enterovirus infections (Clercq, 2019). Clinical trials have been conducted to examine the efficacy of favipiravir for the treatment of COVID-19. However, one meta-analysis revealed no significant difference in fatality rate and mechanical ventilation requirement between favipravir treatment and standard of care in patients with moderate and severe COVID-19 (Ozlusen *et al.*, 2021).

Oseltamivir is another antiviral agent used for preventing and treating influenza. Among the clinical trials to evaluate the efficacy of oseltamivir for the treatment of COVID-19, one study showed no statistical difference in hospitalization duration between the oseltamivir treatment group (9 days) versus the untreated group (12 days) (Tan *et al.*, 2020).

1.5.1.4. *Chloroquine and hydroxychloroquine*

Chloroquine is an antimalarial drug which has been reported to possess antiviral activity. There have been a number of registered clinical trials investigating the efficacy of chloroquine and hydroxychloroquine (a less toxic analog of chloroquine) for the treatment of COVID-19. However, due to the cardiac and retinal toxicity of this drug, close monitoring of patients is strongly advised during chloroquine administration. WHO strongly recommends against chloroquine and hydroxychloroquine in COVID-19 patients of any severity (WHO, 2021b).

1.5.2. *Convalescent plasma therapy*

Prior to the availability of effective drugs and vaccines against SARS-CoV-2, convalescent plasma therapy (CPT) was investigated as an approach for the management of COVID-19. CPT involves the direct injection or transfusion of plasma from donors who have previously been diagnosed with SARS-CoV-2 infection. The donor plasma contains neutralizing antibodies against SARS-CoV-2, and is expected to reduce disease severity in COVID-19 as well as to suppress the inflammatory response by conferring passive immunity (Bozzo and Jorquera, 2017; Pang *et al.*, 2021). CPT has previously been successfully employed to treat a broad range of novel respiratory viral illnesses, including those caused by influenza A virus and other Coronaviruses (Alghamdi and Abdel-Moneim, 2020; Arabi *et al.*, 2016; Cheng *et al.*, 2005; Luke *et al.*, 2006).

One study reported that patients with severe or life-threatening COVID-19 required less oxygen support, and also had improved survival after CPT (Liu *et al.*, 2020). However, there are also contradicting studies suggesting the ineffectiveness of CPT in treating COVID-19 (Pathak, 2020). Therefore, further robust randomized control studies with adequate statistical power are needed to better understand the efficacy and implications of CPT in COVID-19 management (NIH, 2021b).

1.5.3. *Novel drug development: Some examples*

Viruses are obligate parasites that hijack the host cellular mechanisms for replication. Virus entry into host cells is a key step in the viral life-cycle, and is often a multi-step process involving many virus–host interactions. Targeting of processes conserved across a broad range of CoV species may aid in the development of broad-spectrum antivirals that may be effective against currently circulating CoVs and those that may emerge in the future. Moreover, given that viral entry inhibitors prevent the first step of viral replication, they may be deployed as prophylaxis, and may also reduce drug toxicity since membrane permeability may not be required (Vellingiri *et al.*, 2020; Zhou and Simmons, 2012).

The CoV spike protein is known to facilitate viral entry into the host cell. The spike protein consists of the S1 and S2 subunits. The S1 subunit contains the *N*-terminal domain and *C*-terminal domain, with the RBD being located within the latter. Virus entry into the host cell is initiated by binding of the RBD to the human ACE2, a well-documented receptor for SARS-CoV and SARS-CoV-2 entry (Tai *et al.*, 2020). Subsequently, the S2 subunit — which comprises the internal membrane fusion peptide

(FP), two 7-peptide repeats (HR), a membrane-proximal external region (MPER), and a transmembrane domain (TM) — facilitates viral membrane fusion and release of viral genetic material into the host cell (Li *et al.*, 2020). The S1 and S2 subunits are separated by a cleavage site that is recognized by human proteases, such as TMPRSS2.

Highly specific neutralizing monoclonal antibodies have also been developed for COVID-19 treatment. Two recombinant human IgG1 monoclonal antibodies (casirivimab and imdevimab) bind non-competitively to distinct epitopes of the SARS-CoV-2 spike RBD, and inhibit viral entry into host cells. In November 2020, the combination of casirivimab–imdevimab was granted emergency use authorization by FDA for the treatment of high-risk patients with mild to moderate COVID-19. This combination could reduce hospitalization rates among patients with mild to moderate COVID-19 (Razonable *et al.*, 2021). WHO (2021b) conditionally recommends treatment using a combination of neutralizing monoclonal antibodies (casirivimab and imdevimab) in: (a) severe and critically ill COVID-19 patients with seronegative status; and (b) non-severe COVID-19 patients at the highest risk of severe disease (who do not meet criteria for severe or critical infection). Sotrovimab is another spike-targeting human neutralizing monoclonal antibody which is indicated for treating patients with mild to moderate COVID-19 who do not require supplemental oxygen and who are at increased risk of progressing to severe disease (European Medicines Agency, 2021).

The proteolytic activity of TMPRSS2 is indispensable for viral entry as well as for viral and host membrane fusion. Azouz *et al.* (2021) identified two small molecules — 4-(2-aminomethyl) benzenesulfonyl fluoride (AEBSF) and the human anti-inflammatory protein alpha 1 antitrypsin (A1AT) — as protease inhibitors capable of inhibiting TMPRSS2 activity. Further studies are suggested to investigate the potential of these molecules (particularly A1AT, an FDA-approved drug) in limiting SARS-CoV-2 pathogenesis and for treating COVID-19 (Yang *et al.*, 2020). In addition, there are also studies targeting the ACE2 functional receptor to prevent SARS-CoV-2 entry into the host cell. Vero cells pre-treated with anti-human ACE2 antibodies to block spike-ACE2 binding can successfully inhibit SARS-CoV-2 spike protein-mediated viral entry (Hoffmann *et al.*, 2020). Hence, the spike protein and the processes required for successful viral entry serve as excellent targets for the development of therapeutic viral entry inhibitors.

Merck has developed an oral antiviral agent designated molnupiravir. This compound is a nucleoside analog that is incorporated into viral RNA strands by mimicking cytidine and uridine to generate faulty viral genomes leading to viral population collapse or "lethal mutagenesis" (Kabinger *et al.*, 2021; Painter *et al.*, 2021). In November 2021, this drug received approval from the UK Medicines and Healthcare products Regulatory Agency for treatment of COVID-19.

Pfizer has developed an oral antiviral therapeutic against SARS-CoV-2 — a SARS-CoV-2 3CL protease inhibitor that showed promising antiviral activity against SARS-CoV-2 *in vitro*. Interim analysis of phase 2/3 clinical trials of the drug PF-07321332 combined with oral ritonavir (named "paxlovid") reduced the risk of hospitalization or death by ~90% compared with placebo in non-hospitalized high-risk adult patients with COVID-19 (Mahase, 2021b).

1.5.4. *Indirect therapeutic agents and candidates for COVID-19*

1.5.4.1. *Corticosteroids*

Numerous studies provide evidence of excessive cytokine responses in COVID-19 patients (Gao *et al.*, 2021; Kumar *et al.*, 2020). Chemokine and cytokine analysis of COVID-19 patients reveal elevated proinflammatory cytokines in the serum (e.g. IL-1β, IL-6, IL-8, IL-12, IFN-γ). Patients admitted to the intensive care unit (ICU) have higher concentrations of cytokines compared to those not requiring ICU admission — thus suggesting an association between cytokine storm and disease severity (Huang *et al.*, 2020). In addition, cytokine storm is also documented to be the cause of acute respiratory distress syndrome (ARDS) in COVID-19 patients (Domingo *et al.*, 2020).

Since September 2020, WHO strongly recommends systemic corticosteroids such as dexamethasone (rather than no corticosteroids) for patients with severe and critical COVID-19 (WHO, 2021b).

1.5.4.2. *Tocilizumab and IL-6 inhibitors*

Tocilizumab is an IL-6 inhibitor primarily used for the treatment of autoimmune diseases, such as rheumatoid arthritis and juvenile idiopathic arthritis (Ogata and Tanaka, 2012). This drug is a monoclonal antibody designed to bind competitively to IL-6 receptors, thereby preventing the IL-6 signal transduction from eliciting the activation of B and T lymphocytes. Therefore, tocilizumab has been evaluated for its effectiveness in treating COVID-19 (Sinha *et al.*, 2020). A retrospective observational cohort study indicated that intravenous administration of tocilizumab to COVID-19 patients in ICU significantly reduced their mortality rate (Biran *et al.*, 2020). Other clinical trials also suggest positive effects of tocilizumab in treating COVID-19 patients with elevated IL-6 levels and extensive infiltrating lesions in the lungs (Xu *et al.*, 2020; Zhang *et al.*, 2020b). WHO strongly recommends IL-6 blockers (tocilizumab or sarilumab) for treating patients with severe or critical COVID-19 (WHO, 2021b).

1.5.4.3. *Inhibitors of NLRP3 inflammasome receptor*

The high fatality rate of COVID-19 is contributed by severe lung inflammation, notable tissue injury, and a high risk of bacterial superinfections (Domingo *et al.*, 2020). While treatment using drugs that target virus-associated host receptors represent a direct and straightforward strategy, these may inadvertently enhance inflammation and cytokine storm, and cause more harm than good during SARS-CoV-2 infection. Hence, modulating exaggerated inflammation is also crucial for host survival. For instance, the NLRP3 (NOD, LRR, and pyrin domain-containing-3) inflammasome receptor is associated with cell death (pyroptosis) via pore formation and lysosomal disruption upon SARS-CoV infection. Thus, the NLRP3 inflammasome is proposed to be a potential drug target for ameliorating tissue inflammation in COVID-19 patients (Shah, 2020). Parthenolide and Bay 11-7082 (both NLRP3 inhibitors) can reduce lung inflammation and improve survival in SARS-CoV-infected animals — thereby alluding to potential treatment options against the SARS-CoV-2-associated cytokine storm (e.g. IL-1β, IL-6, TNF-α) that often contributes to mortality in COVID-19 patients (Shah, 2020).

1.5.4.4. *Type III interferon lambda*

Interferon (IFN) has been used as an antiviral treatment for chronic hepatitis C and hepatitis B virus infections. This is achieved by the type I interferons (IFN-α, IFN-β) via the engagement of the IFN α/β receptor complex (IFNAR1/IFNAR2 subunits). However, the administration of type I IFN-based drugs led to ubiquitous expression of IFNARs (a hetero-meric receptor complex) in all cells — thereby triggering a pro-inflamma-tory systemic response via the recruitment and activation of immune cells (Prokunina-Olsson *et al.*, 2020). This resulted in unpredictable tissue damage and adverse effects.

Innate IFN responses are critical for restricting SARS-CoV-2 replica-tion and COVID-19 disease progression (Yoshida *et al.*, 2022). Type III interferon lambda (IFN-λ) is a protein involved in virus control and elimi-nation upon viral infection, and has been proposed as a potential treatment against SARS-CoV-2 (Prokunina-Olsson *et al.*, 2020). In contrast to the type I IFNs, type III IFNs target the IFNL complex (IFNLR1/IL10R2 sub-units) whose expression is restricted to epithelial cells and certain immune cells — thus providing more specific treatment of lung epithelial cells and eliminating the risk of developing severe side-effects (Broggi *et al.*, 2020; Prokunina-Olsson *et al.*, 2020). While yet to be fully validated as an alter-native treatment for SARS-CoV-2, this therapeutic approach has exhibited potency against SARS-CoV and MERS-CoV in previous *in vitro* studies.

1.6. Conclusion

The high genetic similarity between SARS-CoV-2 and SARS-like Coronaviruses in bats and other intermediate animal hosts underscores the importance of zoonotic viral transmission to human hosts. The occur-rence of cross-species viral epidemics can be substantially reduced by enforcing stricter laws that ban the slaughter and trade of wild and endan-gered species, and even shifting to a more vegetarian diet (Reddy and Saier, 2020).

While RT-PCR and ARTs have contributed immensely to SARS-CoV-2 detection for diagnosis and contact tracing — faster, cheaper and more informative testing methods (such as next generation sequencing and breathalyzer) are needed in view of the relentless viral mutation and spread. Furthermore, serologic assays can offer rapid yet informative data on the immune status of infected or vaccinated individuals.

Although multiple life-saving COVID-19 vaccines have been devel-oped and deployed with unprecedented speed, many challenges remain, including vaccine efficacy, hesitancy and inequality. The continuous emergence of significant viral variants also necessitates research and development of updated vaccines as well as universal vaccines to target and address immune-escape mutants.

In addition to current promising treatments and drug repurposing, it is imperative to design and develop more efficacious direct antivirals, immunomodulatory agents and other novel drugs for therapeutic and prophylactic purposes.

Finally, much remains for humanity to discover and learn as the world must continue to respond, adapt and live with endemic COVID-19 and SARS-CoV-2 evolutionary dynamics (Callaway, 2021; Global Condition for Post-Pandemic Policy, 2021; Global Health Security Index, 2021; Petersen *et al.*, 2021; Wang and Powell, 2021).

References

Ai J *et al*. Omicron variant showed lower neutralizing sensitivity than other SARS-CoV-2 variants to immune sera elicited by vaccines after boost. *Emerg Microbes Infect* 2021; 11:337–343.

Alghamdi AN, Abdel-Moneim AS. Convalescent plasma: A potential life-saving therapy for Coronavirus disease 2019 (COVID-19). *Front Public Health* 2020; 8:437.

Amanat F *et al*. A serological assay to detect SARS-CoV-2 seroconversion in humans. *Nat Med* 2020; 26:1033–1036.

Arabi YM *et al*. Feasibility of using convalescent plasma immunotherapy for MERS-CoV infection, Saudi Arabia. *Emerg Infect Dis* 2016; 22: 1554–1561.

Azouz NP *et al*. Alpha 1 antitrypsin is an inhibitor of the SARS-CoV-2-priming protease TMPRSS2. *Pathog Immun* 2021; 6:55–74.

Biran N *et al*. Tocilizumab among patients with COVID-19 in the intensive care unit: A multicentre observational study. *Lancet Rheumatol* 2020; 2: e603–e612.

Bozzo J, Jorquera JI. Use of human immunoglobulins as an anti-infective treatment: The experience so far and their possible re-emerging role. *Expert Rev Anti Infect Ther* 2017; 15:585–604.

Broggi A *et al*. Type III interferons: Balancing tissue tolerance and resistance to pathogen invasion. *J Exp Med* 2020; 217:e20190295.

Broughton J *et al*. CRISPR-Cas12-based detection of SARS-CoV-2. *Nat Biotechnol* 2020; 38:870–874.

Cai XF *et al*. A peptide-based magnetic chemiluminescence enzyme immunoassay for serological diagnosis of Coronavirus disease 2019. *J Infect Dis* 2020; 222:189–193.

Callaway E. Beyond Omicron: What's next for COVID's viral evolution. *Nature* 2021; 600:204–207.

Cao B *et al*. A trial of lopinivir-ritonavir in adults hospitalized with severe COVID-19. *N Engl J Med* 2020; 382:1787–1799.

CDC (Centers for Disease Control and Prevention, USA), 2021a. Interim Guidelines for Collecting and Handling of Clinical Specimens for COVID-19 Testing. https://www.cdc.gov/coronavirus/2019-ncov/lab/guidelines-clinical-specimens.html (accessed 25 October 2021).

CDC (Centers for Disease Control and Prevention, USA), 2021b. COVID-19. How to Protect Yourself & Others. https://www.cdc.gov/coronavirus/2019-ncov/prevent-getting-sick/prevention.html (accessed 29 November 2021).

CEPI (Coalition for Epidemic Preparedness and Innovations), 2021. Priority Diseases. https://cepi.net/research_dev/priority-diseases/ (accessed 21 December 2021).

Chen C *et al*. MINERVA: A facile strategy for SARS-CoV-2 whole-genome deep sequencing of clinical samples. *Mol Cell* 2020; 80:1123–1134.

Cheng Y *et al*. Use of convalescent plasma therapy in SARS patients in Hong Kong. *Eur J Clin Microbiol Infect Dis* 2005; 24:44–46.

Clercq ED. New nucleoside analogues for the treatment of hemorrhagic fever virus infections. *Chem Asian J* 2019; 14:3962–3968.

Coleman KK *et al*. Viral load of SARS-CoV-2 in respiratory aerosols emitted by COVID-19 patients while breathing, talking, and singing. *Clin Infect Dis* 2021; Aug 6:ciab691.

Di L *et al*. RNA sequencing by direct tagmentation of RNA/DNA hybrids. *Proc Natl Acad Sci USA* 2020; 117:2886–2893.

Dinnes J *et al*. Rapid, point-of-care antigen and molecular-based tests for diagnosis of SARS-CoV-2 infection. *Cochrane Database Syst Rev* 2021; 3:CD013705.

Domingo P *et al*. The four horsemen of a viral apocalypse: The pathogenesis of SARS-CoV-2 infection (COVID-19). *EBioMedicine* 2020; 58:102887.

Drozdzal S *et al*. FDA approved drugs with pharmacotherapeutic potential for SARS-CoV-2 (COVID-19) therapy. *Drug Resist Updat* 2020; 53:100719.

Du YX, Chen XP. Favipiravir: Pharmacokinetics and concerns about clinical trials for 2019-nCoV infection. *Clin Pharmacol Ther* 2020; 108:242–247.

Eastman RT *et al*. Remdesivir: A review of its discovery and development leading to emergency use authorization for treatment of COVID-19. *ACS Cent Sci* 2020; 6:672–683.

European Medicines Agency, 2021. COVID-19: EMA Recommends Authorisation of Antibody Medicine Xevudy. https://www.ema.europa.eu/en/news/covid-19-ema-recommends-authorisation-antibody-medicine-xevudy (accessed 16 December 2021).

FDA (Food and Drug Administration, USA), 2020. Coronavirus (COVID-19) Update: FDA Issues Emergency Use Authorization for Potential COVID-19 Treatment. https://www.fda.gov/news-events/press-announcements/coronavirus-covid-19-update-fda-issues-emergency-use-authorization-potential-covid-19-treatment (accessed 1 May 2020).

Ferguson N *et al.*, 2021. Report 49 — Growth, Population Distribution and Immune Escape of Omicron in England. https://www.imperial.ac.uk/mrc-global-infectious-disease-analysis/covid-19/report-49-Omicron/ (accessed 16 December 2021).

Ferner RE, Aronson JK. Remdisivir in COVID-19. *BMJ* 2020; 369:m1610.

Gao YM *et al.* Cytokine storm syndrome in coronavirus disease 2019: A narrative review. *J Intern Med* 2021; 289:147–161.

GitHub, 2021. COVID-19 Data Repository by the Center for Systems Science and Engineering (CSSE) at Johns Hopkins University. https://github.com/CSSEGISandData/COVID-19 (accessed 31 December 2021).

Global Condition for Post-Pandemic Policy, 2021. Our Global Condition: An assessement by the Global Condition for Post-Pandemic Policy After 18 Months of COVID-19. https://globalcommissionforpostpandemicpolicy.org/home/our-global-condition-report/ (accessed 23 December 2021).

Global Health Security Index, 2021. Report & Data. https://www.ghsindex.org/report-model/ (accessed 24 December 2021).

Gootenberg JS *et al.* Nucleic acid detection with CRISPR-Cas13a/C2c2. *Science* 2017; 356:438–442.

Grein J *et al.* Compassionate use of remdesivir for patients with severe COVID-19. *N Engl J Med* 2020; 382:2327–2336.

Hagen A, 2021. How Ominous is the Omicron Variant (B.1.1.529)? https://asm.org/Articles/2021/December/How-Ominous-is-the-Omicron-Variant-B-1-1-529 (accessed 16 December 2021).

Hoffmann M *et al.* SARS-CoV-2 cell entry depends on ACE2 and TMPRSS2 and is blocked by a clinically proven protease inhibitor. *Cell* 2020; 181:271–280.e8.

Hong TC *et al.* Development and evaluation of a novel loop-mediated isothermal amplification method for rapid detection of severe acute respiratory syndrome coronavirus. *J Clin Microbiol* 2004; 42:1956–1961.

Huang C, *et al.* Clinical features of patients infected with 2019 novel coronavirus in Wuhan, China. *Lancet* 2020; 395:497–506.

Hui KPY et al. SARS-CoV-2 Omicron variant replication in human bronchus and lung ex vivo. *Nature* 2022; 603:715–720.

Kabinger F *et al.* Mechanism of molnupiravir-induced SARS-CoV-2 mutagenesis. *Nat Struct Mol Biol* 2021; 28:740–746.

Kashir J, Yaqinuddin A. Loop mediated isothermal amplification (LAMP) assays as a rapid diagnostic for COVID-19. *Med Hypotheses* 2020; 141:109786.

Kellner MJ *et al*. SHERLOCK: Nucleic acid detection with CRISPR nucleases. *Nat Protoc* 2019; 14:2986–3012.

Khailany RA *et al*. Genomic characterization of a novel SARS-CoV-2. *Gene Rep* 2020; 19:100682.

Kim D *et al*. The architecture of SARS-CoV-2 transcriptome. *Cell* 2020; 181:914–921.e10.

Kraljevic S *et al*. Accelerating drug discovery. *EMBO Rep* 2004; 5:837–842.

Kumar R *et al*. Pathophysiology and potential future therapeutic targets using preclinical models of COVID-19. *ERJ Open Res* 2020; 6:00405–2020.

Kumar S *et al*. Omicron and delta variant of SARS-CoV-2: A comparative computational study of spike protein. *J Med Virol* 2022; 94:1641–1649.

Kwon KT *et al*. Drive-through screening center for COVID-19: A safe and efficient screening system against massive community outbreak. *J Korean Med Sci* 2020; 35:e123.

Lee E *et al*. Bonuses and pitfalls of a paperless drive-through screening and COVID-19: A field report. *J Microbiol Immunol Infect* 2021; 54:85–88.

Li J *et al*. Targeting the entry step of SARS-CoV-2: A promising therapeutic approach. *Signal Transduct Target Ther* 2020; 5:98.

Liu STH *et al*. Convalescent plasma treatment of severe COVID-19: A propensity score-matched control study. *Nat Med* 2020; 26:1708–1713.

Lou B *et al*. Serology characteristics of SARS-CoV-2 infection after exposure and post-symptom onset. *Eur Respir J* 2020; 56:2000763.

Low ZY *et al*. SARS coronavirus outbreaks past and present — A comparative analysis of SARS-CoV-2 and its predecessors. *Virus Genes* 2021; 57:307–317.

Lu L *et al*. Neutralization of SARS-CoV-2 Omicron variant by sera from BNT162b2 or Coronavac vaccine recipients. *Clin Infect Dis* 2021; Dec 16:ciab1041.

Lu R *et al*. Genomic characterisation and epidemiology of 2019 novel coronavirus: Implications for virus origins and receptor binding. *Lancet* 2020; 395:565–574.

Luke TC *et al*. Meta-analysis: Convalescent blood products for Spanish influenza pneumonia: A future H5N1 treatment? *Ann Intern Med* 2006; 145:599–609.

Lurie N *et al*. Developing COVID-19 vaccines at pandemic speed. *N Engl J Med* 2020; 382:1969–1973.

Lv Z *et al*. HIV protease inhibitors: A review of molecular selectivity and toxicity. *HIV AIDS (Auckl)* 2015; 7:95–104.

Mahase E. COVID-19: How many variants are there, and what do we know about them? *BMJ* 2021a; 374:n1971.

Mahase E. COVID-19: Pfizer's paxlovid is 89% effective in patients at risk of serious illness, company reports. *BMJ* 2021b; 375:n2713.

Morens DM *et al*. Universal coronavirus vaccines — An urgent need. *N Engl J Med* 2022; 386:297–299.

Naqvi AAT *et al*. Insights into SARS-CoV-2 genome, structure, evolution, pathogenesis and therapies: Structural genomics approach. *Biochim Biophys Acta Mol Basis Dis* 2020; 1866:165878.

Neuman MG *et al*. HIV-antiretroviral therapy induced liver, gastrointestinal, and pancreatic injury. *Int J Hepatol* 2012; 2012:760706.

NIH (National Institutes of Health, USA), 2021a. Therapeutic Management of Hospitalized Adults With COVID-19. https://www.covid19treatment guidelines.nih.gov/management/clinical-management/hospitalized-adults--therapeutic-management/ (accessed 16 December 2021).

NIH (National Institutes of Health, USA), 2021b. Convalescent Plasma. https://www.covid19treatmentguidelines.nih.gov/therapies/anti-sars-cov-2-antibody-products/convalescent-plasma/ (accessed 16 December 2021).

Nishiura H *et al*. Relative reproduction number of SARS-CoV-2 Omicron (B.1.1.529) compared with Delta variant in South Africa. *J Clin Med* 2022; 11:30.

Ogata A, Tanaka T. Tocilizumab for the treatment of rheumatoid arthritis and other systemic autoimmune diseases: Current perspectives and future directions. *Int J Rheumatol* 2012; 2012:946048.

Ozlusen B *et al*. Effectiveness of favipiravir in COVID-19: A live systematic review. *Eur J Clin Microbiol Infect Dis* 2021; 40:2575–2583.

Painter GR *et al*. Developing a direct acting, orally available antiviral agent in a pandemic: The evolution of molnupiravir as a potential treatment for COVID-19. *Curr Opin Virol* 2021; 50:17–22.

Pal M *et al*. Severe acute respiratory syndrome coronavirus-2 (SARS-CoV-2): An update. *Cureus* 2020; 12:e7423.

Pan Y *et al*. Serological immunochromatographic approach in diagnosis with SARS-CoV-2 infected COVID-19 patients. *J Infect* 2020; 81:e28–e32.

Pang NY *et al*. Understanding neutralising antibodies against SARS-CoV-2 and their implications in clinical practice. *Mil Med Res* 2021; 8:47.

Patchsung M *et al*. Clinical validation of a Cas13-based assay for the detection of SARS-CoV-2 RNA. *Nat Biomed Eng* 2020; 4:1140–1149.

Pathak EB. Convalescent plasma is ineffective for COVID-19. *BMJ* 2020 Oct 22; 371:m4072.

Peeri NC *et al*. The SARS, MERS and novel coronavirus (COVID-19) epidemics, the newest and biggest global health threats: What lessons have we learned? *Int J Epidemiol* 2020; 49:717–726.

Petersen E *et al*. Emergence of new SARS-CoV-2 Variant of Concern Omicron (B.1.1.529) — highlights Africa's research capabilities, but exposes major knowledge gaps, inequities of vaccine distribution, inadequacies in global COVID-19 response and control efforts. *Int J Infect Dis* 2021; 114:268–272.

Prokunina-Olsson L *et al*. COVID-19 and emerging viral infections: The case for interferon lambda. *J Exp Med* 2020; 217:e20200653.

Razonable RR *et al*. Casirivimab-Imdevimab treatment is associated with reduced rates of hospitalization among high-risk patients with mild to moderate coronavirus disease-19. *EClinicalMedicine* 2021; 40:101102.

Reardon S. How the Delta variant achieves its ultrafast spread. *Nature* 2021; Jul 21.

Reddy BL, Saier MHJ. The causal relationship between eating animals and viral epidemics. *Microb Physiol* 2020; 30:2–8.

Regulatory Affairs Professionals Society, 2021. COVID-19 Vaccine Tracker. https://www.raps.org/news-and-articles/news-articles/2020/3/covid-19-vaccine-tracker (accessed 20 December 2021).

Rothan HA, Byrareddy SN. The epidemiology and pathogenesis of coronavirus disease (COVID-19) outbreak. *J Autoimmun* 2020; 109:102433.

Samrat SK *et al*. Prospect of SARS-CoV-2 spike protein: Potential role in vaccine and therapeutic development. *Virus Res* 2020; 288:198141.

Scavone C *et al*. Current pharmacological treatments for COVID-19: What's next? *Br J Pharmacol* 2020; 177:4813–4824.

Scobie HM *et al*. Monitoring incidence of COVID-19 cases, hospitalizations, and deaths, by vaccination status — 13 U.S. Jurisdictions, April 4–July 17, 2021. *MMWR Morb Mortal Wkly Rep* 2021; 70:1284–1290.

Shah A. Novel coronavirus-induced NLRP3 inflammasome activation: A potential drug target in the treatment of COVID-19. *Front Immunol* 2020; 11:1021.

Sharma A *et al*. COVID-19: A review on the novel coronavirus disease evolution, transmission, detection, control and prevention. *Viruses* 2021a; 13:202.

Sharma A *et al*. Comparative transcriptomic and molecular pathway analyses of HL-CZ human pro-monocytic cells expressing SARS-CoV-2 spike S1, S2, NP, NSP15 and NSP16 genes. *Microorganisms* 2021b; 9:1193.

Sherlock Biosciences, 2020. Sherlock Biosciences Receives FDA Emergency Use Authorization for CRISPR SARS-CoV-2 Rapid Diagnostic. https://sherlock.bio/sherlock-biosciences-receives-fda-emergency-use-authorization-for-crispr-sars-cov-2-rapid-diagnostic/ (accessed 7 May 2020).

Shi Y *et al*. Diagnosis of severe acute respiratory syndrome (SARS) by detection of SARS coronavirus nucleocapsid antibodies in an antigen-capturing enzyme-linked immunosorbent assay. *J Clin Microbiol* 2003; 41:5781–5782.

Shin MD *et al*. COVID-19 vaccine development and a potential nanomaterial path forward. *Nat Nanotechnol* 2020; 15:646–655.

Shirato K *et al*. Development of fluorescent reverse transcription loop-mediated isothermal amplification (RT-LAMP) using quenching probes for the detection of the Middle East respiratory syndrome coronavirus. *J Virol Methods* 2018; 258:41–48.

Shoukat A *et al*. Lives saved and hospitalizations averted by COVID-19 vaccination in New York City: A modeling study. *Lancet Reg Health Am* 2022; 5:100085.

Singh AK *et al*. Remdesivir in COVID-19: A critical review of pharmacology, pre-clinical and clinical studies. *Diabetes Metab Syndr* 2020a; 14:641–648.

Singh TU, *et al*. Drug repurposing approach to fight COVID-19. *Pharmacol Rep* 2020b; 72:1479–1508.

Sinha P *et al*. Is a "cytokine storm" relevant to COVID-19? *JAMA Intern Med* 2020; 180:1152–1154.

Su B *et al*. Efficacy and tolerability of lopinavir/ritonavir- and efavirenz-based initial antiretroviral therapy in HIV-1 infected patients in a tertiary care hospital in Beijing, China. *Front Pharmacol* 2019; 10:1472.

Tai W *et al*. Characterization of the receptor-binding domain (RBD) of 2019 novel coronavirus: Implication for development of RBD protein as a viral attachment inhibitor and vaccine. *Cell Mol Immunol* 2020; 17:613–620.

Tan Q *et al*. Is oseltamivir suitable for fighting against COVID-19: In silico assessment, *in vitro* and retrospective study. *Bioorg Chem* 2020; 104:104257.

Tan YL *et al*. Combination treatment with remdesivir and ivermectin exerts highly synergistic and potent antiviral activity against murine coronavirus infection. *Front Cell Infect Microbiol* 2021; 11:700502.

Tang X *et al*. On the origin and continuing evolution of SARS-CoV-2. *Natl Sci Rev* 2020; 7:1012–1023.

Vellingiri B *et al*. COVID-19: A promising cure for the global panic. *Sci Total Environ* 2020; 725:138277.

Wang D *et al*. Clinical characteristics of 138 hospitalized patients with 2019 novel coronavirus-infected pneumonia in Wuhan, China. *JAMA* 2020a; 323:1061–1069.

Wang H *et al*. The genetic sequence, origin, and diagnosis of SARS-CoV-2. *Eur J Clin Microbiol Infect Dis* 2020b; 39:1629–1635.

Wang X, Powell CA. How to translate the knowledge of COVID-19 into the prevention of Omicron variants. *Clin Transl Med* 2021; 11:e680.

WHO (World Health Organization), 2020. WHO Discontinues Hydroxy-chloroquine and Lopinavir/ritonavir Treatment Arms for COVID-19. https://www.who.int/news/item/04-07-2020-who-discontinues-hydroxychloroquine-and-lopinavir-ritonavir-treatment-arms-for-covid-19 (accessed 4 July 2020).

WHO (World Health Organization), 2021a. Q&As on COVID-19 and Related Health Topics. https://www.who.int/emergencies/diseases/novel-coronavirus-2019/question-and-answers-hub (accessed 22 December 2021).

WHO (World Health Organization), 2021b. Therapeutics and COVID-19: Living Guideline. https://www.who.int/publications/i/item/WHO-2019-nCoV-therapeutics-2021.3 (accessed 24 September 2021).

WHO (World Health Organization), 2021c. Enhancing Readiness for Omicron (B.1.1.529): Technical Brief and Priority Actions for Member

States. https://www.who.int/publications/m/item/enhancing-readiness-for-omicron-(b.1.1.529)-technical-brief-and-priority-actions-for-member-states (accessed 23 December 2021).

Wu R *et al*. An update on current therapeutic drugs treating COVID-19. *Curr Pharmacol Rep* 2020; May 11:1–15.

Xu X *et al*. Effective treatment of severe COVID-19 patients with tocilizumab. *Proc Natl Acad Sci USA* 2020; 117:10970–10975.

Yang C *et al*. Alpha-1 antitrypsin for COVID-19 treatment: Dual role in antiviral infection and anti-inflammation. *Front Pharmacol* 2020; 11:615398.

Yoshida M *et al*. Local and systemic responses to SARS-CoV-2 infection in children and adults. *Nature* 2022; 602:321–327.

Zanin L *et al*. SARS-CoV-2 can induce brain and spine demyelinating lesions. *Acta Neurochir (Wien)* 2020; 162:1491–1494.

Zhang Y *et al*. Rapid molecular detection of SARS-CoV-2 (COVID-19) virus RNA using colorimetric LAMP. *medRxiv* 2020a; 2020.02.26.20028373.

Zhang Y *et al*. Current targeted therapeutics against COVID-19: Based on first-line experience in China. *Pharmacol Res* 2020b; 157:104854.

Zhou P *et al*. A pneumonia outbreak associated with a new coronavirus of probable bat origin. *Nature* 2020; 579:270–273.

Zhou Y, Simmons G. Development of novel entry inhibitors targeting emerging viruses. *Expert Rev Anti Infect Ther* 2012; 10:1129–1138.

Zhu N *et al*. A novel coronavirus from patients with pneumonia in China, 2019. *N Engl J Med* 2020; 382:727–733.

Chapter 2

Insights into Molecular Evolution and Increased Transmissibility of SARS-CoV-2

Rohit Verma[*,‡], **Milan Surjit**[*,§], **Ramandeep Kaur**[†,‖], **and Sunil K. Lal**[†,**]

*Virology Laboratory,
Translational Health Science and Technology Institute,
NCR Biotech Science Cluster,
Faridabad Haryana, India*

†*School of Science, Tropical Medicine and Biology Platform,
Monash University, Bandar Sunway, Selangor, Malaysia*

‡*rohitverma@thsti.res.in*
§*Milan@thsti.res.in*
‖*ramandeepkaur@monash.edu*
****sunil.lal@monash.edu*

Abstract

The never-ending race for survival between the virus and its host continues to be a major challenge for biologists as well as healthcare professionals. Owing to their simple genome organization, capacity for replication, mutation and adaptation — viruses can evolve rapidly, thereby posing a constant threat to human and other animal hosts.

The animal-human species barrier constitutes a considerable hurdle for zoonotic viruses, and often shields humans from the risk of new out-breaks. However, modern lifestyles and advanced technology have diminished geographic barriers, exposing humans to outbreaks initiated in one part of the world, and amplifying the associated health risks and economic losses across the globe. The novel SARS-CoV-2 outbreak that originated from Wuhan, China at the end of 2019 highlights that humans are continuously living under the threat of emerging zoonotic viruses. The Coronavirus disease 2019 (COVID-19) pandemic continues unabated despite the availability and deployment of multiple approved vaccines and supportive therapies. Moreover, SARS-CoV-2 variants have emerged which contain mutations that promote viral transmissibility and/or viru-lence. Furthermore, these new variants have raised concerns over the pro-tective efficacy of current vaccines and the susceptibility of unvaccinated individuals. This chapter discusses the potential causes and factors that influence viral fitness and host selection leading to the emergence of eas-ily transmissible and highly pathogenic SARS-CoV-2 variants.

Keywords: Human Coronavirus; SARS-CoV-2; Coronavirus evolution; transmission; SARS-CoV-2 variants; recombination; mutations; mutation rate

2.1. Introduction

Coronaviruses (CoV) are enveloped, single-stranded, positive-sense RNA viruses known to cause respiratory and intestinal dysfunction in animals and humans. At least seven Coronaviruses are known to cause infections in humans (Cui *et al.*, 2019) (Figure 2.1). Until the emergence of severe acute respiratory syndrome Coronavirus (SARS-CoV) in 2002–2003, these viruses were not considered to be a significant threat to humans as they caused mild infections in immunocompetent individuals. The SARS-CoV outbreak that started in the Guangdong province of China high-lighted the huge impact a zoonotic human-to-human infection can cause — resulting in 755 deaths and 8,273 clinical cases worldwide (Ksiazek *et al.*, 2003). Another highly pathogenic Coronavirus, the Middle East respiratory syndrome CoV (MERS-CoV) emerged approxi-mately 10 years after the SARS-CoV outbreak, and claimed 858 deaths with 2,494 reported cases (Zaki *et al.*, 2012).

On 30 December 2019, a highly pathogenic Coronavirus was identi-fied in Wuhan, China, which was subsequently named as the

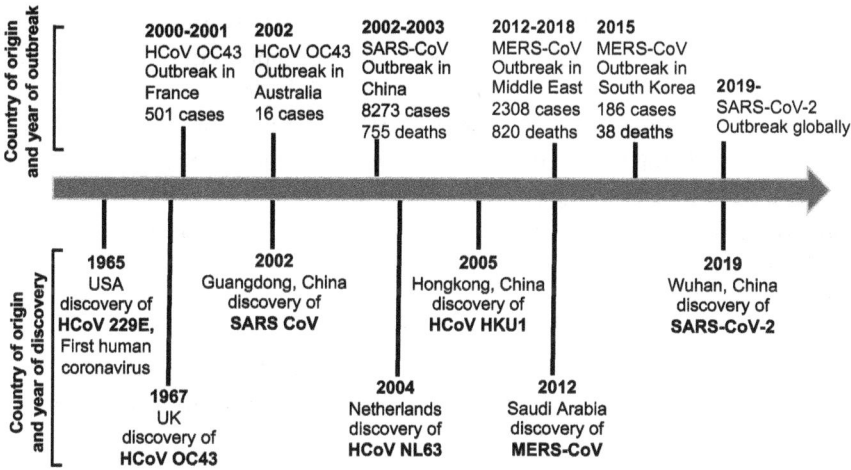

Figure 2.1.   Timeline of discovery and outbreaks of human Coronaviruses.

SARS-CoV-2 (Xu *et al.*, 2020). Several studies indicated that the virus originated in bats, and was subsequently transmitted to humans through intermediate animal host(s). Since the World Health Organization (WHO) designated COVID-19 as a pandemic on 11 March 2020, SARS-CoV-2 continues to spread globally at an alarming speed, in contrast to SARS-CoV and MERS-CoV. Moreover, although initial genome sequencing studies did not reveal much variation in the sequences of different geographical isolates of the virus, several variants have been reported to date, indicating rapid evolution of the virus. Multiple independent studies have attempted to uncover the unique properties of SARS-CoV-2 that enable it to evolve rapidly and to transmit at a higher rate while retaining its virulence. In the following sections, we consolidate the relevant findings, and discuss the unique features of this virus that enable it to retain and enhance its fitness inside the host.

2.2. Zoonosis and Host Range Expansion of SARS-CoV-2

SARS-CoV-2 is a beta-Coronavirus belonging to the family of *Coronaviridae*. Coronaviruses are zoonotic. Phylogenetic analysis of the SARS-CoV-2 genome indicated that it originated from bats, which are known to be a natural host for other human Coronaviruses as well (Lu *et al.*, 2020). In early 2020, sequence analysis of the complete or partial viral genomes isolated from nine patients revealed 99.98% genetic similarity among the different samples. By comparing with the genome sequences of other Coronaviruses, SARS-CoV-2 was found to be closely related to two SARS-like Coronaviruses (SARSl-CoV) of bat origin, i.e. bat-SL-CoVZC45 and bat-SL-CoVZXC21 (88% sequence homology). Further, SARS-CoV-2 shares 79% and 50% sequence homology with SARS-CoV and MERS-CoV, respectively (Lu *et al.*, 2020). The bat origin of SARS-CoV-2 is also supported by another independent study, which compared the genome sequence of SARS-CoV-2 with that of the bat-SARS-like CoVs and the bat-CoV RaTG13. SARS-CoV-2 and RaTG13 share 96.3% sequence homology, indicating the latter to be the likely source that involves a complex natural selection process during zoonotic transfer (Paraskevis *et al.*, 2020). Both studies support the fact that the SARS-CoV-2 originated in bats and recently emerged to infect humans.

Coronaviruses usually depend on an intermediate host that mediates transmission from bat to human. After acquiring the required modifications for infection and replication, viruses in bat can expand their host range and eventually infect humans. By synonymous codon usage analysis, Ji *et al.* (2020) initially suggested the snake to be an intermediate host for SARS-CoV-2. However, that proposition remains to be experimentally validated. Malayan pangolins (*Manis javanica*) are endangered mammals which are highly sought after for their meat and medicinal value of their scales. Metagenomic analysis of diseased Malayan pangolins from China identified them to be infected with the Sendai virus as well as several Coronaviruses, including SARS-CoV (Liu *et al.*, 2019). A study from the South China Agricultural University in Guangzhou, China revealed 99% genetic similarity between the Coronavirus isolated from pangolins and COVID-19 patients (Cyranoski, 2020). Considering their mammalian origin and high demand for human use, pangolins may be another possible intermediate host for SARS-CoV-2 (Figure 2.2). Additionally, the possible existence of an incidental host has also been proposed by some studies. Seroprevalence of SARS-CoV-2 in pet cats indicates the cat as an incidental host. Using RT-PCR-based diagnostic assay, independent reports have confirmed SARS-CoV-2-positive pet cats. Even tigers and lions in New York City zoo have displayed the symptoms of respiratory illness and decreased appetite, suggesting their susceptibility to infection by SARS-CoV-2. However, only the tiger was confirmed to be positive for SARS-CoV-2 infection (Latif and Mukaratirwa, 2020). This raises the possibility of human-to-animal transmission of the SARS-CoV-2 virus. Further, farm-raised minks in the Netherlands were positive for

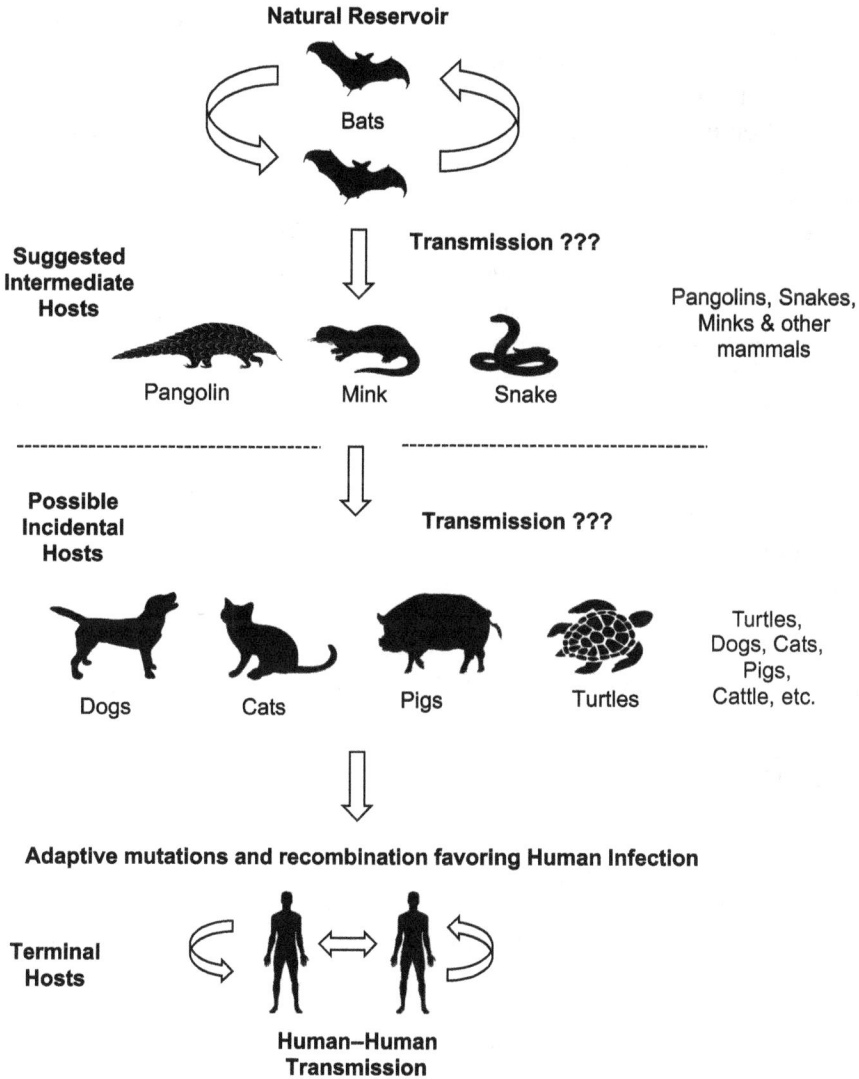

Figure 2.2. Host range and proposed host transmission routes for SARS-CoV-2.

SARS-CoV-2. The possible source of transmission was proposed to be human-to-mink followed by mink-to-mink. However, another report claimed the presence of SARS-CoV-2 infection in farm-raised minks in Denmark since March 2019, thereby suggesting the mink to be a possible intermediate host for transmission of the virus to humans (Latif and Mukaratirwa, 2020).

Once the virus adapts to the human host, direct transmission occurs from human to human. In addition to the transmission via direct contact with infected material or fomites, the virus mainly spreads through respiratory droplets from coughing and sneezing, similar to other airborne pathogens. This further amplifies the infection risk. The first indication of possible human-to-human transmission of SARS-CoV-2 came from the analysis of a family of six patients, who traveled to Wuhan during the early days of initiation of the outbreak, i.e. between 29 December 2019 and 4 January 2020 (Chan *et al.*, 2020). Another case of possible human–human transmission was reported in Vietnam, where a 27-year old man was identified to be infected with the 2019-nCoV. Although he did not travel to China, his parents visited several cities across Vietnam and came in contact with many people before staying with their son for 3 days. His father was believed to be the source of human–human transmission. However, his infection status was not confirmed as he was asymptomatic (Phan *et al.*, 2020). In a larger study involving 138 hospitalized patients infected with SARS-CoV-2, hospital-related transmission was suspected in 41% of patients out of whom 29% were healthcare professionals (Wang *et al.*, 2020a). Subsequent studies have confirmed human-to-human transmission of SARS-CoV-2 (Kutter *et al.*, 2021).

2.3. Evolution and Transmission of SARS-CoV-2

SARS-CoV-2 is an enveloped virus, with a non-segmented positive-strand RNA genome of around 30 kb. The viral genome is capped at the 5′-end and poly(A)-tailed at the 3′-end. The 5′-untranslated region (UTR) RNA folds into a secondary structure similar to that seen in other beta-Coronaviruses. It contains a leader sequence and a transcriptional regulatory sequence (TRS) which are essential regulatory elements for synthesis of virus-encoded proteins. TRS helps in the process of template switching during the synthesis of the negative-strand RNA by base-pairing between the TRS-L and nascent TRS-B by the viral transcriptase/replicase complex (Yang and Leibowitz, 2015). The 5′-end cap of the SARS-CoV-2 genome protects it from host nucleases (Romano *et al.*, 2020). The 5′-cap is also important for cap-dependent translation of the viral RNA by exploiting the host translation machinery. The 3′-UTR of the viral RNA also contains multiple stem loops that regulate the viral replication process. Studies have highlighted the importance of virus–host RNA-protein interactions in the replication and pathogenesis of SARS-CoV-2 (Banerjee *et al.*, 2020; Schmidt *et al.*, 2021; Verma *et al.*, 2021).

The life-cycle of SARS-CoV-2 begins with its entry into the respiratory epithelial cells (primary site of infection). Virus entry relies on two types of host peptidase, i.e. carboxypeptidase and serine/cysteine elastase peptidase (Fuentes-Prior *et al.*, 2021; Shang *et al.*, 2020). First, pre-activation of the spike (S) protein in the incoming viruses occurs by furin cleavage of the S protein at Arg685-Ser686, which separates the S protein into S1 and S2 subunits. The S1subunit contains the receptor-binding domain (RBD), while the S2 subunit mediates fusion of the virus. Second, the carboxypeptidase ACE2 interacts with the RBD of the S1 subunit. Third, the S2 subunit harbors a cleavage site for the membrane-bound serine protease known as transmembrane protease serine 2 (TMPRSS2) that cleaves the S2 subunit at position Arg815-Ser816, resulting in exposure of the highly antigenic Ser816-Phe833 fusion peptide that facilitates membrane fusion in a manner similar to the SNARE-mediated fusion (Bayati *et al.*, 2021; Fuentes-Prior *et al.*, 2021; Shang *et al.*, 2020). Plasma membrane fusion of SARS-CoV-2 results in clathrin-mediated endocytosis of the virus, and subsequent release of the viral RNA into the cytoplasm (Bayati *et al.*, 2021) (Figure 2.3).

Viral genomic RNA contains 14 open reading frames (ORFs) that include ORF1a and ORF1b, which produce polyproteins that are proteolytically processed to produce non-structural proteins essential for viral transcription and replication (Wu *et al.*, 2020a). Transcription of the viral genome is mediated by the viral RNA-dependent RNA polymerase (RdRp)-associated protein complex that leads to generation of multiple sub-genomic RNAs. In the case of SARS-CoV-2, nine sub-genomic RNAs are produced through the canonical pathway, while three sub-genomic RNAs are produced through the non-canonical pathways (Kim *et al.*, 2020). Structural proteins such as spike (S) glycoprotein, matrix (M), envelope (E), nucleocapsid (N) are produced from independent sub-genomic RNAs. Compared to SARS-CoV, SARS-CoV-2 encodes an additional ORF, called ORF10 (Michel *et al.*, 2020). Overall, there are many similarities between the genomes, proteomes and life-cycles of SARS-CoV and SARS-CoV-2. Despite that, SARS-CoV-2 differs from SARS-CoV in terms of higher transmissibility and infectivity. The following sections summarize our current understanding of the mechanisms contributing to rapid evolution and increased transmissibility of the SARS-CoV-2.

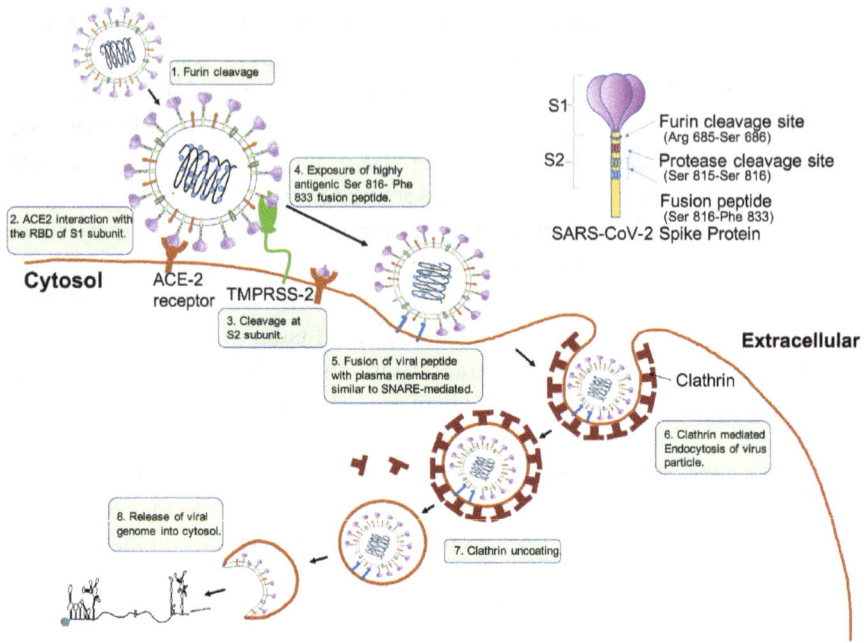

Figure 2.3.   Mechanism of SARS-CoV-2 entry into the host cell.

2.3.1. *Enhanced infectivity*

Multiple independent studies have revealed some unique characteristics of SARS-CoV-2 that enhance its infectivity compared to SARS-CoV. SARS-CoV-2 transcripts are found in broncho-alveolar lavage fluid, sputum, nasal swabs, bronchoscopy brush biopsies, pharyngeal swabs, feces, and blood of COVID-19 patients, at proportions of 93%, 72%, 63%, 46%, 32%, 29%, and 1%, respectively (Wang *et al.*, 2020b). Further, autopsy reports from 27 COVID-19 patients (aged above 50 years) confirm SARS-CoV-2 infection in pharynx, heart, kidney, liver, brain, lymphocytes, submucous gland, spleen, and blood (in addition to lungs). Specifically, different compartments of the kidney were found to be positive for SARS-CoV-2 infection. The primary target site for renal infection was identified as the glomerular cells (Bradley *et al.*, 2020; Puelles *et al.*, 2020). Gastrointestinal symptoms and presence of virus in rectal swabs imply SARS-CoV-2 infection of intestine in COVID-19 patients. SARS-CoV-2 infection has also been demonstrated in human small intestine organoids which exhibited virus replication, mainly in the enterocyte progenitor cells (Lamers *et al.*, 2020). Placental infection and vertical transmission of SARS-CoV-2 has also been reported (Algarroba *et al.*, 2020; Baud *et al.*, 2020; Hosier *et al.*, 2020). Several proteases are known to regulate the life-cycle of human Coronaviruses. These proteases have tissue-specific expression patterns which may explain the higher cell tropism of SARS-CoV-2. In the case of SARS-CoV and SARS-CoV-2, during entry to the host cell, a host membrane-associated serine protease (MASP) known as TMPRSS2, plays a vital role in facilitating fusion and endocytosis of the virus — by proteolytically cleaving both the spike and ACE2 proteins (Fuentes-Prior *et al.*, 2021). In addition, SARS-CoV-2 S protein also harbors a furin cleavage site preceding the TMPRSS2 cleavage site, which enables the incoming virions to remain in a pre-activated state to facilitate rapid entry of the virus into host cells. Pre-activation by furin provides an advantage to SARS-CoV-2 by allowing them to be less dependent on the target cells for their life-cycle, and enhances their entry into other target cells which have lower expression of TMPRSS2 (Shang *et al.*, 2020). It is noteworthy that ACE2, TMPRSS2 and furin are co-expressed in a subset of bronchial cells in the lungs, that may explain severe lung dysfunction and pneumonia in many COVID-19 patients.

Studies also show that additional MASPs may synergize or substitute TMPRSS2 during the course of SARS-CoV-2 infection. Recognition sites for 11 out of 13 known MASPs have been reported in the SARS-CoV-2 S protein, out of which 10 are accessible (Chakraborty *et al.*, 2021). In addition to lungs, heart and intestine, certain MASPs are expressed at high levels in the liver, skin, esophagus, stomach, kidney, placenta, testis, vagina, and brain. For example, TMPRSS5 and TMPRSS7 are highly expressed in brain; TMPRSS6 and TMPRSS1 are expressed in the liver; TMPRSS10 is expressed in the cardiomyocytes; and TMPRSS12, TMPRSS6, TMPRSS7 are expressed highly the prostate and testis (Fuentes-Prior *et al.*, 2021). *In vitro* studies have shown the ability of several MASPs in promoting fusion of SARS-CoV-2 (Shang *et al.*, 2020). Notably, TMPRSS2 and TMPRSS4 have been shown to synergistically promote viral fusion (Bertram *et al.*, 2010; Zang *et al.*, 2020). Further, TMPRSS11D, TMPRSS11E and TMPRSS11F have been shown to activate viral fusion (Hoffmann *et al.*, 2020). Contrasting results have been shown regarding the ability of TMPRSS11A in activating viral fusion. TMPRSSB has been proposed to be involved in an alternate viral entry pathway (Zhang *et al.*, 2020).

Involvement of multiple MASPs in the SARS-CoV-2 entry process suggests the possible existence of virus reservoirs in different organs of COVID-19 patients, which may further amplify the infection cycle. Immune-privileged organs such as testis, placenta, eyes, and brain may be potential reservoirs of SARS-CoV-2. A study on the host–virus interactome revealed the testis as the second most prominent tissue for interaction between SARS-CoV-2 and host proteins (Gordon *et al.*, 2020). Further, reports of patients displaying persistent COVID-19 symptoms warrant the need for functional characterization of such virus reservoirs (Counotte *et al.*, 2018; Siemann *et al.*, 2017; Xu *et al.*, 2006).

In addition, inhibitors of MASPs have also been proposed for controlling SARS-CoV-2 infection. Kunitz or serpin family protease inhibitors control the activity of MASPs *in vivo*. HAI-2 (a Kunitz-type protease inhibitor) has been shown to inhibit TMPRSS2 or matriptase activity, and to reduce the replication of influenza viruses (Chen *et al.*, 1998). Moreover, *in vitro* studies have demonstrated inhibition of SARS-CoV-2 infection by alpha-1-antitrypsin (AAT), a member of the serpin family of protease inhibitors — AAT acts by inhibiting the activity of TMPRSS2 and elastase-like proteases (Yan *et al.*, 2020). Interestingly, the D614G mutation of the SARS-CoV-2 spike protein creates a cleavage site for neutrophil elastase, leading to enhanced activation of spike protein (Bhattacharyya *et al.*, 2021). CD209L/L-SIGN and CD209/D-SIGN have been identified as alternative receptors for SARS-CoV-2 entry into human cells. Ectopic expression of CD209L/L-SIGN and CD209/D-SIGN was found to mediate SARS-CoV-2 S-pseudotyped virus entry into human endothelial cells. Further, soluble CD209L-Fc prevented virus entry. These studies demonstrate the use of an alternate receptor by SARS-CoV-2 which may further expand its cell tropism (Amraei *et al.*, 2021).

2.3.2. *Recombination efficiency of the viral genome*

Coronaviruses are notorious for their ability to generate new variants through frequent RNA recombination. Homologous RNA recombination is achieved by random template switching during RNA replication (van der Most *et al.*, 1992). The high tendency for recombination may aid in the emergence of new variants that are more pathogenic and/or show a wider host range. Among the highly pathogenic human CoVs, SARS-CoV and MERS-CoV have been extensively studied. Initial studies on the origin of SARS-CoV led to identification of SARS-related CoVs (SARSr-CoVs) in horseshoe bats in 2005 (Lau *et al.*, 2005; Li *et al.*, 2005). Subsequent studies identified many SARSr-CoVs in bats from different provinces of China as well as many other countries. Further studies discovered the co-existence of diverse SARSr-CoVs among the bat population from single habitat in a cave in the Yunnan province of China (Hu *et al.*, 2017). The viruses isolated from these caves contained all the genetic variants found in the SARS-CoVs. Recombination analysis revealed S and ORF8 genes to be involved in frequent recombination (Hu *et al.*, 2017). Since RNA recombination is common in CoVs, it is believed that SARS-CoV originally emerged through RNA recombination from the bat-derived SARSr-CoVs found in Yunnan. However, since there were no SARS cases in Yunnan during the 2002–2003 SARS outbreak, it was proposed that the progenitor of SARS-CoV was generated by recombination in bats, which was then transmitted to an intermediate host such as masked palm civets. These infected civets probably spread the virus in the Guangdong market where the virus acquired additional mutations in the genome to become competent to infect humans (Hu *et al.*, 2017).

In the case of SARS-CoV-2, two independent studies suggest bats to be the natural host (Lu *et al.*, 2020; Paraskevis *et al.*, 2020). Comparison of the genome sequences of SARS-CoV-2 with those of the bat-SARS-like CoVs and the bat-CoV RaTG13 revealed the discordant phylogenetic relationship between SARS-CoV-2 and RaTG13 clade with the bat-SARS-like CoVs. Bat-SARS-like CoV sequences were found to cluster in different positions in the tree, indicating that they were recombinants, distant from the SARS-CoV-2 and RaTG13 (Paraskevis *et al.*, 2020). Thus, it appears that SARS-CoV-2 did not emerge due to any recent recombination event. As mentioned earlier, the pangolin has been suggested to be a possible intermediate host for human transmission of SARS-CoV-2. However, direct evidence in support of this claim remains to be shown. A study of 26,312 SARS-CoV-2 genomic sequences found three different unrelated recombination events in humans, pangolins, and bats — and also identified putative recombination among the bat-CoV-RaTG13 and pangolin-CoV-2019. This recombination site is located in the RBD region of the S protein. This recombination event followed by directional evolution may have led to the adaptation of the virus in the human host (Zhu *et al.*, 2020). Moreover, co-expression analysis of MERS-CoV and SARS-CoV-2 suggests that recombination events may be the main player for potential future outbreaks (Banerjee *et al.*, 2020).

In support of the role of recombination events in driving the evolution of the virus, another study claims that evolution of an ancestor of SARS CoV-2 may have begun 11 years ago, which included two insertions in the RBD region (at positions 432–436 and 460–472) of the S protein (Patino-Galindo *et al.*, 2021).

2.3.3. *Mutation rate of the viral genome*

Coronaviruses are RNA viruses which rely on the viral RdRp to replicate. Compared to DNA polymerases, RdRp has lower fidelity and is therefore more prone to introduce mutations in the viral genome (Steinhauer *et al.*, 1992). Multiple rounds of replication thus generate a considerable number of genetic variants in a short time span. These variants may offer several benefits to the progeny viruses, including increased virulence, transmissibility, and/or broader host range. The mutation rate for SARS-CoV-2 has been estimated to be 33 genomic mutations per year. The estimated R0 of SARS-CoV-2 ranges between 1.4 and 6.5 — which is a much higher transmission rate compared to SARS-CoV and MERS-CoV (Li *et al.*, 2020; Liu *et al.*, 2020b; Wu *et al.*, 2020b). Mutations in the viral genome have resulted in the emergence of numerous variants of SARS-CoV-2. Initially, six major lineages of SARS-CoV-2 were classified as A, B, B.1, B.1.1., B.1.177, and B.1.1.7 (Rambaut *et al.*, 2020). Subsequently, to further simplify the nomenclature, WHO recommended the use of a distinct classification system based on the Greek alphabets. According to the WHO classification, all SARS-CoV-2 variants are distributed into two major categories, namely variants of interest (VOI) and variants of concern (VOC). VOI refers to a variant of SARS-CoV-2 which causes significant community transmission and possesses genetic changes that are likely to affect its transmissibility, disease severity, diagnostic detection, therapeutic management, or immune escape. VOC refers to a VOI that has been experimentally demonstrated to possess the characteristics of VOI, and shown to be a major public health hazard. So far, VOCs have been classified as Alpha, Beta, Gamma, Delta and Omicron variants; while VOIs have been classified as Eta, Iota, Kappa, Lambda and Epsilon variants (Table 2.1) (Otto *et al.*, 2021; Wang and Powell, 2021).

The B.1.1.7 or Alpha variant was first detected in October 2020 in the UK. It accumulated 23 mutations with reference to the Wuhan lineage A. Among these 23 mutations, 14 mutations are lineage-specific, while three

Table 2.1. List of key circulating and emerging SARS-CoV-2 variants with their defining mutations and subsequent impact on viral transmission and infectivity.

Variant Name	First Detection	WHO Classification	Spread	Defining Mutations	Gene/ORF	Advantages of Mutations to Virus	References
Variants of Concern (VOCs)							
B.1.1.7 "UK variant"	October 2020, UK	Alpha	Reported mainly in UK, USA, Germany, Italy (over 114 countries worldwide).	del 69/70 HV, del 144/145 Y, E484K, N501Y, A570D, P681H, T716I, S982A, D1118H (S). T10011, A1708D, I2230T (ORF1ab). Q27*, R52I, Y73C (ORF8). D3L, S235F (N).	S ORF1ab ORF8 N	Enhanced transmission potential (~70%) and virulence compared to initially emerged SARS-CoV-2. Enhanced death in infected individuals by 64%. del 69/70 and del 144/145 potentially alter the shape of spike protein, rendering available antibodies ineffective. E484K is located in RBD, influencing viral entry via its interaction with	Challen *et al.* (2021). Davies *et al.* (2021). Grint *et al.* (2021). Hoffmann *et al.*, (2020). Liu *et al.*, 2021. Peacock *et al.* (2021). Rambaut *et al.* (2020). Resende *et al.* (2021). Starr *et al.* (2020). Tang *et al.* (2021). Tarke *et al.* (2021). Volz *et al.* (2021).

(Continued)

Table 2.1.   *(Continued)*

Variant Name	First Detection	WHO Classification	Spread	Defining Mutations	Gene/ORF	Advantages of Mutations to Virus	References
						ACE2 receptor; may favor immune evasion. N501Y in RBD enhances its affinity to human and murine ACE2 receptor. P681H may potentially affect viral replication and infectivity. P681H proximity to furin cleavage site confers advantage to virus by promoting viral entry and transmission.	Davies *et al.* (2021). Liu *et al.* (2021). Rees-Spear *et al.* (2021). Tegally *et al.* (2021). Wibmer *et al.* (2021). Zhou *et al.* (2021).
B.1.351 or 20H501Y.V2 "South African variant"	October 2020, South Africa	Beta	Prevalent mainly in South Africa, Belgium, Germany (over 68 countries).	L18F, D80A, D215G (S NTD). K417N, E484K, N501Y, A701V (S RBD). K1655N (ORF1a). P71L (E). T205I (N).	S (NTD, RBD) ORF1a E N	Enhances immune or vaccine induced evasion. Transmission enhanced by ~50%. NTD deletion near furin cleavage site abrogates	

Name	Origin	WHO	Prevalence	Mutations	Gene	Effects	References
B.1.1.28.1 or P.1 or 20J/501Y.V3 "Brazil variant"	November-December 2020, Brazil	Gamma	Prevalent mainly in Brazil, Belgium, USA, Italy (over 36 countries).	L18F, T20N, P26S, D138Y, R190S, K417N/T, E484K, N501Y, H655Y, T1027I (S). del 11288-11296 (3675-3677) in ORF1b. G174C (ORF3a). E92K (ORF8). P80R (N).	S ORF1b ORF3a ORF8 N	protection conferred by neutralizing human monoclonal antibodies. Increased transmission potential by 2.5 fold as compared to the parental strain. Overall reduction against neutralizing antisera.	Coutinho et al. (2021). Faria et al. (2021). Franceschi et al. (2021). Kupferschmidt (2021). Naveca et al. (2021). Nonaka et al. (2021). Voloch et al. (2021).
B.1.617.2 AY.1 AY.2 AY.3	October 2020, India.	Delta	Mainly in India. Seen in USA during March 2021.	T19R, G142D, del 156, del 157, R158G, L452R, T478K, D614G, P681R, D950N (S).	S	Increased transmission than B.1.1.7 by 64%. T478K is mainly responsible for greater spike protein stability, and higher positive	Otto et al. (2021). Pascarella et al. (2021).

(Continued)

Table 2.1.   (*Continued*)

Variant Name	First Detection	WHO Classification	Spread	Defining Mutations	Gene/ ORF	Advantages of Mutations to Virus	References
						electrostatic potential between spike and ACE2 proteins.	
B.1.1.529	November 2021, South Africa	Omicron	Very rapid spread to least 90 countries by mid-December 2021.	At least 50 mutations, with 36 in S and RBD.	S	In early infection, about 4 times more transmissible than Delta. Over 5-fold higher risk of reinfection than Delta.	Kumar *et al.* (2021).
					Others	Mutations S371L, S373P, S375F, T478K, Q493R, Q498R, 501Y contribute significantly to stronger binding affinity for ACE2 than Delta variant.	
Variants of Interest (VOIs)							
B.1.427 or B.1.429 diverged from CAL.20C "California variant"	July 2020, USA	Epsilon	USA, Australia, Denmark, Singapore, New Zealand, Israel, UK.	B.1.429: S131, W152C, L452R, S477N, Q677H (S). I4205V (ORF1a). D1183Y (ORF1b).		L452R was first detected in minks. L452R confers resistance to neutralizing monoclonal antibodies	Annavajhala *et al.* (2021). Deng *et al.* (2021). Otto *et al.* (2021). Zhang *et al.* (2021).

Lineage	Date, Location	WHO label	Countries	Mutations	Genes	Notes	References
				B.1.427: L452R (S).	S, ORF1a, ORF1b	generated against spike antigen (by 4 to 6.7 fold), but does not affect sensitivity to convalescent plasma. L452R enhances receptor binding. Transmission potential enhanced by ~20%. Evidence of increased disease severity is not reported.	Chand et al. (2020). McNally et al. (2021).
B.1.525	December 2020, USA	Eta	USA, Canada, Denmark, Britain, France, Belgium, Spain, Finland, Nigeria, Ghana, Jordan, Australia, Singapore, UK (over 23 countries).	A67V, del 69/70, del 144, E484K, D614G, Q677H, F888L (S). T20071 (ORF1a). P314F (ORF1b). I82T (M). A12G, T205I (N).	S, ORF1a, ORF1b, M, N	E484K facilitates immune evasion. Q677H/P may enhance viral entry and infectivity. Overall advantage conferred to virus is not characterized.	

(Continued)

Table 2.1.   *(Continued)*

Variant Name	First Detection	WHO Classification	Spread	Defining Mutations	Gene/ORF	Advantages of Mutations to Virus	References
B.1.526	November 2020, USA	Iota	Mainly in USA, Mexico, Australia, New Zealand, Singapore, Thailand, Taiwan, Poland and Israel with few reports in Aruba, UK, Ireland, Croatia.	L5F, T95I, D253G, S477N, E484K, N501Y, D614G, A701V (S). T265I, L3201P, del 3675/3677 (ORF1a). P314L, Q1011H (ORF1b). P42L, Q57H (ORF3a). T111 (ORF8).	S (RBD, NTD) ORF1a ORF1b ORF3a ORF8	D253G is located in antigen supersite, rendering neutralizing antibodies ineffective. E484K is located in RBD, influences viral entry. E484K lowers activity of convalescent plasma or vaccine sera (by 7.7 or 3.4 fold).	Annavajhala et al. (2021). Cerutti et al. 2021 West et al. (2021).
B.1.617.1	October 2020	Kappa	Mainly in India	T95I, G142D, E154K, L452R, E484Q, D614G, P681R, Q1071H (S). T1567I, T3646A, M5753I, K6711R (ORF1ab). V82A (ORF7a). R203M (N).	S ORF1ab ORF3a ORF7a N	Transmission rate is similar to B.1.1.7.	Otto et al. (2021). Zella et al. (2021).
C.37	December 2020	Lambda	Peru, Chile, USA, and over 41 countries.	G75V, T76I, L452Q, F490S, D614G, T859N, del RSYLTPGD246-253N (Δ246–252).	S	Over 80% of COVID-19 cases replaced with this variant in Peru. Mutations T76I,	Kimura et al. (2021).

Lineage	Date	Name	Location	Mutations	Gene	Description	References
						L452Q (S); and seven amino acid deletion in NTD of spike protein (RSYLTPGD246-253N) responsible for evasion from neutralizing antibodies.	
P2	April 2020	Zeta	Brazil	E484K, D614G, V1176F.	S	—	Otto *et al.* (2021).
B.1.617.3	October 2020	Not applicable	India	T19R, G142D, L452R, E484Q, D614G, P681R, D950N.	S	—	Otto *et al.* (2021).
Other Emerging Variants							
A.23.1 (originated from A.23 lineage)	December 2020, Uganda	Not applicable	UK, Rwanda, Uganda, Canada, Belgium (over 15 countries in Africa, Asia, Europe, North America, Oceania)	R102I, F157L, L367F, V367F, Q613H, P681R (S). Multiple changes in S, NSP6, ORF8, ORF9.	S NSP6 ORF8 ORF9	V367F is thought to promote infectivity. Q613H shows similar attributes to D614G by enhancing spike trimer stability, infectivity and furin cleavage.	Bugembe *et al.* (2021). Hoffmann *et al.* (2020). Ou *et al.* (2021).

(Continued)

Table 2.1. *(Continued)*

Variant Name	First Detection	WHO Classification	Spread	Defining Mutations	Gene/ ORF	Advantages of Mutations to Virus	References
B.1.2 20C-US	October 2020, USA	Not applicable	USA, with cases in Canada, Mexico, Germany, Denmark	Q677H (S). M26061 (ORF1a). N1653D, R2613C (ORF1b).	S (RBD) ORF1a ORF1b	P681R adds a basic residue adjacent to the cleavage site; linked to enhanced cleavage by cellular proteases *in vitro*. Proximity of Q677H/P to S1/S2 cleavage site in spike protein may promote viral entry, and confer evolutionary advantage in transmission. N1653D is thought to alter potential protein-RNA interactions and viral translation. R2613C may manipulate local protein stability. Biological function of this variant needs further characterization.	Lauring and Hodcroft (2021). Pater *et al.* (2021).

Abbreviations: S = Spike protein, E = Envelope protein, M = Membrane protein, N = Nucleocapsid protein, * = Stop codon, del = Deletion, NTD = N-terminal domain, RBD = Receptor-binding domain.

mutations are in the S protein (substitutions N501Y, P681H; and deletion at positions 69–70) (Figure 2.4). It shows 40–80% increased transmissibility (with the R0 between 1.4 and 1.8), and around 60% increased lethality. It had caused a significant increase in the rate of COVID-19 in the UK. The N501Y mutation is considered to be crucial for the increased transmissibility of this variant (Davies *et al.*, 2021; Volz *et al.*, 2021). A variant of B.1.1.7 that contains an additional E484K mutation was identified in February 2021 in Oregon, and it is believed to be a locally emerged variant.

Another notable variant, the B.1.351 or Beta variant, was identified in October 2020 in South Africa — it contains K417N, E484K, N501Y mutations (Tegally *et al.*, 2021), and shows about 50% increased transmissibility (Figure 2.4). A third variant (B1.1.28.1 or Gamma) was identified in Brazil and Japan in December 2020 (Tegally *et al.*, 2021), and possesses 12 mutations that includes eight lineage-specific mutations and three substitution mutations at K417T, E484K, and N501Y (Figure 2.4). Gamma shows more than 100% increased transmissibility, and about 40–50% increased lethality (ECDC (European Centre for Disease Prevention and Control), 2021; PANGO Lineages, 2021). Another notable variant prevalent in the USA, the Cal.20C (B.1.429 or Epsilon) variant was identified in June 2020 — it contains five lineage-specific mutations including two mutations in ORF1a and ORF1b (I4205V, D1183Y), and three mutations in S protein (S13I, W152C, L452C) (Table 2.1). However, Epsilon marginally increases transmissibility (Li *et al.*, 2020; Zhang *et al.*, 2021).

It is noteworthy that the N501Y mutation is present in all variants associated with significantly increased transmissibility and lethality (Tegally *et al.*, 2021). Considering its location in the RBD, the N501Y mutation appears to enhance the affinity of interaction between RBD and ACE2. Another notable mutation is the D614G missense mutation, which first appeared in June 2020. The frequency of this mutation is high in COVID-19 patients — it moderately increases transmissibility but does not significantly increase lethality (Tiwari and Mishra, 2020; Saha *et al.*, 2020). The D614G mutation destroys the hydrogen-bond interaction with its neighbor monomer T859, and increases the interaction between RBD and ACE2 protein (Hu *et al.*, 2020).

In late 2020, the emergence of a new B.1.617+ lineage was reported from Maharashtra, India. This variant shows higher transmission, not seen with any other identified variants. It harbors E484Q and L452R mutations for its increased transmissibility (Vaidyanathan, 2021).

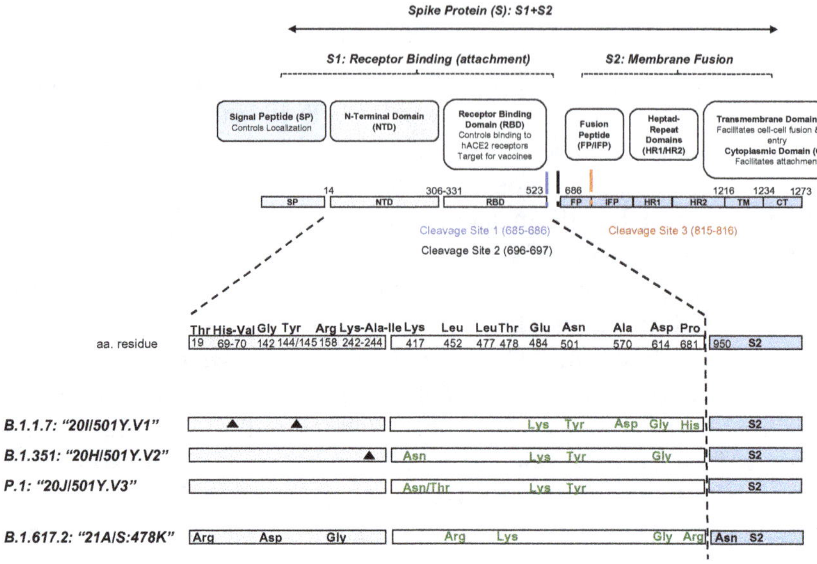

Figure 2.4.   Characteristics of SARS-CoV-2 spike (S) protein within four variants of concern. Alpha variant (B1.1.7), Beta variant (B1.351), Gamma variant (B.1.1.28.1 or P.1), and Delta variant (B.1.617.2) with their key mutations. Abbreviations: hACE2 = human angiotensin-converting enzyme-2, aa = amino acid residue, ▲= deletion, Ala = Alanine, Arg = Arginine, Asn = Asparagine, Asp = Aspartic acid, Glu = Glutamic acid, Gly = Glycine, His = Histidine, Ile = Isoleucine, Leu = Leucine, Lys = Lysine, Pro = Proline, Thr = Threonine, Tyr = Tyrosine, Val = Valine.

Examples of advantageous mutations in the spike protein of SARS-CoV-2 variants:

Asp614Gly (D614G) — missense mutation enhances transmission rate and viral infectivity.

Glu484Lys (E484K), del H69-V70, del Y144-145 — associated with host immune evasion.

Asn501Tyr (N501Y) — enhances binding affinity of RBD to hACE2 receptor.

Pro681His (P681H) — potentially affects viral replication and infectivity.

Lys417Asn/Thr (K417N/T) — may affect initial binding of the virus.

Thr478Lys (T478K) — enhances binding of RBD to hACE2 receptor by increasing the positive electrostatic potential.

In addition, triple mutations of E484Q, L452R, and P681R have been reported from other parts of India (first seen in West Bengal) — which was assigned as the B.1.618 lineage. Further, the variants of the B lineage have been classified into sub-lineages such as B.1.617.1, B.1.617.2, and B.1.617.3. Lineage B.1.617.1 and B.1.617.3 were proposed as VOIs by

WHO (Cherian *et al.*, 2021). These two VOIs contain 7–8 mutations in the S protein, of which five mutations (G142D, L452R, E484Q, D614G, P681R) are common in both variants. Mutations E154K and Q1071H are found in B.1.617.1 only. One of the sub-lineages of B.1.617 was designated as VOC in April 2021 because of its increased transmissibility, i.e. 64% higher transmission than B.1.1.7 or Alpha variant (Otto *et al.*, 2021). Based on WHO guidelines, it is now designated as the Delta variant. The Delta variant transmits with ten mutations in its spike protein, of which four mutations (G142D, L452R, D614G, P681R) are common with the other sub-lineages of B.1.617, while mutations T19R and D950N are similar to the B.1.617.3 sub-lineage. Mutations T478K, E484Q, and L452R are thought to increase binding strength of ACE2 and spike protein (Cherian *et al.*, 2021). Pascarella *et al.* (2021) investigated the role of mutant sites using surface and interface analysis, and suggested a possible role of T478K mutation in augmenting the stability and binding strength of spike protein by providing higher positive electrostatic potential between ACE2 and spike protein. Another study measured the energy required to detach ACE2 and spike protein binding in all the identified variants, and found that N501Y required highest energy, while RBD of Epsilon variant (L452R) easily detached from ACE2 (Kim *et al.*, 2021). Mutation P681R has been shown to promote furin-mediated cleavage in some of the variants (Lubinski *et al.*, 2021). On 26 November 2021, WHO identified another VOC, the Omicron variant B.1.1.529 which is considerably more transmissible than Delta. Omicron has about 50 mutations, of which 36 are in the spike protein and its RBD. Computational docking studies indicate that Omicron mutations Q493R, N501Y, S371L, S373P, S375F, Q498R and T478K contribute significantly to stronger binding affinity for ACE2 than the Delta variant (Kumar *et al.*, 2021) (Table 2.1).

The relationship between pathogenicity and evolution has not yet been clearly established for SARS-CoV-2. Several factors may support the continuous evolution of SARS-CoV-2 in humans, such as immunodeficiency and transient exposure to antibodies. In a case study, accelerated evolution has been observed in the case of immunocompromised patients with cancer (Avanzato *et al.*, 2020). In another *in vitro* study, sequential exposure of patient's plasma resulted in accumulation of mutations in the RBD region of SARS-CoV-2 S protein, ultimately causing resistance to neutralizing antibody (Andreano *et al.*, 2021; Li *et al.*, 2021). Additionally, SARS-CoV-2 evolution leads to infection in the incidental host and expansion of host range. For example, Y453F mutation in the S protein was first found in the mink, followed by increased transmission of the virus to humans (Oude Munnink *et al.*, 2021).

2.3.4. *Ability of the virus to survive in harsh environments*

The magnitude of viral infection is directly influenced by the structural integrity of the virus and quality of viral RNA. Several studies have shown the ability of human Coronaviruses to survive under harsh environmental conditions. HCoV-229E can survive for 6 days at 50% relative humidity or in phosphate-buffered saline solution. In contrast to the standard practice of inactivation of viruses in fetal calf serum at 56°C for 30 minutes, SARS-CoV needs 60°C for 30 minutes, and SARS-CoV-2 requires 70°C for 5 minutes for their inactivation (Kitajima *et al.*, 2020). SARS-CoV can also survive for 3–4 days after drying in different kinds of materials. Based on the structural characteristics of SARS-CoV-2, long survival time is estimated in waters and on different surfaces (Bogler *et al.*, 2020). The presence of SARS-CoV-2 RNA in feces, rectal swabs, and urine has been confirmed using reverse transcription-quantitative PCR (RT-qPCR), while cell-culturable viruses have been successfully isolated from feces. In some cases, feces and rectal swabs were found to be positive on day 11 from the onset of infection. Thus, the presence of SARS-CoV-2 in feces, urine, saliva ultimately leads to viral discharge in the sewer system. SARS-CoV-2 has been detected in various forms of waters such as municipal sewage, hospital wastewater, river water, non-potable water, secondary treated wastewater, domestic sewer, wastewater treatment derived sludge, etc. — it ranges between 22–100% depending upon the status of wastewater. In case of SARS-CoV-2, 90% decay (T90) of viral RNA requires 1.7 days at room temperature in water and wastewater, while decay time is reduced to 15 minutes and 2 minutes with increase in the temperature to 50°C and 70°C, respectively (Bivins *et al.*, 2020). The pH of wastewater also influences the stability of the virus. According to one report, SARS-CoV was found to be stable at slightly acidic to basic pH, whereas SARS-CoV-2 was found to be stable at pH 3–10 at room temperature.

Surprisingly, lower stability of SARS-CoV-2 has been reported in culture media (e.g. DMEM) in comparison to SARS-CoV. At 56°C, it takes 30 minutes for complete decay of SARS-CoV-2, and 1–1.5 hour in the case of SARS-CoV. However, complete decay time in media is reduced to 30 minutes and 5 minutes when the temperature is raised to 70°C in the case of SARS-CoV and SARS-CoV-2, respectively (Aboubakr *et al.*, 2021). Increased infection with SARS-CoV-2 has been observed during the winter season, which may be due to the fact that lower temperature promotes the stability to the virus and enhances its environmental survival.

2.3.5. *Easy access to reach susceptible hosts*

Avoiding exposure through "geographical isolation" is perhaps the easiest and most effective mode of preventing cross-species as well as intra-species transmission of any infectious agent. In the evolutionary process, humans were not the natural host of many viruses that pose significant threats for humanity in recent times. Notable examples include the human immunodeficiency virus and the SARS-CoV. These pathogens crossed the species barrier as a consequence of human activities. An increase in global population has reduced the per-capita availability of land. Overcrowding and higher demand for food and other supplements have resulted in the aggregation of wild and farm animals in close proximity, thereby exposing animals as well as their handlers to new and emerging pathogens. An increased demand for exotic food also contributes to the above situation (Reddy and Saier, 2020). In addition to that, the availability of faster and multimodal means of transport has further augmented the accessibility of infectious agents to cross geographic and environmental barriers, and perhaps reach more favorable conditions and hosts for better infection and replication. Once the pathogen adapts to the human host and becomes competent for human-to-human transmission, it is very difficult to control its spread. In the case of SARS-CoV-2, pangolins and/or other animals are believed to the intermediate host(s), through which the virus was subsequently transmitted to humans. It is unclear how the virus reached humans from these animals. In the current scenario, there should be emphasis on identifying the source(s) as well as the intermediate host(s) for SARS-CoV-2 in order to mitigate cross-species infections in the future.

2.4. Conclusion

Although Coronaviruses are known to infect animals and humans for a long time, highly pathogenic human Coronaviruses were first reported only in 2002. The recurring inter-species transmission of viruses from their natural reservoir to intermediate hosts and humans is primarily due to human interference. Within the last two decades, three major Coronavirus outbreaks have occurred. Therefore, there is a pressing need to formulate long-term global action plans to confront future outbreaks and emergencies of this nature. In the past decades, the role of environmental changes in influencing the evolution of these Coronaviruses cannot be ruled out. Destruction of habitats of wild animals also contributes to the spread of zoonotic pathogens and cross-species transmission. Strict measures need to be employed to prevent the mixing of wildlife, backyard and reared animals for human consumption. Given that Coronaviruses appear to be quite resistant to environmental conditions, special care and awareness should be promoted for ensuring personal hygiene as well as disinfection of contact points and surrounding areas.

It is a significant achievement for the entire scientific community that within a very short time span, multiple vaccines have been developed against SARS-CoV-2. However, the emergence of newer virus variants, and increased transmissibility and/or lethality associated with some of the SARS-CoV-2 variants (such as the Delta and Omicron variants) raise concerns regarding the long-term efficacy of existing vaccines. Therefore, there is an urgent need for innovative research into the molecular evolution and transmissibility of the SARS-CoV-2 so that crucial future mutations in the virus can be predicted with confidence, while the course of virus evolution can be monitored in advance (Wang and Powell, 2021). This information will help in designing better vaccines, e.g. formulating suitable "cocktails" of multivalent vaccines that offer long-term protective immunity against the newly emerging variants of the rapidly evolving SARS-CoV-2.

Acknowledgments

Rohit Verma is supported by a senior research fellowship from the Council of Scientific and Industrial Relations, Government of India. Milan Surjit is supported by grants from the Science and Engineering Research Board, Department of Science and Technology, Government of India (IPA/2020/000233) and Biotechnology Industry Research Assistance Council, Department of Biotechnology, Government of India (BT/COVID0081/01/20). Ramandeep Kaur and Sunil Lal are supported by internal funds from the School of Science, Monash University Malaysia.

References

Aboubakr HA *et al*. Stability of SARS-CoV-2 and other Coronaviruses in the environment and on common touch surfaces and the influence of climatic conditions: A review. *Transbound Emerg Dis* 2021; 68:296–312.

Algarroba GN *et al*. Visualization of severe acute respiratory syndrome Coronavirus 2 invading the human placenta using electron microscopy. *Am J Obstet Gynecol* 2020; 223:275–278.

Amraei R *et al*. CD209L/L-SIGN and CD209/DC-SIGN act as receptors for SARS-CoV-2. *ACS Cent Sci* 2021; 7:1156–1165.

Andreano E *et al*. SARS-CoV-2 escape from a highly neutralizing COVID-19 convalescent plasma. *Proc Natl Acad Sci USA* 2021; 118:e2103154118.

Annavajhala MK *et al*. Emergence and expansion of SARS-CoV-2 B.1.526 after identification in New York. *Nature* 2021; 597:703–708.

Avanzato VA *et al*. Case Study: Prolonged infectious SARS-CoV-2 shedding from an asymptomatic immunocompromised individual with cancer. *Cell* 2020; 183:1901–1912.e9.

Banerjee A *et al*. Predicting the recombination potential of severe acute respiratory syndrome Coronavirus 2 and Middle East respiratory syndrome Coronavirus. *J Gen Virol* 2020; 101:1251–1260.

Baud D *et al*. Second-trimester miscarriage in a pregnant woman with SARS-CoV-2 infection. *JAMA* 2020; 323:2198–2200.

Bayati A *et al*. SARS-CoV-2 infects cells after viral entry via clathrin-mediated endocytosis. *J Biol Chem* 2021; 296:100306.

Bertram S *et al*. TMPRSS2 and TMPRSS4 facilitate trypsin-independent spread of influenza virus in Caco-2 cells. *J Virol* 2010; 84:10016–10025.

Bhattacharyya C *et al*. SARS-CoV-2 mutation 614G creates an elastase cleavage site enhancing its spread in high AAT-deficient regions. *Infect Genet Evol* 2021; 90:104760.

Bivins A *et al*. Persistence of SARS-CoV-2 in water and wastewater. *Environ Sci Technol Lett* 2020; 7:937–942.

Bogler A *et al*. Rethinking wastewater risks and monitoring in light of the COVID-19 pandemic. *Nat Sustainability* 2020; 3:981–990.

Bradley BT *et al*. Histopathology and ultrastructural findings of fatal COVID-19 infections in Washington State: A case series. *Lancet* 2020; 396:320–332.

Bugembe DL *et al*. Emergence and spread of a SARS-CoV-2 lineage A variant (A.23.1) with altered spike protein in Uganda. *Nat Microbiol* 2021; 6:1094–1101.

Cerutti G *et al*. Potent SARS-CoV-2 neutralizing antibodies directed against spike N-terminal domain target a single supersite. *Cell Host Microbe* 2021; 29:819–833.e7.

Chakraborty C *et al*. SARS-CoV-2 and other human Coronaviruses: Mapping of protease recognition sites, antigenic variation of spike protein and their grouping through molecular phylogenetics. *Infect Genet Evol* 2021; 89:104729.

Challen R *et al*. Risk of mortality in patients infected with SARS-CoV-2 variant of concern 202012/1: Matched cohort study. *BMJ* 2021; 372:n579.

Chan JF *et al*. A familial cluster of pneumonia associated with the 2019 novel Coronavirus indicating person-to-person transmission: A study of a family cluster. *Lancet* 2020; 395:514–523.

Chand GB *et al*. Identification of twenty-five mutations in surface glycoprotein (Spike) of SARS-CoV-2 among Indian isolates and their impact on protein dynamics. *Gene Rep* 2020; 21:100891.

Chen J *et al*. Structure of the hemagglutinin precursor cleavage site, a determinant of influenza pathogenicity and the origin of the labile conformation. *Cell* 1998; 95:409–417.

Cherian S *et al*. SARS-CoV-2 Spike Mutations, L452R, T478K, E484Q and P681R, in the Second Wave of COVID-19 in Maharashtra, India. *Microorganisms* 2021; 9:1542.

Counotte MJ *et al*. Sexual transmission of Zika virus and other flaviviruses: A living systematic review. *PLoS Med* 2018; 15:e1002611.

Coutinho RM *et al*. Model-based estimation of transmissibility and reinfection of SARS-CoV-2 P.1 variant. *Commun Med* 2021; 1:48.

Cui J *et al*. Origin and evolution of pathogenic Coronaviruses. *Nat Rev Microbiol* 2019; 17:181–192.

Cyranoski D. Did pangolins spread the China Coronavirus to people? *Nature* 2020; Feb 7.

Davies NG *et al*. Estimated transmissibility and impact of SARS-CoV-2 lineage B.1.1.7 in England. *Science* 2021; 372:eabg3055.

Deng X *et al*. Transmission, infectivity, and neutralization of a spike L452R SARS-CoV-2 variant. *Cell* 2021; 184:3426–3437.e8.

ECDC (European Centre for Disease Prevention and Control), 2021. Risk Assessment: Risk related to the spread of new SARS-CoV-2 variants of concern in the EU/EEA- first update. https://www.ecdc.europa.eu/en/publications-data/covid-19-risk-assessment-spread-new-variants-concern-eueea-first-update (accessed 21 January 2021).

Faria NR *et al*. Genomics and epidemiology of the P.1 SARS-CoV-2 lineage in Manaus, Brazil. *Science* 2021; 372:815–821.

Franceschi VB *et al*. Genomic epidemiology of SARS-CoV-2 in Esteio, Rio Grande do Sul, Brazil. *BMC Genomics* 2021; 22:371.

Fuentes-Prior P. Priming of SARS-CoV-2 S protein by several membrane-bound serine proteinases could explain enhanced viral infectivity and systemic COVID-19 infection. *J Biol Chem* 2021; 296:100135.

Gordon DE *et al*. A SARS-CoV-2 protein interaction map reveals targets for drug repurposing. *Nature* 2020; 583:459–468.

Grint DJ *et al*. Case fatality risk of the SARS-CoV-2 variant of concern B.1.1.7 in England, 16 November to 5 February. *Euro Surveill* 2021; 26:2100256.

Hoffmann M *et al*. A multibasic cleavage site in the spike protein of SARS-CoV-2 is essential for infection of human lung cells. *Mol Cell* 2020; 78:779–784.e5.

Hoffmann M *et al*. Camostat mesylate inhibits SARS-CoV-2 activation by TMPRSS2-related proteases and its metabolite GBPA exerts antiviral activity. *EBioMedicine* 2021; 65:103255.

Hosier H *et al*. SARS-CoV-2 infection of the placenta. *J Clin Invest* 2020; 130:4947–4953.

Hu, B *et al*. Discovery of a rich gene pool of bat SARS-related Coronaviruses provides new insights into the origin of SARS Coronavirus. *PLoS Pathogens* 2017; 13:e1006698.

Hu J *et al*. D614G mutation of SARS-CoV-2 spike protein enhances viral infectivity. *bioRxiv* 2020; 2020.06.20.161323.

Ji W *et al*. Homologous recombination within the spike glycoprotein of the newly identified Coronavirus may boost cross-species transmission from snake to human. *J Med Virol* 2020; 92:433–440.

Kim D *et al*. The architecture of SARS-CoV-2 transcriptome. *Cell* 2020; 181:914–921.

Kim S *et al*. Differential interactions between human ACE2 and spike RBD of SARS-CoV-2 variants of concern. *J Chem Theory Comput* 2021; 17:7972–7979.

Kimura I *et al*. SARS-CoV-2 Lambda variant exhibits higher infectivity and immune resistance. *bioRxiv* 2021; 2021.07.28.454085.

Kitajima M *et al*. SARS-CoV-2 in wastewater: State of the knowledge and research needs. *Sci Total Environ* 2020; 739:139076.

Ksiazek TG *et al*. A novel Coronavirus associated with severe acute respiratory syndrome. *N Engl J Med* 2003; 348:1953–1966.

Kumar S *et al*. Omicron and delta variant of SARS-CoV-2: A comparative computational study of spike protein. *J Med Virol* 2021 Dec 15. https://doi.org/10.1002/jmv.27526Citations.

Kupferschmidt K. New mutations raise specter of "immune escape". *Science* 2021; 371:329–330.

Kutter JS *et al*. SARS-CoV and SARS-CoV-2 are transmitted through the air between ferrets over more than one meter distance. *Nat Commun* 2021; 12:1653.

Lamers MM *et al*. SARS-CoV-2 productively infects human gut enterocytes. *Science* 2020; 369:50–54.

Latif AA, Mukaratirwa S. Zoonotic origins and animal hosts of Coronaviruses causing human disease pandemics: A review. *Onderstepoort J Vet Res* 2020; 87:e1–e9.

Lau SK *et al*. Severe acute respiratory syndrome Coronavirus-like virus in Chinese horseshoe bats. *Proc Natl Acad Sci USA* 2005; 102:14040–14045.

Lauring AS, Hodcroft EB. Genetic variants of SARS-CoV-2-what do they mean? *JAMA* 2021; 325:529–531.

Li R *et al*. Substantial undocumented infection facilitates the rapid dissemination of novel Coronavirus (SARS-CoV-2). *Science* 2020; 368:489–493.

Li R *et al*. Differential efficiencies to neutralize the novel mutants B.1.1.7 and 501Y.V2 by collected sera from convalescent COVID-19 patients and RBD nanoparticle-vaccinated rhesus macaques. *Cell Mol Immunol* 2021; 18:1058–1060.

Li W *et al*. Bats are natural reservoirs of SARS-like Coronaviruses. *Science* 2005; 310:676–679.

Liu H *et al*. The basis of a more contagious 501Y.V1 variant of SARS-CoV-2. *Cell Res* 2021; 31:720–722.

Liu L *et al*. Potent neutralizing antibodies against multiple epitopes on SARS-CoV-2 spike. *Nature* 2020a; 584:450–456.

Liu P *et al*. Viral metagenomics revealed sendai virus and Coronavirus infection of Malayan Pangolins (Manis javanica). *Viruses* 2019; 11:979.

Liu Y *et al*. The reproductive number of COVID-19 is higher compared to SARS Coronavirus. *J Travel Med* 2020b; 27:taaa021.

Lu R *et al*. Genomic characterisation and epidemiology of 2019 novel Coronavirus: Implications for virus origins and receptor binding. *Lancet* 2020; 395:565–574.

Lubinski B *et al*. Functional evaluation of the P681H mutation on the proteolytic activation the SARS-CoV-2 variant B.1.1.7 (Alpha) spike. *iScience* 2021; Dec 10:103589.

McNally A. What makes new variants of SARS-CoV-2 concerning is not where they come from, but the mutations they contain. *BMJ* 2021; 372:n504.

Michel CJ *et al*. Characterization of accessory genes in Coronavirus genomes. *Virol J* 2020; 17:131.

Naveca FG *et al*. COVID-19 in Amazonas, Brazil, was driven by the persistence of endemic lineages and P.1 emergence. *Nat Med* 2021; 27:1230–1238.

Nonaka CKV *et al*. Genomic evidence of SARS-CoV-2 reinfection involving E484K spike mutation, Brazil. *Emerg Infect Dis* 2021; 27:1522–1524.

Otto SP *et al*. The origins and potential future of SARS-CoV-2 variants of concern in the evolving COVID-19 pandemic. *Curr Biol* 2021; 31:R918–R929.

Ou J *et al*. V367F mutation in SARS-CoV-2 spike RBD emerging during the early transmission phase enhances viral infectivity through increased human ACE2 receptor binding affinity. *J Virol* 2021; 95:e0061721.

Oude Munnink BB *et al*. Transmission of SARS-CoV-2 on mink farms between humans and mink and back to humans. *Science* 2021; 371:172–177.

PANGO Lineages, 2021. Latest Epidemiological Lineages of SARS-CoV-2. https://cov-lineages.org/index.html (accessed 1 December 2021).

Paraskevis D *et al*. Full-genome evolutionary analysis of the novel corona virus (2019-nCoV) rejects the hypothesis of emergence as a result of a recent recombination event. *Infect Genet Evol* 2020; 79:104212.

Pascarella S *et al*. SARS-CoV-2 B.1.617 Indian variants: Are electrostatic potential changes responsible for a higher transmission rate? *J Med Virol* 2021; 93:6551–6556.

Pater AA *et al*. Emergence and evolution of a prevalent new SARS-CoV-2 variant in the United States. *bioRxiv* 2021; 2021.01.11.426287.

Patino-Galindo JA *et al*. Recombination and lineage-specific mutations linked to the emergence of SARS-CoV-2. *Genome Med* 2021; 13:124.

Peacock TP *et al*. The furin cleavage site in the SARS-CoV-2 spike protein is required for transmission in ferrets. *Nat Microbiol* 2021; 6:899–909.

Phan LT *et al*. Importation and human-to-human transmission of a Novel coronavirus in Vietnam. *N Engl J Med* 2020; 382:872–874.

Public Health England, 2020. Investigation of SARS-CoV-2 Variants of Concern: Technical Briefings. https://www.gov.uk/government/publications/investigation-of-novel-sars-cov-2-variant-variant-of-concern-20201201 (accessed 21 December 2021).

Puelles VG *et al*. Multiorgan and renal tropism of SARS-CoV-2. *N Engl J Med* 2020; 383:590–592.

Rambaut A *et al*. A dynamic nomenclature proposal for SARS-CoV-2 lineages to assist genomic epidemiology. *Nat Microbiol* 2020; 5:1403–1407.

Reddy BL, Saier MH. The causal relationship between eating animals and viral epidemics. *Microb Physiol* 2020; 30:2–8.

Rees-Spear C *et al*. The effect of spike mutations on SARS-CoV-2 neutralization. *Cell Rep* 2021; 34:108890.

Resende PC *et al*. A potential SARS-CoV-2 variant of interest (VOI) harboring mutation E484K in the spike protein was identified within lineage B.1.1.33 circulating in Brazil. *Viruses* 2021; 13:724.

Romano M *et al*. A structural view of SARS-CoV-2 RNA replication machinery: RNA synthesis, proofreading and final capping. *Cells* 2020; 9:1267.

Saha I *et al*. Inferring the genetic variability in Indian SARS-CoV-2 genomes using consensus of multiple sequence alignment techniques. *Infect Genet Evol* 2020; 85:104522.

Schmidt N *et al*. The SARS-CoV-2 RNA-protein interactome in infected human cells. *Nat Microbiol* 2021; 6:339–353.

Shang J *et al*. Cell entry mechanisms of SARS-CoV-2. *Proc Natl Acad Sci USA* 2020; 117:11727–11734.

Siemann DN *et al*. Zika virus infects human sertoli cells and modulates the integrity of the *in vitro* blood-testis barrier model. *J Virol* 2017; 91:e00623–17.

Starr TN *et al*. Deep mutational scanning of SARS-CoV-2 receptor binding domain reveals constraints on folding and ACE2 binding. *Cell* 2020; 182:1295–1310.e20.

Steinhauer DA *et al.* Lack of evidence for proofreading mechanisms associated with an RNA virus polymerase. *Gene* 1992; 122:281–288.

Tang JW *et al.* Emergence of a new SARS-CoV-2 variant in the UK. *J Infect* 2021; 82:e27–e28.

Tarke A *et al.* Impact of SARS-CoV-2 variants on the total CD4+ and CD8+ T cell reactivity in infected or vaccinated individuals. *Cell Rep Med* 2021; 2:100355.

Tegally H *et al.* Detection of a SARS-CoV-2 variant of concern in South Africa. *Nature* 2021; 592:438–443.

Tiwari M, Mishra D. Investigating the genomic landscape of novel Coronavirus (2019-nCoV) to identify non-synonymous mutations for use in diagnosis and drug design. *J Clin Virol* 2020; 128:104441.

Vaidyanathan G. Coronavirus variants are spreading in India — What scientists know so far. *Nature* 2021; 593:321–322.

van der Most RG *et al.* Homologous RNA recombination allows efficient introduction of site-specific mutations into the genome of Coronavirus MHV-A59 via synthetic co-replicating RNAs. *Nucleic Acids Res* 1992; 20:3375–3381.

Verma R *et al.* RNA-protein interaction analysis of SARS-CoV-2 5' and 3' untranslated regions reveals a role of lysosome-associated membrane protein-2a during viral infection. *mSystems* 2021; 6:e0064321.

Voloch CM *et al.* Genomic characterization of a novel SARS-CoV-2 lineage from Rio de Janeiro, Brazil. *J Virol* 2021; 95:e00119–21.

Volz E *et al.* Assessing transmissibility of SARS-CoV-2 lineage B.1.1.7 in England. *Nature* 2021; 593:266–269.

Wang D *et al.* Clinical characteristics of 138 hospitalized patients with 2019 novel Coronavirus-infected pneumonia in Wuhan, China. *JAMA* 2020a; 323:1061–1069.

Wang W *et al.* Detection of SARS-CoV-2 in different types of clinical specimens. *JAMA* 2020b; 323:1843–1844.

Wang X, Powell CA. How to translate the knowledge of COVID-19 into the prevention of Omicron variants. *Clin Transl Med* 2021; 11:e680.

West AP *et al.* Detection and characterization of the SARS-CoV-2 lineage B.1.526 in New York. *Nat Commun* 2021; 12:4886.

Wibmer CK *et al.* SARS-CoV-2 501Y.V2 escapes neutralization by South African COVID-19 donor plasma. *Nat Med* 2021; 27:622–625.

Wu J *et al.* Severe acute respiratory syndrome Coronavirus 2: From gene structure to pathogenic mechanisms and potential therapy. *Front Microbiol* 2020a; 11:1576.

Wu JT *et al.* Nowcasting and forecasting the potential domestic and international spread of the 2019-nCoV outbreak originating in Wuhan, China: A modelling study. *Lancet* 2020b; 395:689–697.

Xu J *et al.* Orchitis: A complication of severe acute respiratory syndrome (SARS). *Biol Reprod* 2006; 74:410–416.

Xu X *et al*. Evolution of the novel Coronavirus from the ongoing Wuhan outbreak and modeling of its spike protein for risk of human transmission. *Sci China Life Sci* 2020; 63:457–460.

Yan R *et al*. Structural basis for the recognition of SARS-CoV-2 by full-length human ACE2. *Science* 2020; 367:1444–1448.

Yang D, Leibowitz JL. The structure and functions of Coronavirus genomic 3′ and 5′ ends. *Virus Res* 2015; 206:120–133.

Zaki AM *et al*. Isolation of a novel Coronavirus from a man with pneumonia in Saudi Arabia. *N Engl J Med* 2012; 367:1814–1820.

Zang R *et al*. TMPRSS2 and TMPRSS4 promote SARS-CoV-2 infection of human small intestinal enterocytes. *Sci Immunol* 2020; 5:eabc3582.

Zella D *et al*. The variants question: What is the problem? *J Med Virol* 2021; 93:6479–6485.

Zhang C *et al*. Intracellular autoactivation of TMPRSS11A, an airway epithelial transmembrane serine protease. *J Biol Chem* 2020; 295:12686–12696.

Zhang W *et al*. Emergence of a novel SARS-CoV-2 variant in Southern California. *JAMA* 2021; 325:1324–1326.

Zhou D *et al*. Evidence of escape of SARS-CoV-2 variant B.1.351 from natural and vaccine-induced sera. *Cell* 2021; 184:2348–2361.e6.

Zhu Z *et al*. Genomic recombination events may reveal the evolution of Coronavirus and the origin of SARS-CoV-2. *Sci Rep* 2020; 10:21617.

Chapter 3

Clinical Features and Management of COVID-19

Sean Wei Xiang Ong[†] and Shawn Vasoo[*]

*National Centre for Infectious Diseases,
and Department of Infectious Diseases,
Tan Tock Seng Hospital, Singapore*

[*]*shawn_vasoo@ncid.sg*
[†]*sean_ongwx@ttsh.com.sg*

Abstract

Much has been learnt about severe acute respiratory syndrome Coronavirus 2 (SARS-CoV-2) since the beginning of the Coronavirus disease 2019 (COVID-19) pandemic, including its clinical manifestations, diagnosis, and management. Unlike its zoonotic predecessor SARS-CoV which was largely a symptomatic disease where fever was a hallmark, a significant proportion of SARS-CoV-2 infections can be asymptomatic (40%), while severe disease (requiring oxygen supplementation or ventilatory support) occurs in approximately 20%, and mortality in about 2% of infected patients. Extra-pulmonary COVID-19 manifestations are also more protean, compared to SARS. Supportive care is the mainstay of treatment for most patients, but for those who progress to severe COVID-19, antivirals such as remdesivir and immunomodulatory treatment (such as corticosteroids or the JAK-inhibitor, baricitinib) may improve outcomes. While further advances in the management of

COVID-19 are anticipated (including novel therapies), prevention of infection through public health measures (including vaccination), will remain as vital facets in confronting this pandemic.

Keywords: COVID-19; SARS-CoV-2; clinical features; symptoms; severity; complications; management; treatment; antivirals; immuno-modulators

3.1. Clinical Features

3.1.1. *Introduction*

The collective scientific and medical understanding of Coronavirus disease 2019 (COVID-19) has evolved at a breath-taking pace since its first emergence at the end of 2019, with first recognition and sequencing of the causative virus, evaluation of effective therapeutics, and even development and implementation of multiple vaccine candidates all within the span of a year. Similarly, the broad spectrum of clinical features of COVID-19 infection has been well-described in the literature.

The clinical presentation of COVID-19, similar to other respiratory viruses, has a wide spectrum of severity, ranging from asymptomatic infection or a mild upper respiratory tract illness to severe pneumonia with fulminant multiple organ failure and acute respiratory distress syndrome (ARDS). However, there have been several characteristic features in the symptomatology of COVID-19 that distinguish it from the clinical illness caused by other seasonal respiratory viruses and its zoonotic Coronavirus predecessors, severe acute respiratory syndrome Coronavirus (SARS-CoV) and Middle East respiratory syndrome Coronavirus (MERS-CoV). In addition, numerous atypical complications and post-infective sequelae have been reported across multiple organ systems, making COVID-19 a varied and fascinating disease to study.

3.1.2. *Asymptomatic infection*

Asymptomatic infections have been well-reported in the literature (Bi *et al.*, 2020; Ng *et al.*, 2021; Plucinski *et al.*, 2021). However, the proportion of all infections that are truly asymptomatic is difficult to accurately determine, due to inherent limitations in study methodology. For example, point prevalence population-based testing may not have adequate follow-up to determine interval symptom development after initial diagnostic testing, and smaller cohort studies vary significantly in their study population demographics and hence susceptibility to development of symptomatic disease. Keeping these caveats in mind, large population and contact tracing studies have reported asymptomatic infection rates ranging from 30% to 40% (Lavezzo *et al.*, 2020; Ng *et al.*, 2021). Of significant public health concern, and a continuing challenge to outbreak control, is the fact that asymptomatic individuals infected with SARS-CoV-2 remain infectious and capable of transmission to susceptible individuals (Plucinski *et al.*, 2021; Wei *et al.*, 2020). In one study, infectivity was found to be 3.85 times higher for close contacts of a symptomatic versus asymptomatic index case (Sayampanathan *et al.*, 2021).

3.1.3. *Clinical symptoms*

The initial presenting symptoms of COVID-19 resemble those of other respiratory viruses, with variable proportions of cough, fever, coryza, sore throat, myalgia, headache, and dyspnea. These vary significantly in severity between patients, and the reported frequency of each of these presenting symptoms differs between study cohorts. For example, the frequency of fever as a presenting symptom has ranged from as low as 30% to as high as 98% in different settings (Guan *et al.*, 2020; Huang *et al.*, 2020a; Richardson *et al.*, 2020). The range of potential presenting symptoms is summarized in Table 3.1.

Table 3.1. Presenting symptoms of COVID-19.

Respiratory
Cough
Dyspnea
Coryza or nasal congestion
Sore throat
Chest pain or tightness
Constitutional
Fever
Chills/rigors
Myalgia
Fatigue/lethargy

(Continued)

Table 3.1.   (*Continued*)

Headache
Arthralgia
Olfactory/Gustatory
Anosmia (diminished sense of smell)
Ageusia (diminished sense of taste)
Dysgeusia (altered sense of taste)
Gastrointestinal
Diarrhea
Abdominal pain
Nausea/vomiting
Dermatologic
Rash (maculopapular, vesicular, urticarial, erythema multiforme-like)
Vascular eruptions (livedo reticularis, purpura, necrosis)
Pseudo-chilblains ("COVID toes")
Others
Conjunctivitis

While several atypical symptoms have been described, no single symptom or combination of symptoms has been shown to be adequately sensitive or specific to reliably distinguish COVID-19 from other respiratory infections (Struyf *et al.*, 2020), and hence all patients with any symptoms and an epidemiologic risk of COVID-19 should be evaluated.

3.1.3.1. *Olfactory and gustatory dysfunction*

Smell disorders, in the form of anosmia (diminished sense of smell), and taste disorders, in the form of ageusia (diminished sense of taste) or dysgeusia (altered sense of taste) were reported as a potentially distinguishing feature of COVID-19 early on in the outbreak (Giacomelli *et al.*, 2020; Spinato *et al.*, 2020). A meta-analysis and systematic review found a prevalence of 53% and 44% of olfactory and gustatory dysfunction, respectively — however, the reported prevalence differed significantly among the included studies (Tong *et al.*, 2020). While these appear to be symptoms unique to COVID-19 infection, they are not adequately discriminatory to be reliably used in the clinical setting for diagnosis or exclusion of COVID-19. Nevertheless, the presence of acute olfactory or gustatory dysfunction, even in the absence of other respiratory or constitutional symptoms, should prompt further evaluation for COVID-19.

3.1.3.2. *Gastrointestinal symptoms*

Gastrointestinal symptoms such as diarrhea, abdominal pain, nausea, or vomiting have also been observed in COVID-19, even in the absence of concomitant respiratory symptoms (Jin *et al.*, 2020). Another systematic review and meta-analysis found a pooled prevalence of gastrointestinal symptoms of 17.6% (Cheung *et al.*, 2020). Importantly, stool shedding of SARS-CoV-2 has been reported in patients with and without gastrointestinal symptoms (Cheung *et al.*, 2020; Tian *et al.*, 2020), although the significance of stool shedding as a route of transmission remains unclear (Ong *et al.*, 2020).

3.1.3.3. *Dermatologic manifestations*

A wide range of dermatologic manifestations has been reported with varying frequencies, though most studies are limited to case reports and small case series (Daneshgaran *et al.*, 2020). However, the strength of association of these findings with COVID-19 is difficult to establish in some cases, given potentially numerous confounders such as co-administered medical treatments or experimental therapies (Tursen *et al.*, 2020). Reported patterns of skin involvement are protean, and include erythematous maculopapular eruptions, vesicular rashes, urticarial rashes, vascular rashes (e.g. livedo reticularis, purpura, necrosis), and erythema multiforme-like eruptions (Daneshgaran *et al.*, 2020; Galvan Casas *et al.*, 2020). A notable manifestation is that of pseudo-chilblains or pernio-like lesions of the extremities, colloquially known as "COVID toes", presenting with erythematous or purpuric macules over the fingers or toes (Freeman *et al.*, 2020; Galvan Casas *et al.*, 2020).

3.1.4. *Spectrum of disease severity*

Most individuals with COVID-19 display only a mild respiratory illness without developing severe disease. However, an entire spectrum of disease severity has been observed. Table 3.2 provides consensus definitions

Table 3.2.   Proposed definitions of disease severity categorization.

Severity	Features
Asymptomatic or presymptomatic	Positive nucleic acid test for SARS-CoV-2 without symptoms consistent with COVID-19
Mild	Presence of any signs or symptoms consistent with COVID-19, without dyspnea, or clinical signs or abnormal chest imaging consistent with pneumonia
Moderate	Presence of clinical signs or abnormal chest imaging consistent with pneumonia, without hypoxia (defined as oxygen saturation <94% on ambient air)
Severe	Hypoxia (oxygen saturation <94% on ambient air), P/F ratio of <300 mmHg, respiratory rate of >30 breaths per minute, or lung infiltrates occupying >50% of lung fields on chest imaging
Critical	Presence of respiratory failure, septic shock, or multiple organ dysfunction

Note: Adapted from NIH (National Institutes of Health, USA). COVID-19 Treatment Guidelines (2020).

for the various categories of disease severity, adapted from the National Institutes of Health and World Health Organization (NIH, 2020; WHO, 2020). In one of the largest cohort studies which analyzed 44,672 PCR-confirmed infections in the early course of the outbreak in China, 81% of patients had only mild disease, while severe and critical disease was reported in 14% and 5%, respectively, with a reported case fatality rate (CFR) of 2.3% (Wu and McGoogan, 2020). These relative proportions of mild and severe disease, as well as reported CFR, have varied widely across different settings, largely due to variations in demographics, testing and detection rates, and resource availabilities (Cummings *et al.*, 2020; Ji *et al.*, 2020b; Onder *et al.*, 2020; Sudharsanan *et al.*, 2020).

3.1.4.1. *Risk factors for developing severe illness*

Numerous risk factors have been associated with an increased risk of developing severe illness, of which the most well-recognized are age and presence of medical comorbidities (Chen *et al.*, 2020; Huang *et al.*, 2020a; Richardson *et al.*, 2020; Verity *et al.*, 2020). These risk factors are sum-marized in Table 3.3. Presence of these risk factors can be used in a risk

Table 3.3. Risk factors for developing severe COVID-19.

Demographic	Comorbidities	Possible Risk Factors
Age >60 years old	Obesity (BMI >30 kg/m^2)	Overweight (BMI 25–30 kg/m^2)
Male gender	Diabetes mellitus	Ethnic minority (e.g. African, Hispanic,
Smoking	Hypertension	South Asian)
	Cardiac disease	Poorer social economic status
	Chronic lung disease	Genetic polymorphisms
	Cerebrovascular disease	Type O Rh-negative blood type
	Chronic kidney disease	
	Cancer	
	Immunosuppression use	

stratification algorithm to determine disposition or to inform treatment decisions. However, it is worth noting that while many predictive tools or risk scores combining risk factors and laboratory indices have been developed to attempt risk stratification and prediction of severe disease (Galloway *et al.*, 2020; Ji *et al.*, 2020a; Liang *et al.*, 2020), none to date has been prospectively evaluated in multiple international cohorts or sufficiently validated for routine clinical use across all settings, and clinical decision making has to be made on an individualized basis.

3.1.4.2. *Biphasic pattern of illness*

It has been well-recognized that COVID-19 patients pass through distinct phases of illness. The first week of illness after symptom onset is when viral load is at its highest, and is associated with significant upper respiratory tract symptoms (Lee *et al.*, 2020; Young *et al.*, 2021; Zou *et al.*, 2020). Deterioration or development of severe illness, if it occurs, typically sets in at the end of the first week or beginning of the second week of illness — this distinctive temporal evolution has been demonstrated multiple cohorts (Huang *et al.*, 2020a; Wang *et al.*, 2020a). This progression has been described as a hyperinflammatory phase, whereby a dysregulated host immune response or "cytokine storm" accounts for the predominant pathophysiology in severe disease (Lucas *et al.*, 2020; Qin *et al.*, 2020; Siddiqi *et al.*, 2020; Young *et al.*, 2021).

3.1.5. *Disease complications*

A wide range of complications associated with COVID-19 have been reported, across almost all organ systems. These are summarized in Table 3.4. Some of these complications are more frequent and have a clear direct causal link to COVID-19 (e.g. respiratory failure) — however for some, the association is less clear and further investigation is required.

Table 3.4.   Potential complications of COVID-19.

Respiratory

Hypoxemic respiratory failure/acute respiratory distress syndrome

Cardiovascular

Myocardial injury

Cardiac arrhythmias

Myocardial infarction

Neurologic

Encephalopathy

Stroke

Meningoencephalitis

Guillain-Barré syndrome

Acute disseminated encephalomyelitis (ADEM)

Acute hemorrhagic necrotizing encephalopathy

Thrombosis

Deep venous thrombosis

Pulmonary embolism

Acute limb ischemia

Multiple Organ Dysfunction Syndrome

Acute kidney injury

Acute liver failure

Septic shock

Coagulopathy

Secondary Infections

Ventilator-associated pneumonia

Secondary nosocomial bacterial infections

COVID-19 associated pulmonary aspergillosis (CAPA)

Mucormycosis

Table 3.4. (*Continued*)

Long-term Sequelae
Functional limitation
Chronic fatigue syndrome/myalgic encephalomyelitis
Cardiomyopathy
Lung fibrosis and chronic lung disease

3.1.5.1. *Respiratory failure*

Given that the primary site of infection is the respiratory tract, it is natural that the most common complication of severe COVID-19 is widespread bilateral pneumonitis resulting in respiratory failure in the form of ARDS. The proportion of patients developing ARDS and respiratory failure requiring mechanical ventilation has varied across different cohort studies from 10% to 20% (Richardson *et al.*, 2020; *et al.*, 2020; Wang *et al.*, 2020a; Wu and McGoogan, 2020). The primary respiratory pathology is that of a profound acute hypoxemia, or type 1 respiratory failure, resulting from impaired alveolar gas exchange (Chand *et al.*, 2020). Intubation and mechanical ventilation is often required, and the period of ventilatory support required may be prolonged for up to several weeks. In severe cases, respiratory failure may be refractory to ventilatory support and patients may require extra-corporeal membrane oxygenation or ECMO (Matthay *et al.*, 2020).

Critically ill patients with ARDS may progress further to develop multiple organ dysfunction syndrome (MODS) resembling severe sepsis. This can present with widespread organ dysfunction including acute kidney injury requiring dialysis, elevated liver enzymes or liver failure, septic shock with hypotension requiring vasopressors.

3.1.5.2. *Thrombotic events*

A hypercoagulable state with resultant pro-thrombotic tendency has been observed in COVID-19 patients, with resultant arterial and venous thromboses, even in young patients without pre-existing risk factors for thrombosis (Bilaloglu *et al.*, 2020; Cui *et al.*, 2020; Klok *et al.*, 2020). The underlying pathophysiologic mechanism appears to be a combination of direct endothelial injury and inflammation induced by SARS-CoV-2 (Libby and Luscher, 2020; Varga *et al.*, 2020), as well as increased circulating levels of pro-thrombotic factors as a result of the dysregulated immune response triggered by infection (Panigada *et al.*, 2020; Ranucci *et al.*, 2020). Laboratory derangements in coagulation profiles are frequently observed, including alterations in prothrombin time (PT), activated partial thromboplastin time (aPTT), D-dimer, and fibrinogen (Helms *et al.*, 2020a; Medcalf *et al.*, 2020). These features are in contrast to disseminated intravascular coagulation (DIC) seen in other critically ill states such as severe sepsis due to other bacterial or viral infections, which typically results in a bleeding tendency rather than a pro-thrombotic tendency.

Venous thromboembolism (VTE) is commonly observed in patients admitted to the intensive care unit (ICU), likely as a result of the additional immobility caused by critical illness and resultant venous stasis. Up to 20% to 25% of ICU patients have been reported to develop VTE in the form of deep venous thrombosis (DVT) or pulmonary embolism (PE), even in the presence of routine VTE chemoprophylaxis (Cui *et al.*, 2020; Middeldorp *et al.*, 2020). The incidence of symptomatic VTE is lower in non-ICU patients, ranging from 2% to 3% (Bilaloglu *et al.*, 2020; Hill *et al.*, 2020), although smaller studies have found higher rates using active surveillance, finding a high frequency of asymptomatic DVT (Artifoni *et al.*, 2020).

Arterial thromboses have also been frequently reported in COVID-19, manifesting as myocardial infarction, stroke, or acute limb ischemia. Underlying comorbidities such as age, smoking, and pre-existing atherosclerotic disease may increase this risk (Bilaoglu *et al.*, 2020). However, acute large vessel thromboses have been reported in young ambulant patients without comorbidities or known risk factors for thrombosis (Fan *et al.*, 2021). It remains unclear whether these can be directly attributed to COVID-19, or are a function of COVID-19 unmasking undiagnosed thrombophilic states.

3.1.5.3. *Cardiac complications*

Cardiac complications of COVID-19 are common, ranging from 7% to 17% in various cohort studies. Elevated troponin levels can be seen in acute myocardial injury as part of MODS, and may be contributed by stress cardiomyopathy, ischemic or hypoxic injury, and the exaggerated inflammatory response seen in the hyperinflammatory phase of

COVID-19 (Guo *et al.*, 2020). An increased frequency of cardiac arrhyth-mias has been reported — however, the strength of this association with COVID-19 remains unclear (Bhatla *et al.*, 2020; Guo *et al.*, 2020). Furthermore, this may have be confounded by other factors such as off-label use of therapeutics that affect the QT interval — e.g. hydroxychlo-roquine and azithromycin, both of which were used frequently in the initial phase of the pandemic (Chorin *et al.*, 2020). Lastly, as discussed above, COVID-19 may have an associated increased risk of arterial thrombosis manifesting in myocardial infarction.

3.1.5.4. *Neurologic complications*

Encephalopathy has been commonly observed among critically ill COVID-19 patients, with reported frequencies of up to 32% (Liotta *et al.*, 2020). This may variably present in the form of delirium, agitation, altered sensorium, and less commonly, seizures (Helms *et al.*, 2020b; Mao *et al.*, 2020; Somani *et al.*, 2020). The pathophysiologic mechanism underlying this appears to be due to systemic dysfunctions such as hypoxemia, metabolic derangements, and pro-inflammatory cytokine responses, rather than direct central nervous system invasion by SARS-CoV-2 (Matschke *et al.*, 2020; Pezzini and Padovani, 2020). Frank meningoencephalitis has been reported, with isolation of SARS-CoV-2 in cerebrospinal fluid (CSF) — however, this is limited to isolated case reports, and this presentation is likely very rare (Huang *et al.*, 2020b; Moriguchi *et al.*, 2020).

Similar to other viral or bacterial infections, sporadic cases of Guillain-Barré syndrome (GBS) have been reported in association with COVID-19, though this appears to be infrequent (Paterson *et al.*, 2020; Toscano *et al.*, 2020). The clinical picture of COVID-19-associated GBS is similar to GBS caused by other precipitants, with a typical progressive ascending paralysis, and consistent diagnostic features on CSF analysis and nerve conduction studies. Other subtypes such as Miller-Fisher syn-drome, cranial neuropathies, and ophthalmoplegia have also been reported (Gutierrez-Ortiz *et al.*, 2020). Respiratory muscle weakness may necessitate mechanical ventilation (Toscano *et al.*, 2020).

Rarer neurologic complications include acute disseminated encepha-lomyelitis (ADEM) and acute hemorrhagic necrotizing encephalopathy, with protean clinical, radiologic, and pathologic findings, and associated with significant morbidity and mortality (Koralnik *et al.*, 2020; Reichard *et al.*, 2020; Paterson *et al.*, 2020).

Lastly, as discussed above, a hypercoagulable pro-thrombotic state has been described in COVID-19, although the direct causality between COVID-19 and an increased stroke risk has not been firmly established (Bekelis *et al.*, 2020). Data from multiple hospital systems have shown decreases in stroke admission associated with the COVID-19 pandemic, although this may be confounded by decreased health-seeking behavior due to fear of acquiring infection (Jasne *et al.*, 2020; Zhao *et al.*, 2020a).

3.1.5.5. *Secondary infections*

Compared to other severe respiratory viral infections such as influenza, secondary bacterial pneumonia and infection appears to be less frequent in COVID-19 (Lansbury *et al.*, 2020; Rawson *et al.*, 2020). A systematic review and meta-analysis identified a bacterial co-infection rate (defined as being diagnosed on presentation) of 3.5% and a secondary bacterial infection rate of 14.3%, the latter being more common in critically ill patients (Langford *et al.*, 2020). Nevertheless, patients with severe COVID-19 requiring mechanical ventilation are at risk of ventilator-associated pneumonia, and due vigilance should be exercised, balancing the need for rational antibiotic use and stewardship.

A separate entity of COVID-19-associated pulmonary aspergillosis (CAPA) has been proposed, with several studies describing a clinical picture of invasive pulmonary aspergillosis developing in intubated COVID-19 patients, even without underlying immunocompromising conditions. In one multi-center study, a diagnosis of probable CAPA using serum or bronchoalveolar lavage galactomannan antigen and cultures was made in 27.7% of patients (Bartoletti *et al.*, 2021). This is analogous to invasive aspergillosis complicating patients with severe influenza, and further studies are required to determine the prevalence and to identify predictors for CAPA (Schauwvlieghe *et al.*, 2018). Thousands of cases of mucormycosis (dubbed "black fungus") were reported in COVID-19 patients during India's second wave in 2021 (Stone *et al.*, 2021). Some reasons for the sharp increase in this severe and often fatal invasive fungal infection include widespread use of steroids, uncontrolled diabetes, and viral-induced mucosal injury.

3.1.6. *Clinical manifestations in pediatric populations*

COVID-19 presents similarly in children and adults, with a similar spectrum of presenting symptoms. However, children typically have milder disease, and there may be a greater proportion of asymptomatic infection (Liguoro *et al.*, 2020; Mehta *et al.*, 2020). Nonetheless, a small minority of children can still develop severe disease, with ~2% requiring admission to a pediatric ICU in one large systematic review, although the mortality rate was much lower at 0.08% (Liguoro *et al.*, 2020).

3.1.6.1. *Multisystem inflammatory syndrome*

Although disease severity is lower, children and adolescents can develop a unique complication rarely observed in adults, termed multisystem inflammatory syndrome in children (MIS-C), which bears resemblance to Kawasaki disease or KD (Feldstein *et al.*, 2020; Verdoni *et al.*, 2020; Whittaker *et al.*, 2020). MIS-C typically develops as a post-infectious sequela 2–4 weeks after acute COVID-19 infection, suggesting an immune-mediated mechanism. Case definitions are evolving and differ between the CDC and WHO, although both have common features of persistent fever, elevated inflammatory markers (including ESR, C-reactive protein, or procalcitonin), multisystemic involvement (cardiovascular, respiratory, coagulopathy, gastrointestinal, or dermatologic), and documentation of recent or current SARS-CoV-2 infection. Although not fully understood, there appears to be a genetic predisposition as reports of this clinical entity only emerged later on when the pandemic affected Europe and North America heavily; there had been no prior reports from Asia earlier.

3.1.7. *Laboratory and radiologic findings*

Typical laboratory findings seen in COVID-19 include decreased white blood cell count and absolute lymphocyte count. Mild to moderate elevations in liver enzymes are commonly observed as well. Severe disease is associated with a typical biochemical picture with markedly elevated inflammatory markers including C-reactive protein, lactate dehydrogenase, D-dimer, troponin, and ferritin (Guan *et al.*, 2020; Huang *et al.*, 2020a; Ruan *et al.*, 2020; Wu and McGoogan, 2020). However, no specific laboratory index is specific or sensitive enough to reliably distinguish COVID-19 from other respiratory infections. Similarly, while numerous risk scores have been developed utilizing various combinations of these biochemical markers, none have been sufficiently validated to recommend routine use.

Chest radiography (CXR) is typically used as first-line radiographic investigation in the evaluation for COVID-19 pneumonia, which develops in about 20% of patients. CXR findings typically demonstrate lung consolidation with varying distributions and patterns. However, CXR may be normal early in the illness course, with radiographic changes only subsequently detected on computed tomography (CT) imaging (Cleverley *et al.*, 2020). CT imaging is more sensitive than CXR in detection of pulmonary abnormalities, with the most common finding being that of bilateral ground-glass opacities (Ai *et al.*, 2020; Yang *et al.*, 2020). Other findings may include septal or pleural thickening, consolidation, air bronchograms, or a "crazy-paving" pattern. Pleural effusions are relatively infrequent.

3.1.8. *Long-term sequelae*

Anecdotal reports of persistent symptoms post-COVID-19 recovery, colloquially termed "long COVID", have been reported extensively in the media, describing a clinical phenotype resembling myalgic encephalomyelitis or chronic fatigue syndrome (ME/CFS) (Mahase, 2020; Marshall, 2020). However, there are limited data to fully understand the frequency of such symptoms, or the pathophysiologic mechanisms driving them (Yelin *et al.*, 2020). Several cohort studies tracking confirmed COVID-19 patients post-recovery have described a high frequency (55–87.6%) of persistent symptoms (most commonly fatigue and dyspnea) for up to several months, with an associated decrease in quality of life measured using quantitative questionnaires (Carfi *et al.*, 2020; Garrigues *et al.*, 2020; Halpin *et al.*, 2021).

COVID-19 survivors have exhibited chronic respiratory and cardiac impairment. In a small cohort study of 55 patients, 71% showed persistent radiographic abnormalities on CT scans, and 25% had persistent lung function abnormalities at 3 months (Zhao *et al.*, 2020b). Persistent cardiac involvement post-COVID-19 recovery has also been demonstrated, with a cohort of 100 patients showing myocardial involvement in 78% and ongoing inflammation in 60% on cardiac magnetic resonance imaging beyond 2 months (Puntmann *et al.*, 2020).

As the COVID-19 pandemic progresses, this field of knowledge will continue to evolve as more data emerges.

3.2. Management

3.2.1. *Introduction*

The management of COVID-19, as with numerous other aspects of this disease, has evolved significantly within a compressed period of time. More so than many other infectious diseases, it has generated significant controversy and elicited strong political and cultural opinions (Berlivet and Lowy, 2020). The rapid turnover of evidence from innumerable clinical trials and a veritable avalanche of publications, both peer-reviewed and not, has revealed both the promise of international collaboration in the form of multi-center international platform trials and the danger of acting upon premature findings with potentially damaging results (Gianola *et al.*, 2020; Odone *et al.*, 2020).

Numerous lessons can be gained from studying the process of therapeutic drug identification during this pandemic. Firstly, the lack of concurrence between *in vitro* and *in vivo* findings, and the need to be cautious in extrapolation of data. Early in the pandemic, drugs such as lopinavir-ritonavir, hydroxychloroquine, and chloroquine were widely touted due to their purported efficacy *in vitro* (Wang *et al.*, 2020b; Yao *et al.*, 2020b) — although therapeutic outcomes in clinical trials were eventually dismal (Cavalcanti *et al.*, 2020; Self *et al.*, 2020). Numerous therapeutic decisions were also made extrapolating data from previous Coronavirus pandemics, namely SARS and MERS, though in retrospect these were erroneous (Cao *et al.*, 2020; Young *et al.*, 2020). Secondly, the importance of incorporating a rigorous clinical trial structure into future pandemic planning — numerous treatment decisions early in the course of the pandemic were made on scant data using off-label experimental therapeutics. If these were all channelled into a clinical trial, evidence may have been accrued more quickly, saving time, effort, and lives.

The stumbling blocks notwithstanding, it is reassuring that within less than a year of the emergence of this novel disease, we have at our disposal an array of therapeutic options backed by high quality evidence, with significant differences in outcomes. Future research questions will relate to better stratification and risk-prediction of who will benefit from treatment, and a more individualized approach to therapy.

3.2.2. *Disposition*

Given that the majority of COVID-19 patients develop only mild illness and remain well, with a minority progressing onward to develop severe illness, the mainstay of care for most COVID-19 patients is watchful observation and symptomatic treatment. Patients with only mild upper respiratory tract infection will only require symptomatic management with antipyretics, antitussives, and analgesia, and can be managed on an outpatient basis if there is adequate access to medical facilities should their condition deteriorate. However, decision-making regarding disposition of patients should be made on an individualized basis taking into account the patient's risk factors for disease severity (as previously discussed). A suggested risk-stratification table is summarized in Table 3.5, although this will ultimately depend on the attending physician's assessment.

National guidelines, with a public health viewpoint and broad aim to limit transmission, will often influence disposition policy. For example, in some countries, all patients with confirmed COVID-19 are isolated either

Table 3.5.   Risk stratification to guide patient disposition in confirmed COVID-19.[a]

Low Risk (fulfilling all criteria below)	High Risk (fulfilling any of the criteria below)
Age <30	Age ≥30, particularly >50
No chronic comorbidities	Chronic comorbidities (chronic lung, heart or kidney disease, diabetes mellitus, immunosuppression, obesity)
Reassuring clinical features • No dyspnea • Respiratory rate ≤20 breaths/min • Normal SpO_2 • Not requiring oxygen therapy	Worrisome clinical features • Dyspnea • Respiratory rate >20 breaths/min • Abnormal SpO_2 (≤94%) • Requiring oxygen therapy
Normal Chest X-ray	Chest X-ray with pneumonia
Reassuring laboratory results • CRP ≤20 mg/L • LDH ≤550 U/L • Lymphocytes ≥1 × 10⁹/L • Neutrophils ≤3 × 10⁹/L	Worrisome laboratory results • CRP >20 mg/L • LDH >550 U/L • Lymphocytes <1.0 × 10⁸/L • Neutrophils >3 × 10⁹/L

Note: [a]From: National Centre for Infectious Diseases and Chapter of Infectious Disease Physicians, College of Physicians, Singapore. Treatment Guidelines for COVID-19 (version 5.0, 4 January 2021).

in hospitals or dedicated isolation facilities to prevent onward transmission in the community, whereas in other countries well ambulatory patients are allowed to remain in self-isolation at home. This policy-making depends on a balance of resource availabilities, case numbers, and risk-benefit analysis, and is beyond the scope of this chapter.

3.2.3. *Critical care in COVID-19*

While there is an increasingly broad array of pharmaceutical interventions that may benefit patients with severe COVID-19, good supportive intensive care remains the mainstay in their management. Patients with severe COVID-19 and progressive hypoxia should thus be considered for early transfer to an ICU to be managed by an ICU multi-disciplinary team with expertise in management of patients with ARDS. The technical details of ICU management including ventilatory parameters and daily monitoring parameters are beyond the scope of this chapter, and best left to intensive care physicians — however several broad principles and concepts will be covered.

Most patients with respiratory failure and ARDS from severe COVID-19 will require intubation and mechanical ventilation, and we have a low threshold to intubate patients. Elective intubation is preferable to emergency intubation for two major reasons: (a) a more controlled setting will allow optimization of infection control precautions, and (b) avoiding acute respiratory decompensation which may be harmful to the patient.

Prone positioning in non-intubated patients has been suggested as a potential intervention to reduce the need for intubation. While small studies have shown some benefit in terms of improvement in oxygenation, there are no data to show that it can delay or prevent eventual need for intubation (Coppo *et al.*, 2020; Elharrar *et al.*, 2020; Sartini *et al.*, 2020). Nonetheless, as this is a relatively safe and non-invasive intervention, it can be considered in patients requiring low-flow oxygen supplementation.

Other non-invasive ventilatory modalities such as high-flow nasal cannula (HFNC) and non-invasive positive pressure ventilation (NIV) may be used as a bridge in hypoxemic patients to avoid mechanical ventilation. HFNC has been used extensively in COVID-19 patients, with some small studies reporting good outcomes (Guy *et al.*, 2020). While they have been shown to be beneficial in terms of mortality reduction and progression to intubation in hypoxemic respiratory failure of all causes (Ferreyro *et al.*, 2020), good large cohort or randomized-controlled trial (RCT) data specific to COVID-19 remain lacking (Schunemann *et al.*, 2020). While concern has been raised regarding potentially increased aerosol dispersion or environmental contamination, there has been data to demonstrate the safety of HFNC from an infection control perspective — as long as carried out within airborne isolation infection rooms or AIIRs (Ong *et al.*, 2021). Nonetheless, as use of these modalities may alleviate pressure on limited ventilator or intensive care resources, they can be used in a closely monitored environment, with the necessary infection control precautions and a view to intubation and mechanical ventilation should patients further deteriorate.

3.2.4. *Antivirals*

3.2.4.1. *Remdesivir*

Doses and key points about commonly-used drugs are summarized in Table 3.6. Remdesivir is a novel antiviral that was originally developed for Ebola and Marburg virus infections. It is a prodrug that is metabolized intracellularly to an adenosine triphosphate analog, inhibiting the viral RNA-dependent RNA polymerase involved in viral replication.

The clinical utility of remdesivir in COVID-19 was demonstrated in a large double-blind placebo-controlled RCT, ACTT-1, which recruited 541 patients who received remdesivir and 521 patients who received placebo (Beigel *et al.*, 2020). Remdesivir was associated with a shortened time to recovery, although there was no statistically significant impact on mortality in the entire study population. Sub-group analysis revealed the greatest benefit in patients requiring supplemental oxygen, but not those on non-invasive or invasive ventilation.

In contrast, another large randomized open-label trial, the SOLIDARITY trial, found no significant difference in mortality between patients treated with remdesivir and patients receiving standard of care only, although this was limited by its open-label study design and pragmatic nature with limited data collection focusing on a smaller set of primary end-points (WHO Solidarity Trial Consortium *et al.*, 2021).

Taken together, the data suggest that even if remdesivir has a therapeutic effect, its impact on the disease course in severe COVID-19 is

Table 3.6. Summary of medications approved for the treatment of COVID-19 with dosing regimens.[a]

Medication	Adult Dose	Notes
Dexamethasone	6 mg PO or IV, for up to 10 days	If dexamethasone is unavailable, may consider substitution with equivalent daily doses of another corticosteroid (e.g. hydrocortisone 15 mg, methylprednisolone 40 mg, prednisolone 40 mg daily in divided doses). Do NOT use dexamethasone in patients without hypoxemia, or not requiring oxygen. Caution in patients with concurrent infections. Monitor for hyperglycaemia, psychiatric effects, gastrointestinal bleeding, sepsis and heart failure.
Remdesivir	200 mg IV loading, 100 mg IV daily, for 5 to 10 days	Timing of antiviral initiation may be important, as administration with high viral loads seen after peak viral titre has been found to fail in reducing lung damage despite reducing viral loads. Early therapy may be more beneficial compared to later therapy. May cause liver function abnormalities. Monitor liver function tests prior to initiation and regularly while on remdesivir.
Baracitinib	4 mg PO once daily, for up to 14 days	Not recommended for patients with known active tuberculosis infections, who are on dialysis, have end-stage renal disease, or have acute kidney injury.

Note: [a]National Centre for Infectious Diseases and Chapter of Infectious Disease Physicians, College of Physicians, Singapore. Treatment Guidelines for COVID-19 (version 5.0, dated 4 Jan 2021).

modest, and further studies should focus on identifying characteristics of patients who will benefit most from antiviral treatment, the efficacy of combination therapies, as well as the cost-effectiveness of remdesivir use in the real-world clinical setting. Antivirals are likely to be most effective earlier on in the illness during the viral replicative phase, before the immune phase sets in and becomes the major driver of inflammation.

Remdesivir is generally well-tolerated, and most side-effects are minor including infusion-related reactions such as diaphoresis, nausea, vomiting, or chills. Reversible transaminase elevations have been observed while on treatment, though this was seen in both treatment and placebo arms in the ACTT-1 trial. Nonetheless, patients receiving remdesivir should have regular monitoring of liver function tests.

3.2.5. *Anti-inflammatories*

As previously discussed, the significant pathophysiologic mechanism driving severe illness in the second week of COVID-19 infection appears to be largely due to a dysregulated hyperinflammatory immune response. For this reason, anti-inflammatory drugs have been postulated to be beneficial by ameliorating this immune response.

3.2.5.1. *Corticosteroids*

The best evidence for this is for corticosteroids, with dexamethasone being the most well-studied drug. This was demonstrated in the large open-label randomized-controlled RECOVERY trial, with 2,104 patients receiving dexamethasone (oral or intravenously, 6 mg daily for up to 10 days) and 4,321 patients receiving standard of care (RECOVERY Collaborative Group *et al.*, 2021). Dexamethasone resulted in significantly lower mortality, with the greatest benefit seen in patients on mechanical ventilation or receiving supplemental oxygen in a sub-group analysis. This benefit was not seen in patients not receiving either respiratory support, with a non-statistically significant trend towards higher mortality in this group.

This finding was echoed in a meta-analysis of seven RCTs evaluating different corticosteroid formulations (including dexamethasone, hydrocortisone, and methylprednisolone), which found that corticosteroid treatment was associated with a lower 28-day all-cause mortality for critically ill patients with COVID-19 (WHO REACT Working Group *et al.*, 2020). While dexamethasone has the best data to support its use, other corticosteroid formulations can be considered if dexamethasone is not available, with equivalent dosing (e.g. hydrocortisone 150 mg/day, methylprednisolone 40 mg/day, or prednisolone 40 mg/day).

The evidence is clear that corticosteroids are a significant life-saving intervention in severe COVID-19. While advantageous in terms of its cost and availability, especially in resource-limited settings, corticosteroids are not without their adverse effects. Secondary infections or reactivation of latent infections remain significant concerns, and pre-emptive treatment of strongyloidiasis should be considered in regions that are endemic. Even short-course corticosteroids have been associated with increased rates of bleeding, heart failure, and secondary infections or sepsis (Yao *et al.*, 2020a). The decision to start a COVID-19 patient on corticosteroids will thus need to take into account an individualized risk-benefit analysis weighing the potential benefits of corticosteroids against their deleterious effects, especially in elderly patients with multiple comorbidities.

3.2.5.2. *Baricitinib*

Baricitinib is an oral Janus kinase (JAK) inhibitor used in the treatment of autoimmune inflammatory diseases such as rheumatoid arthritis. Its anti-viral activity lies in its affinity for adaptor-associated kinase-1 (AAK1) which is a regulator of viral endocytosis, thereby preventing SARS-CoV-2 from entering and infecting pulmonary cells. It also blunts the downstream inflammatory cascade by the inhibition of JAK1/JAK2 and IL-6-induced STAT3 phosphorylation.

A double-blind RCT, ACTT-2, evaluated the use of baricitinib in com-bination with remdesivir as combination therapy, compared with remdesi-vir and placebo (Kalil *et al.*, 2021). This showed a marginal reduction in median time to recovery across the entire study population. However, a sub-group analysis showed that the impact of treatment was greatest in patients who were on high-flow nasal oxygen or non-invasive ventilation, with a greater difference in time to clinical recovery. Combination therapy also decreased the proportion of patients who died or progressed to inva-sive mechanical ventilation.

Although baricitinib has been associated with increased rates of thromboembolism when used in autoimmune disease (Taylor *et al.*, 2019), this association was not observed in the clinical trials conducted to evalu-ate its use in COVID-19. Nonetheless, since COVID-19 itself already elevates thrombotic risk, patients should be closely monitored and pro-phylactic anticoagulation should be considered.

3.2.5.3. *Targeted immunomodulators*

The role of IL-6 inhibitors such as tocilizumab has had some mixed data, likely due to the heterogeneity in the persons included in the studies and the specific end-points studied. Results from COVACTA trial in hospitalized adults with severe COVID-19 pneumonia found that treatment with tocilizumab compared to placebo did not meet primary endpoint of improved clinical status using a 7-category ordinal scale or 28-day mortality (Rosas *et al.*, 2021). The EMPACTA trial comprising found that tocilizumab decreased the likelihood of a composite outcome of mechanical ventilation or death, but did not improve 28-day survival (Salama *et al.*, 2021). The findings from another trial, REMAP-CAP trial, found that critically ill patients receiving tocilizumab were more likely to improve than patients who received no immunomodulators (odds ratio 1.64) (REMAP-CAP Investigators *et al.*, 2021).

The roles of other agents for hyperinflammation in COVID-19, e.g. IL-1 and BTK inhibitors are currently unclear.

3.2.6. *Passive immune therapies*

3.2.6.1. *Convalescent plasma*

Like tocilizumab, trials on convalescent plasma (CP) have shown mixed results to date. Related to this includes the heterogeneity of studied populations, measurement of antibody titers in CP and determining what is an optimal protective titer. While large cohort data from the US of more than 35,000 hospitalized patients with COVID-19 have indicated that CP treatment is safe and that earlier use of CP (within 3 days of COVID-19 diagnosis) was associated with a survival benefit (7-day and 30-day mortality) compared to the later use of CP (4 or more days after diagnosis), RCT data have been mixed, with several trials not showing differences in disease progression or mortality (Agarwal *et al.*, 2020; Li *et al.*, 2020; Simonovich *et al.*, 2021). However, one trial showed that early administration of high-titer CP to mildly ill infected older adults reduced the progression of COVID-19 (Libster *et al.*, 2021).

3.2.6.2. *Monoclonal antibodies*

Two monoclonal antibody preparations (bamlanivimab and casirivimab-imdevimab) have been received emergency use authorization by the US FDA for non-hospitalized patients with mild to moderate COVID-19 who are at risk for severe disease (e.g. obesity, diabetes, chronic kidney disease, immunosuppression, age ≥65 years, or age ≥55 years with chronic cardiovascular, pulmonary disease or hypertension). Viral loads and hospitalization were diminished, compared to placebo with these monoclonal antibodies, but further studies are needed to fully assess the safety and efficacy of these treatments (Chen *et al.*, 2021).

3.2.6.3. *Immunoglobulins*

There is currently no robust data on the utility of SARS-CoV-2-specific immunoglobulins or hyper-immunoglobulins or non-SARS-CoV-2-specific immunoglobulins for the treatment of COVID-19.

3.2.7. *Anticoagulation*

As outlined previously, COVID-19 has been associated with a pro-thrombotic hypercoagulable state, and both arterial and venous thrombotic complications such as DVT, PE, myocardial infarction, stroke, and limb ischemia have been described even in patients without pre-existing risk factors for atherosclerotic or thrombotic disease. Anticoagulation to prevent such thrombotic complications should be considered in patients with COVID-19 infection, although it is not without risk (e.g. bleeding). Further studies are needed to better delineate the subgroups who would most benefit from prophylactic anticoagulation.

The agent of choice for prophylactic anticoagulation is low molecular-weight heparin (LWMH). This is beneficial over other oral anticoagulation agents as it can be stopped quickly in the event of bleeding complications, as opposed to other agents with a longer washout period. It also obviates the need for therapeutic drug monitoring and titration involved when using oral warfarin.

There are institutional and country-specific differences in approaches to thromboprophylaxis, with some adopting universal thromboprophylaxis for all admitted patients with COVID-19, while others use a risk-stratified approach. As the risk of thrombotic complications is greatest in critically ill patients and those admitted to the ICU, these patients should all receive prophylactic anticoagulation in the absence of contraindications (e.g. active bleeding, or recent significant bleeding in the past 24 to 48 hours, recent intracranial haemorrhage, severe coagulopathy). In Singapore, for example, it is recommended that patients with mild or moderate COVID-19 infection but requiring hospitalization should be risk-stratified for thromboembolism and bleeding using a risk assessment calculator (e.g. the PADUA risk score and the VTE bleed score), and be considered for receiving prophylactic anticoagulation if there is a high risk (NCID, 2021). Anticoagulation can be discontinued after the acute phase of illness or upon discharge from hospital.

3.2.8. *Management of comorbid conditions*

3.2.8.1. *Hypertension*

Hypertension is a common comorbidity seen in COVID-19 patients, and it is thus important to review the effect of anti-hypertensive medications on COVID-19 infection. In the initial phase of the pandemic, there was significant debate on whether chronic treatment with angiotensin-converting enzyme (ACE) inhibitors or angiotensin receptor blockers (ARBs) had an impact on the clinical course of COVID-19, either positively or negatively. The theoretical basis for this is because ACE inhibitor or ARB use may increase levels of ACE2 (Ishiyama *et al.*, 2004) — this is a shared receptor for SARS-CoV-2 binding (Zheng *et al.*, 2020). However, large studies and meta-analyses subsequently found that there was no impact on severity or mortality, supporting the recommendation to continue these medications in patients who were previously receiving them (Flacco *et al.*, 2020; Mackey *et al.*, 2020; Reynolds *et al.*, 2020).

3.2.8.2. *Hyperlipidemia*

Statins have been associated with an immunomodulatory effect, and may thus theoretically be beneficial in acute infections. However, this has to be countered with potential adverse effects of hepatotoxicity. Retrospective studies have showed that statin treatment may be associated with a reduced risk of mortality or severe COVID-19, though this needs to be confirmed in prospective cohorts (Daniels *et al.*, 2020; Zhang *et al.*, 2020). Since COVID-19 has been associated with an increased prothrombotic risk and a higher incidence of cardiovascular and cerebrovascular events, continuation of statins may also proffer benefits from a plaque-stabilization point of view. In the absence of severe liver dysfunction, they should thus be continued.

3.3. Conclusion

Beyond what has been discussed in this chapter, public health measures such as safe-distancing, mask-wearing, accessible diagnostics (which are accurate, and coupled with isolation of infectious persons to prevent further spread) and vaccination are vital facets in dealing with this pandemic. There has been tremendous progress in understanding the pathophysiology, clinical manifestations and treatment of COVID-19 within the short span of time since the initial description of SARS-CoV-2, and it is anticipated that we will learn much more and continue to refine our management of patients with COVID-19 with emerging and evidence-based data.

References

Agarwal A *et al*. Convalescent plasma in the management of moderate covid-19 in adults in India: Open label phase II multicentre randomised controlled trial (PLACID Trial). *BMJ* 2020; 371:m3939.

Ai T *et al*. Correlation of chest CT and RT-PCR testing for Coronavirus disease 2019 (COVID-19) in China: A report of 1014 cases. *Radiology* 2020; 296:E32–E40.

Artifoni M *et al*. Systematic assessment of venous thromboembolism in COVID-19 patients receiving thromboprophylaxis: Incidence and role of D-dimer as predictive factors. *J Thromb Thrombolysis* 2020; 50:211–216.

Bartoletti M *et al*. Epidemiology of invasive pulmonary aspergillosis among intubated patients with COVID-19: A prospective study. *Clin Infect Dis* 2021; 73:e3606–e3614.

Beigel JH *et al*. Remdesivir for the treatment of COVID-19 — Final report. *N Engl J Med* 2020; 383:1813–1826.

Bekelis K *et al*. Ischemic stroke occurs less frequently in patients with COVID-19: A multicenter cross-sectional study. *Stroke* 2020; 51:3570–3576.

Berlivet L, Lowy I. Hydroxychloroquine controversies: Clinical trials, epistemology, and the democratization of science. *Med Anthropol Q* 2020; 34:525–541.

Bhatla A *et al*. COVID-19 and cardiac arrhythmias. *Heart Rhythm* 2020; 17:1439–1444.

Bi Q *et al*. Epidemiology and transmission of COVID-19 in 391 cases and 1286 of their close contacts in Shenzhen, China: A retrospective cohort study. *Lancet Infect Dis* 2020; 20:911–919.

Bilaloglu S *et al*. Thrombosis in hospitalized patients with COVID-19 in a New York City health system. *JAMA* 2020; 324:799–801.

Cao B *et al*. A trial of Lopinavir-Ritonavir in adults hospitalized with severe COVID-19. *N Engl J Med* 2020; 382:1787–1799.

Carfi A *et al*. Persistent symptoms in patients after acute COVID-19. *JAMA* 2020; 324:603–605.

Cavalcanti AB *et al*. Hydroxychloroquine with or without azithromycin in mild-to-moderate COVID-19. *N Engl J Med* 2020; 383:2041–2052.

Chand S *et al*. COVID-19-associated critical illness-report of the first 300 patients admitted to intensive care units at a New York City medical center. *J Intensive Care Med* 2020; 35:963–970.

Chen N *et al*. Epidemiological and clinical characteristics of 99 cases of 2019 novel coronavirus pneumonia in Wuhan, China: A descriptive study. *Lancet* 2020; 395:507–513.

Chen P *et al*. SARS-CoV-2 neutralizing antibody LY-CoV555 in outpatients with COVID-19. *N Engl J Med* 2021; 384:229–237.

Cheung KS *et al*. Gastrointestinal manifestations of SARS-CoV-2 infection and virus load in fecal samples from a Hong Kong cohort: Systematic review and meta-analysis. *Gastroenterology* 2020; 159:81–95.

Chorin E *et al*. The QT interval in patients with COVID-19 treated with hydroxy-chloroquine and azithromycin. *Nat Med* 2020; 26:808–809.

Cleverley J *et al*. The role of chest radiography in confirming COVID-19 pneumonia. *BMJ* 2020; 370:m2426.

Coppo A *et al*. Feasibility and physiological effects of prone positioning in non-intubated patients with acute respiratory failure due to COVID-19 (PRON-COVID): A prospective cohort study. *Lancet Respir Med* 2020; 8:765–774.

Cui S *et al*. Prevalence of venous thromboembolism in patients with severe novel coronavirus pneumonia. *J Thromb Haemost* 2020; 18:1421–1424.

Cummings MJ *et al*. Epidemiology, clinical course, and outcomes of critically ill adults with COVID-19 in New York City: A prospective cohort study. *Lancet* 2020; 395:1763–1770.

Daneshgaran G *et al*. Cutaneous manifestations of COVID-19: An evidence-based review. *Am J Clin Dermatol* 2020; 21:627–639.

Daniels LB *et al*. Relation of statin use prior to admission to severity and recovery among COVID-19 inpatients. *Am J Cardiol* 2020; 136:149–155.

Elharrar X, Trigui Y, Dols AM, *et al*. Use of prone positioning in nonintubated patients with COVID-19 and hypoxemic acute respiratory failure. *JAMA* 2020; 323:2336–2338.

Fan BE *et al*. Delayed catastrophic thrombotic events in young and asymptomatic post COVID-19 patients. *J Thromb Thrombolysis* 2021; 51:971–977.

Feldstein LR *et al*. Multisystem inflammatory syndrome in U.S. children and adolescents. *N Engl J Med* 2020; 383:334–346.

Ferreyro BL *et al*. Association of noninvasive oxygenation strategies with all-cause mortality in adults with acute hypoxemic respiratory failure: A systematic review and meta-analysis. *JAMA* 2020; 324:57–67.

Flacco ME *et al*. Treatment with ACE inhibitors or ARBs and risk of severe/lethal COVID-19: A meta-analysis. *Heart* 2020; 106:1519–1524.

Freeman EE *et al*. Pernio-like skin lesions associated with COVID-19: A case series of 318 patients from 8 countries. *J Am Acad Dermatol* 2020; 83:486–492.

Galloway JB *et al*. A clinical risk score to identify patients with COVID-19 at high risk of critical care admission or death: An observational cohort study. *J Infect* 2020; 81:282–288.

Galvan Casas C *et al*. Classification of the cutaneous manifestations of COVID-19: A rapid prospective nationwide consensus study in Spain with 375 cases. *Br J Dermatol* 2020; 183:71–77.

Garrigues E *et al*. Post-discharge persistent symptoms and health-related quality of life after hospitalization for COVID-19. *J Infect* 2020; 81:e4–e6.

Giacomelli A *et al*. Self-reported olfactory and taste disorders in patients with severe acute respiratory Coronavirus 2 infection: A cross-sectional study. *Clin Infect Dis* 2020; 71:889–890.

Gianola S *et al*. Characteristics of academic publications, preprints, and registered clinical trials on the COVID-19 pandemic. *PLoS One* 2020; 15: e0240123.

Guan WJ *et al*. Clinical characteristics of Coronavirus disease 2019 in China. *N Engl J Med* 2020; 382:1708–1720.

Guo T *et al*. Cardiovascular implications of fatal outcomes of patients with Coronavirus disease 2019 (COVID-19). *JAMA Cardiol* 2020; 5:811–818.

Gutierrez-Ortiz C *et al*. Miller Fisher syndrome and polyneuritis cranialis in COVID-19. *Neurology* 2020; 95:e601–e605.

Guy T *et al*. High-flow nasal oxygen: A safe, efficient treatment for COVID-19 patients not in an ICU. *Eur Respir J* 2020; 56:2001154.

Halpin SJ *et al*. Postdischarge symptoms and rehabilitation needs in survivors of COVID-19 infection: A cross-sectional evaluation. *J Med Virol* 2021; 93:1013–1022.

Helms J *et al*. High risk of thrombosis in patients with severe SARS-CoV-2 infection: A multicenter prospective cohort study. *Intensive Care Med* 2020a; 46:1089–1098.

Helms J *et al*. Neurologic features in severe SARS-CoV-2 infection. *N Engl J Med* 2020b; 382:2268–2270.

Hill JB *et al*. Frequency of venous thromboembolism in 6513 patients with COVID-19: A retrospective study. *Blood Adv* 2020; 4:5373–5377.

Huang C *et al*. Clinical features of patients infected with 2019 novel coronavirus in Wuhan, China. *Lancet* 2020a; 395:497–506.

Huang YH *et al*. SARS-CoV-2 detected in cerebrospinal fluid by PCR in a case of COVID-19 encephalitis. *Brain Behav Immun* 2020b; 87:149.

Ishiyama Y *et al*. Upregulation of angiotensin-converting enzyme 2 after myocardial infarction by blockade of angiotensin II receptors. *Hypertension* 2004; 43:970–976.

Jasne AS *et al*. Stroke code presentations, interventions, and outcomes before and during the COVID-19 pandemic. *Stroke* 2020; 51:2664–2673.

Ji D *et al*. Prediction for progression risk in patients with COVID-19 pneumonia: The CALL score. *Clin Infect Dis* 2020a; 71:1393–1399.

Ji Y *et al*. Potential association between COVID-19 mortality and health-care resource availability. *Lancet Glob Health* 2020b; 8:e480.

Jin X *et al*. Epidemiological, clinical and virological characteristics of 74 cases of coronavirus-infected disease 2019 (COVID-19) with gastrointestinal symptoms. *Gut* 2020; 69:1002–1009.

Kalil AC *et al*. Baricitinib plus remdesivir for hospitalized adults with COVID-19. *N Engl J Med* 2021; 384:795–807.

Klok FA *et al*. Incidence of thrombotic complications in critically ill ICU patients with COVID-19. *Thromb Res* 2020; 191:145–147.

Koralnik IJ, Tyler KL. COVID-19: A global threat to the nervous system. *Ann Neurol* 2020; 88:1–11.

Langford BJ *et al*. Bacterial co-infection and secondary infection in patients with COVID-19: Aa living rapid review and meta-analysis. *Clin Microbiol Infect* 2020; 26:1622–1629.

Lansbury L *et al*. Co-infections in people with COVID-19: A systematic review and meta-analysis. *J Infect* 2020; 81:266–275.

Lavezzo E *et al*. Suppression of a SARS-CoV-2 outbreak in the Italian municipality of Vo'. *Nature* 2020; 584:425–429.

Lee PH *et al*. Associations of viral ribonucleic acid (RNA) shedding patterns with clinical illness and immune responses in Severe Acute Respiratory Syndrome Coronavirus 2 (SARS-CoV-2) infection. *Clin Transl Immunology* 2020; 9:e1160.

Li L *et al*. Effect of convalescent plasma therapy on time to clinical improvement in patients with severe and life-threatening COVID-19: A randomized clinical trial. *JAMA* 2020; 324:460–470.

Liang W *et al*. Development and validation of a clinical risk score to predict the occurrence of critical illness in hospitalized patients with COVID-19. *JAMA Intern Med* 2020; 180:1081–1089.

Libby P, Luscher T. COVID-19 is, in the end, an endothelial disease. *Eur Heart J* 2020; 41:3038–3044.

Libster R *et al*. Early high-titer plasma therapy to prevent severe COVID-19 in older adults. *N Engl J Med* 2021; 384:610–618.

Liguoro I *et al.* SARS-COV-2 infection in children and newborns: A systematic review. *Eur J Pediatr* 2020; 179:1029–1046.

Liotta EM *et al.* Frequent neurologic manifestations and encephalopathy-associated morbidity in COVID-19 patients. *Ann Clin Transl Neurol* 2020; 7:2221–2230.

Lucas C *et al.* Longitudinal analyses reveal immunological misfiring in severe COVID-19. *Nature* 2020; 584:463–469.

Mackey K *et al.* Risks and impact of angiotensin-converting enzyme inhibitors or angiotensin-receptor blockers on SARS-CoV-2 infection in adults: A living systematic review. *Ann Intern Med* 2020; 173:195–203.

Mahase E. COVID-19: What do we know about "long covid"? *BMJ* 2020; 370:m2815.

Mao L *et al.* Neurologic manifestations of hospitalized patients with Coronavirus disease 2019 in Wuhan, China. *JAMA Neurol* 2020; 77:683–690.

Marshall M. The lasting misery of coronavirus long-haulers. *Nature* 2020; 585:339–341.

Matschke J *et al.* Neuropathology of patients with COVID-19 in Germany: A post-mortem case series. *Lancet Neurol* 2020; 19:919–929.

Matthay MA *et al.* Treatment for severe acute respiratory distress syndrome from COVID-19. *Lancet Respir Med* 2020; 8:433–434.

Medcalf RL *et al.* Fibrinolysis and COVID-19: A plasmin paradox. *J Thromb Haemost* 2020; 18:2118–2122.

Mehta NS *et al.* SARS-CoV-2 (COVID-19): What do we know about children? A systematic review. *Clin Infect Dis* 2020; 71:2469–2479.

Middeldorp S *et al.* Incidence of venous thromboembolism in hospitalized patients with COVID-19. *J Thromb Haemost* 2020; 18:1995–2002.

Moriguchi T *et al.* A first case of meningitis/encephalitis associated with SARS-Coronavirus-2. *Int J Infect Dis* 2020; 94:55–58.

NCID (National Centre for Infectious Diseases, Singapore), 2021. Treatment Guidelines for COVID-19. https://www.ncid.sg/Health-Professionals/Diseases-and-Conditions/Documents/Treatment%20Guidelines%20for%20COVID-19%20v7%20Final%20%20%2828-7-2021%29.pdf (accessed 28 July 2021).

Ng OT *et al.* SARS-CoV-2 seroprevalence and transmission risk factors among high-risk close contacts: A retrospective cohort study. *Lancet Infect Dis* 2021; 21:333–343.

NIH (National Institutes of Health, USA), 2020. Clinical Presentation of People with SARS-CoV-2 Infection. https://www.covid19treatmentguidelines.nih.gov/overview/clinical-presentation/ (accessed 16 December 2020).

Odone A *et al.* The runaway science: A bibliometric analysis of the COVID-19 scientific literature. *Acta Biomed* 2020; 91:34–39.

Onder G *et al*. Case-fatality rate and characteristics of patients dying in relation to COVID-19 in Italy. *JAMA* 2020; 323:1775–1776.

Ong SWX *et al*. Transmission modes of severe acute respiratory syndrome coronavirus 2 and implications on infection control: A review. *Singapore Med J* 2020; Jul 30.

Ong SWX *et al*. Environmental contamination in a coronavirus disease 2019 (COVID-19) intensive care unit — What is the risk? *Infect Control Hosp Epidemiol* 2021; 42:669–677.

Panigada M *et al*. Hypercoagulability of COVID-19 patients in intensive care unit: A report of thromboelastography findings and other parameters of hemostasis. *J Thromb Haemost* 2020; 18:1738–1742.

Paterson RW *et al*. The emerging spectrum of COVID-19 neurology: Clinical, radiological and laboratory findings. *Brain* 2020; 143:3104–3120.

Pezzini A, Padovani A. Lifting the mask on neurological manifestations of COVID-19. *Nat Rev Neurol* 2020; 16:636–644.

Plucinski MM *et al*. Coronavirus disease 2019 (COVID-19) in Americans aboard the Diamond Princess Cruise Ship. *Clin Infect Dis* 2021; 72: e448–e457.

Puntmann VO *et al*. Outcomes of cardiovascular magnetic resonance imaging in patients recently recovered from Coronavirus disease 2019 (COVID-19). *JAMA Cardiol* 2020; 5:1265–1273.

Qin C *et al*. Dysregulation of immune response in patients with Coronavirus 2019 (COVID-19) in Wuhan, China. *Clin Infect Dis* 2020; 71:762–768.

Ranucci M *et al*. The procoagulant pattern of patients with COVID-19 acute respiratory distress syndrome. *J Thromb Haemost* 2020; 18:1747–1751.

Rawson TM *et al*. Bacterial and fungal coinfection in individuals with coronavirus: A rapid review to support COVID-19 antimicrobial prescribing. *Clin Infect Dis* 2020; 71:2459–2468.

Reichard RR *et al*. Neuropathology of COVID-19: A spectrum of vascular and acute disseminated encephalomyelitis (ADEM)-like pathology. *Acta Neuropathol* 2020; 140:1–6.

REMAP-CAP Investigators *et al*. Interleukin-6 receptor antagonists in critically ill patients with COVID-19. *N Engl J Med* 2021; 384:1491–1502.

Reynolds HR *et al*. Renin-angiotensin-aldosterone system inhibitors and risk of COVID-19. *N Engl J Med* 2020; 382:2441–2448.

Richardson S *et al*. presenting characteristics, comorbidities, and outcomes among 5,700 patients hospitalized with COVID-19 in the New York City area. *JAMA* 2020; 323:2052–2059.

Rosas IO *et al*. Tocilizumab in hospitalized patients with severe COVID-19 pneumonia. *N Engl J Med* 2021; 384:1503–1516.

Ruan Q *et al*. Clinical predictors of mortality due to COVID-19 based on an analysis of data of 150 patients from Wuhan, China. *Intensive Care Med* 2020; 46:846–848.

Salama C *et al*. Tocilizumab in patients hospitalized with COVID-19 pneumonia. *N Engl J Med* 2021; 384:20–30.

Sartini C *et al*. Respiratory parameters in patients with COVID-19 after using noninvasive ventilation in the prone position outside the intensive care unit. *JAMA* 2020; 323:2338–2340.

Sayampanathan AA *et al*. Infectivity of asymptomatic versus symptomatic COVID-19. *Lancet* 2021; 397:93–94.

Schauwvlieghe AFAD *et al*. Invasive aspergillosis in patients admitted to the intensive care unit with severe influenza: A retrospective cohort study. *Lancet Respir Med* 2018; 6:782–792.

Schunemann HJ *et al*. Ventilation techniques and risk for transmission of coronavirus disease, including COVID-19: A living systematic review of multiple streams of evidence. *Ann Intern Med* 2020; 173:204–216.

Self WH *et al*. Effect of hydroxychloroquine on clinical status at 14 days in hospitalized patients with COVID-19: A randomized clinical trial. *JAMA* 2020; 324:2165–2176.

Siddiqi HK, Mehra MR. COVID-19 illness in native and immunosuppressed states: A clinical-therapeutic staging proposal. *J Heart Lung Transplant* 2020; 39:405–407.

Simonovich VA *et al*. A randomized trial of convalescent plasma in COVID-19 severe pneumonia. *N Engl J Med* 2021; 384:619–629.

Somani S *et al*. De novo status epilepticus in patients with COVID-19. *Ann Clin Transl Neurol* 2020; 7:1240–1244.

Spinato G *et al*. Alterations in smell or taste in mildly symptomatic outpatients with SARS-CoV-2 infection. *JAMA* 2020; 323:2089–2090.

Stone N *et al*. Mucormycosis: Time to address this deadly fungal infection. *Lancet Microbe* 2021; 2:E343–E344.

Struyf T *et al*. Signs and symptoms to determine if a patient presenting in primary care or hospital outpatient settings has COVID-19 disease. *Cochrane Database Syst Rev* 2020; 7:CD013665.

Sudharsanan N *et al*. The contribution of the age distribution of cases to COVID-19 case fatality across countries: A nine-country demographic study. *Ann Intern Med* 2020; 173:714–720.

Taylor PC *et al*. Cardiovascular safety during treatment with baricitinib in Rheumatoid Arthritis. *Arthritis Rheumatol* 2019; 71:1042–1055.

Tian Y *et al*. Review article: Gastrointestinal features in COVID-19 and the possibility of faecal transmission. *Aliment Pharmacol Ther* 2020; 51:843–851.

Tong JY *et al*. The prevalence of olfactory and gustatory dysfunction in COVID-19 patients: A systematic review and meta-analysis. *Otolaryngol Head Neck Surg* 2020; 163:3–11.

Toscano G *et al*. Guillain-Barre syndrome associated with SARS-CoV-2. *N Engl J Med* 2020; 382:2574–2576.

Tursen U *et al.* Cutaneous side-effects of the potential COVID-19 drugs. *Dermatol Ther* 2020; 33:e13476.

Varga Z *et al.* Endothelial cell infection and endotheliitis in COVID-19. *Lancet* 2020; 395:1417–1418.

Verdoni L *et al.* An outbreak of severe Kawasaki-like disease at the Italian epicentre of the SARS-CoV-2 epidemic: An observational cohort study. *Lancet* 2020; 395:1771–1778.

Verity R *et al.* Estimates of the severity of coronavirus disease 2019: A model-based analysis. *Lancet Infect Dis* 2020; 20:669–677.

Wang D *et al.* Clinical characteristics of 138 hospitalized patients with 2019 novel Coronavirus-infected pneumonia in Wuhan, China. *JAMA* 2020a; 323:1061–1069.

Wang M *et al.* Remdesivir and chloroquine effectively inhibit the recently emerged novel coronavirus (2019-nCoV) *in vitro. Cell Res* 2020b; 30: 269–271.

Wei WE *et al.* Presymptomatic transmission of SARS-CoV-2 — Singapore, January 23-March 16, 2020. *MMWR — Morb Mortal Wkly Rep* 2020; 69:411–415.

Whittaker E *et al.* Clinical characteristics of 58 children with a pediatric inflammatory multisystem syndrome temporally associated with SARS-CoV-2. *JAMA* 2020; 324:259–269.

WHO (World Health Organization), 2020. Clinical management of COVID-19. https://www.who.int/teams/health-care-readiness-clinical-unit/covid-19 (accessed 30 November 2021).

WHO REACT Working Group *et al.* Association between administration of systemic corticosteroids and mortality among critically ill patients with COVID-19: A meta-analysis. *JAMA* 2020; 324:1330–1341.

WHO Solidarity Trial Consortium *et al.* Repurposed antiviral drugs for COVID-19 — Interim WHO solidarity trial results. *N Engl J Med* 2021; 384:497–511. RECOVERY Collaborative Group, *et al.* Dexamethasone in hospitalized patients with COVID-19. *N Engl J Med* 2021; 384:693–704.

Wu Z, McGoogan JM. Characteristics of and important lessons from the coronavirus disease 2019 (COVID-19) outbreak in China: Summary of a report of 72 314 cases From the Chinese Center for Disease Control and Prevention. *JAMA* 2020; 323:1239–1242.

Yang Q *et al.* Imaging of coronavirus disease 2019: A Chinese expert consensus statement. *Eur J Radiol* 2020; 127:109008.

Yao TC *et al.* Association between oral corticosteroid bursts and severe adverse events: A nationwide population-based cohort study. *Ann Intern Med* 2020a; 173:325–330.

Yao X *et al. In vitro* antiviral activity and projection of optimized dosing design of hydroxychloroquine for the treatment of severe acute respiratory syndrome Coronavirus 2 (SARS-CoV-2). *Clin Infect Dis* 2020b; 71:732–739.

Yelin D *et al*. Long-term consequences of COVID-19: Research needs. *Lancet Infect Dis* 2020; 20:1115–1117.

Young BE *et al*. Epidemiologic features and clinical course of patients infected with SARS-CoV-2 in Singapore. *JAMA* 2020; 323:1488–1494.

Young BE *et al*. Viral dynamics and immune correlates of Coronavirus disease 2019 (COVID-19) severity. *Clin Infect Dis* 2021; 73:e2932–e2942.

Zhang XJ *et al*. In-hospital use of statins is associated with a reduced risk of mortality among individuals with COVID-19. *Cell Metab* 2020; 32: 176–187.e4.

Zhao J *et al*. Impact of the COVID-19 epidemic on stroke care and potential solutions. *Stroke* 2020a; 51:1996–2001.

Zhao YM *et al*. Follow-up study of the pulmonary function and related physiological characteristics of COVID-19 survivors 3 months after recovery. *EClinicalMedicine* 2020b; 25:100463.

Zheng YY *et al*. COVID-19 and the cardiovascular system. *Nat Rev Cardiol* 2020; 17:259–260.

Zou L *et al*. SARS-CoV-2 viral load in upper respiratory specimens of infected patients. *N Engl J Med* 2020; 382:1177–1179.

https://doi.org/10.1142/9789811254338_0004

Chapter 4

Detection and Diagnosis Technologies for SARS-CoV-2

Wan Ni Chia*, Chee Wah Tan[†], Jinyan Zhang[‡], and Lin-Fa Wang[§]

*Programme in Emerging Infectious Diseases,
Duke-NUS Medical School, Singapore*

*wanni.chia@duke-nus.edu.sg
[†]cheewah.tan@duke-nus.edu.sg
[‡]jyzhang@duke-nus.edu.sg
[§]linfa.wang@duke-nus.edu.sg

Abstract

Detection and diagnosis platforms play key roles in early warning, outbreak control and exit strategy for any pandemic, and they are especially pertinent for the Coronavirus disease 2019 (COVID-19) pandemic. The challenges posed by the speed and extent of severe acute respiratory syndrome Coronavirus-2 (SARS-CoV-2) spread around the globe also offered unprecedented opportunities for the development and deployment of novel strategies and products — not only vaccines and therapeutics, but also diagnostics. This chapter provides a brief summary of the vast array of molecular, serological, cell-based and other diagnostic tools for the specific detection of SARS-CoV-2 infections and immune responses. The focus is on the principles and applications of each platform, while detailed protocols can be found in the cited references.

Keywords: nCoV-2019; COVID-19; SARS-CoV-2; SARS-CoV; next generation sequencing (NGS); polymerase chain reaction (PCR); antigen rapid test (ART); lateral flow assay (LFA); point-of-care test (POC test); enzyme-linked immunosorbent assay (ELISA); virus neutralization test (VNT); surrogate VNT (sVNT); pseudovirus (PV)

4.1. Introduction

The Coronavirus disease 2019 (COVID-19) pandemic, caused by severe acute respiratory syndrome Coronavirus-2 (SARS-CoV-2), started in Wuhan, China in December 2019 (Wang *et al.*, 2020a). Compared with past pandemics, COVID-19 also provided unprecedented opportunities to harness the power of science and technology advancement in responding to a major infectious disease outbreak caused by a previously unknown pathogen.

The best example is the role that next generation sequencing (NGS) played throughout the COVID-19 pandemic. Here are a few important milestones achieved via NGS in the COVID-19 pandemic:

(a) The first warning of a novel Coronavirus as the potential causative agent of the severe pneumonia in Wuhan came from the NGS report provided by commercial NGS service provider to infectious disease doctors in Wuhan who ordered NGS analysis of patient lung lavage samples. This was the first time that a novel pathogen was first discovered by practicing clinicians and not research scientists (Wang *et al.*, 2020b).

(b) The whole genome sequence, determined by NGS, was released to the public on 9 January 2020, which laid the foundation for rapid development of not only diagnostics, but also vaccines, especially the mRNA-based vaccines.

(c) In the same week that the full SARS-CoV-2 genome was released, another important full genome of a bat CoV (RaTG13) was obtained by NGS, which indicated the probable bat origin of severe acute respiratory syndrome Coronavirus 2 (SARS-CoV-2) (Zhou *et al.*, 2020).

(d) By April 2021, there are over 1 million full genome sequences of SARS-CoV-2 deposited in public database (https://www.gisaid.org/). This international effort has not only facilitated the molecular epidemiological investigations, but also played a pivotal role in identifying variants of concerns (VOCs) which may impact the efficacy of currently available vaccines, and hence the exit strategies of the COVID-19 pandemic (WHO, 2020b).

Although NGS is by far the most impactful technology which has not been widely applied in pandemic responses before COVID-19, it is not suitable nor affordable by most users as a routine diagnostic or surveillance tool. This chapter will therefore focus on the more "routine" methodologies and platforms which play key roles in the diagnosis and detection of the virus and immune responses to the virus.

4.2. Molecular Detection

Nucleic acid amplification is the primary method of diagnosing COVID-19 (Carter *et al.*, 2020; Corman *et al.*, 2020; Sethuraman *et al.*, 2020). Among the different molecular platforms deployed, polymerase chain reaction (PCR) is considered the "gold standard" for the detection of viruses with speed, sensitivity, and specificity (Espy *et al.*, 2006; Mackay *et al.*, 2002).

4.2.1. *Real-time reverse transcriptase-PCR (RT-PCR)*

RT-PCR has become the method of choice for rapid diagnosis of RNA viruses, which is also true for SARS-CoV-2. Here, we summarize the workflow of SARS-CoV-2 RT-PCR and the key events in SARS-CoV-2 PCR development.

The generic workflow of RT-PCR for SARS-CoV-2 is as follows:

Sample collection. Upper respiratory tract samples (nasopharyngeal swabs, oropharyngeal swabs, nasopharyngeal washes, nasal aspirates) are broadly recommended. Lower respiratory samples (sputum, bronchoalveolar lavage or BAL fluid, tracheal aspirates) are recommended for patients exhibiting productive cough, but with greater risk of aerosol generation (CDC, 2021b; Wang *et al.*, 2020c). The detectable viral load depends on the days post-symptom onset (dpso). Sputum and nasal swabs are reliable for the first 14 dpso. Throat swabs were unreliable 8 dpso (Pan *et al.*, 2020). RT-PCR on nasopharyngeal swabs is the reference method to detect SARS-CoV-2 (Sethuraman *et al.*, 2020). However, nasopharyngeal swabs require trained healthcare professionals and extensive personal protective equipment. Saliva-based sampling has the potential to address the barriers associated with nasopharyngeal swab sampling. In a systematic review and meta-analysis, data suggested that saliva sampling may be a similarly sensitive and less costly alternative to nasopharyngeal swabs (Bastos *et al.*, 2021).

Primer and probe selection. As soon the SARS-CoV-2 genome was available, a variety of RT-PCR assays utilizing different primer/probe sets targeting different regions of the SARS-CoV-2 genome have been developed (Table 4.1) (CDC, 2020b; China CDC, 2020; Chu *et al.*, 2020; Corman *et al.*, 2020). The selection of the primer/probe set affects the sensitivity of the assay. Etievant *et al.* (2020) assessed the performance of SARS-CoV-2 PCR assays developed by WHO referral laboratories — data suggested that all RT-PCR assays performed well and are specific, except the N Charité and N2 US CDC assays. Vogels *et al.* (2020) demonstrated the US CDC, China CDC, HKU and Charité primer/probe sets can be used to detect SARS-CoV-2 at 500 viral RNA copies per reaction, with the exception of the RdRp-SARSr (Charité) confirmatory primer-probe set which has low sensitivity. This is probably due to a mismatch to circulating SARS-CoV-2 in the reverse primer.

RT-PCR testing. RT-PCR is composed of four steps: (a) lysis, (b) RNA extraction, (c) reverse transcription, and (d) amplification of specific genomic regions. One of the examples is the one-step RT-PCR assay developed by the US Centers for Disease Control and Prevention (CDC) (Table 4.1). Extracted viral RNA is added to a master mix containing primers and probe, reverse transcriptase and polymerase, followed by pre-programmed run in a PCR thermocycler (Figure 4.1). The quantity of the viral RNA in the sample is measured by the cycle threshold (Ct). The Ct is the number of the replication cycles required to produce a fluorescent signal. Low Ct values represent higher viral RNA loads (Espy *et al.*, 2006). A Ct value less than 40 is clinically reported as PCR-positive (Sethuraman *et al.*, 2020).

4.2.2. *Loop-mediated isothermal amplification* (*LAMP*)

Isothermal amplification-based molecular detection methods, best represented by LAMP, is another promising platform used for rapid molecular diagnosis. LAMP can be conducted in less than 1 hour at constant temperature of 60–65°C and does not require a thermocycler, hence

Table 4.1.   List of main RT-PCR tests developed for SARS-CoV-2 detection.

Institute	Target	Primer/Probe	Sequence (5'-3')	Polymerase	Reference
Charité	E	E_Sarbeco_F1	ACAGGTACGTTAATAGTTAATAGCGT	SuperScript III Platinum One-Step Quantitative RT-PCR System (Invitrogen)	Corman et al. (2020)
		E_Sarbeco_R2	ATATTGCAGCAGTACGCACACA		
		E_Sarbeco_P1	FAM-ACACTAGCCATCCTTACTGCGCTTCG-BBQ		
	RdRp	RdRp_SARSr-F2	GTGARATGGTCATGTGTGGCGG		
		RdRp_SARSr-R1	CARATGTTAAASACACTATTAGCATA		
		RdRp_SARSr-P1	FAM-CCAGGTGGWACRTCATCMGGTGATGC-BBQ		
		RdRp_SARSr-P2	FAM-CAGGTGGAACCTCATCAGGAGATGC-BBQ		
Hong Kong University	N	HKU-N-F	TAATCAGACACAAGGAACTGATTA	TaqMan Fast Virus Master Mix (ABI)	Chu et al. (2020)
		HKU-N-R	CGAAGGTGTGACTTCCATG		
		HKU-N-P	FAM-GCAAATTGTGCAATTTGCGG-TAMRA		
	NSP14	HKU-ORF1b-nsp14F	TGGGGYTTTACRGGTAACCT		
		HKU-ORF1b-nsp14R	AACRCGCTTAACAAAGCACTC		
		HKU-ORF1b-nsp14P	FAM-TAGTTGTGATGCWATCATGACTAG-TAMRA		
China CDC	N	CCDC-N-F	GGGGAACTTCTCCTGCTAGAAT	Unspecified	China-CDC (2020)
		CCDC-N-R	CAGACATTTGTCTCAAGCTG		
		CCDC-N-P	FAM-TTGCTGCTGCTTGACAGATT-TAMRA		
	NSP10	CCDC-ORF1-F	CCCTGTGGGTTTTACACTTAA		
		CCDC-ORF1-R	ACGATTGTGCATCAGCTGA		
		CCDC-ORF1-P	FAM-CCGTCTGCGGGTATGTGGAAAGGTTATGG-BHQ1		

(Continued)

Table 4.1. *(Continued)*

Institute	Target	Primer/Probe	Sequence (5'-3')	Polymerase	Reference
US CDC	N	2019-nCoV_N1-F	GACCCCAAAATCAGCGAAAT	TaqPath 1-Step RT-qPCR Master Mix, CG (Thermo Fisher)	CDC (2020b)
		2019-nCoV_N1-R	TCTGGTTACTGCCAGTTGAATCTG		
		2019-nCoV_N1-P	FAM-ACCCCGCATTACGTTTGGTGGACC-BHQ1		
		2019-nCoV_N2-F	TTACAAACATTGGCCGCAAA		
		2019-nCoV_N2-R	GCGCGACATTCCGAAGAA		
		2019-nCoV_N2-P	FAM-ACAATTTGCCCCCAGCGCTTCAG-BHQ1		
		2019-nCoV_N3-F	GGGAGCCTTGAATACACCAAAA		
		2019-nCoV_N3-R	TGTAGCACGATTGCAGCATTG		
		2019-nCoV_N3-P	FAM-AYCACATTGGCACCCGCAATCCTG-BHQ1		
	RNAse P	RP-F	AGATTTGGACCTGCGAGCG		
		RP-R	GAGCGGCTGTCTCCACAAGT		
		RP-P	FAM-TTCTGACCTGAAGGCTCTGCGCG-BHQ1		
NIID, Japan	N	NIID_2019-nCoV_N_F2	AAATTTTGGGGACCAGGAAC	QuantiTech Probe RT-PCR Kit (Qiagen)	Shirato *et al.* (2020)
		NIID_2019-nCoV_N_R2	TGGCAGCTGTGTAGGTCAAC		
		NIID_2019-nCoV_N_P2	FAM-ATGTCGCGCATTGGCATGGA-BHQ1		

NIH, Thailand	N	WH-NIC N-F WH-NIC N-R WH-NIC N-P	CGTTTGGTGGACCCTCAGAT CCCCACTGCGTTCTCCATT FAM-CAACTGGCAGTAACCA-BHQ1	Unspecified	Ministry of Public Health, Thailand (2020)
Institut Pasteur, Paris	RdRp	Pasteur_IP2_F Pasteur_IP2_R Pasteur_IP2_P	ATGAGCTTAGTCCTGTTG CTCCCTTTGTTGTGTTGT HEX-AGATGTCTGTGCTGCCGGTA-BHQ1	SuperScript III Platinum One-Step Quantitative RT-PCR System	Institut Pasteur (2020)
	RdRp	Pasteur_IP4_F Pasteur_IP4_R Pasteur_IP4_P	GGTAACTGGTATGATTTCG CTGGTCAAGGTTAATATAGG FAM-TCATACAAACCACGCCAGG-BHQ1		
	E	Pasteur_E_F Pasteur_E_R Pasteur_E_P	ACAGGTACGTTAATAGTTAATAGCGT ATATTGCAGCAGTACGCACACA FAM-ACACTAGCCATCCTTACTGCGCTTCG-BHQ1		

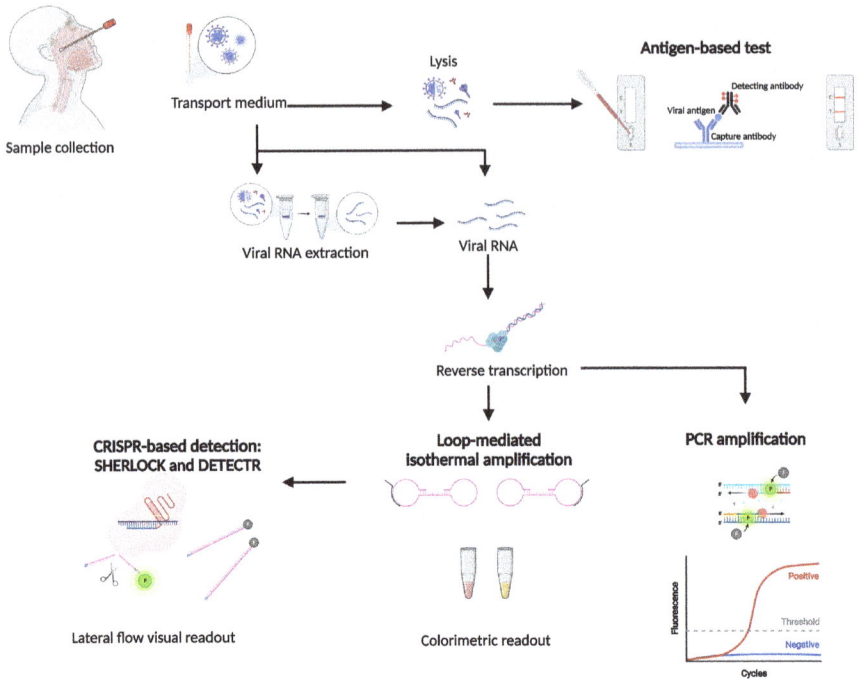

Figure 4.1. Workflow of SARS-CoV-2 molecular detection. Nasopharyngeal or oropharyngeal swab samples are collected in transport medium, lysed, RNA extracted, reverse-transcribed to cDNA, and then amplified through PCR or loop-mediated isothermal amplification.

possessing certain advantages over RT-PCR. The LAMP reaction comprises a DNA polymerase with strong strand displacement activity, and 4–6 primers to bind to 6–8 distinct regions within the target genome for a highly specific amplification. RT-LAMP reactions include a reverse transcriptase for cDNA synthesis. Oligonucleotides act as primers for the reverse transcriptase, and additional oligonucleotides for the DNA polymerase are designed so that DNA products loop back at their ends and form a LAMP dumbbell structure (Notomi *et al.*, 2000). These, in turn, serve as self-priming templates for the DNA polymerase and produce concatemer. In RT-LAMP diagnostic tests, amplified DNA can be visualized and/or quantified by turbidity, color, or fluorescence. For example, pH indicator such as phenol red has been used as an indicator to detect DNA product. As the reaction proceeds, the pH is lowered, resulting in a visible color change from red to yellow, making it an appealing assay for point-of-care diagnosis. The drawbacks to LAMP are the challenges of optimizing primers and reaction conditions, as well as its potential high failure rate due to genetic sequence variants of SARS-CoV-2. Multiple SARS-CoV-2 RT-LAMP systems have been reported (Dao Thi *et al.*, 2020; Dudley *et al.*, 2020; Mautner *et al.*, 2020; Rabe and Cepko, 2020), and some have been commercialized.

4.2.3. *CRISPR-based detection*

A rapid lateral flow-based assay, SARS-CoV-2 DNA Endonuclease-Targeted CRISPR Trans Reporter (DETECTR) for detection of SARS-CoV-2, has been developed which has comparable sensitivity to the US CDC SARS-CoV-2 RT-PCR assay and can be run in 30–40 minutes (Broughton *et al.*, 2020). DETECTR combines RT-LAMP, CRISPR-Cas12a trans-cleavage assay, and a readout on a lateral flow strip. Briefly, input viral RNAs are reversed-transcribed and amplified by RT-LAMP. When Cas12a-cRNA base-pairs with targeted dsDNA of interest, the DNase activity of Cas12a is activated, and surrounding trans-ssDNA including ssDNA-fluorescently quenched probe (/56-FAM/TTATTATT/ 3bio/) are subsequently degraded. The SARS-CoV-2 DETECTR reagent kit by Mammoth Biosciences received emergency use authorization (EUA) by FDA (Food and Drug Administration, USA) in December 2020.

Specific High Sensitivity Enzymatic Reporter UnLOCKing (SHERLOCK) is a detection strategy that uses Cas13a ribonuclease for RNA sensing. Viral RNA targets are reverse-transcribed to cDNA, and isothermally amplified using RT-LAMP. The amplified products are tran-scribed back into RNA. Cas13a can be activated by complexing with an RNA guide sequence that binds with the amplified RNA product. The activated Cas13a will then cleave surrounding fluorophore-quencher probes to produce a fluorescent signal (Joung *et al.*, 2020; Patchsung *et al.*, 2020). The SHERLOCK CRISPR SARS-CoV-2 kit by Sherlock Biosciences has been granted EUA by FDA. Gootenberg *et al.* (2018) developed a multiplexed SHERLOCKv2 which is capable of detecting four targets in a single reaction. This multiplexing is achieved by using distinct cleavage preferences of different Cas13 enzymes on homopoly-mer reporters. Myhrvold *et al.* (2018) established a protocol that can pair with SHERLOCK — Heat Unextracted Diagnostic Samples to Obliterate Nucleases (HUDSON) — for viral detection directly from bodily fluids, thus obviating the need for RNA extraction. In addition, SHERLOCK and

HUDSON Integration to Navigate Epidemics (SHINE) was established to detect SARS-CoV-2 from unextracted nasal swabs and saliva (Arizti-Sanz *et al.*, 2020).

4.2.4. *Emergence of spike gene targeting failure*

The rapid rise of COVID-19 cases in South East England, UK during November 2020 resulted in enhanced epidemiological and virological investigations which led to the discovery of an increase in spike (S) gene RT-PCR dropout for SARS-CoV-2 (Leung *et al.*, 2021; Volz *et al.*, 2021). The ThermoFisher TaqPath system, which targets the S and nucleocapsid (N) genes, was used in the UK national testing system. Genome analysis by the UK COVID-19 Genomics Consortium identified a large proportion (>50%) of cases belonged to a new single phylogenetic cluster, referred as SARS-CoV-2 VUI 202012/01 in UK, which belongs to Nextstrain clade 20B, GISAID clade GR, lineage B.1.1.7. SARS-CoV-2 VUI 202012/01 consists of multiple spike mutations (deletion 69–70, deletion 144, N501Y, A570D, D614G, P681H, T716I, S982A, D1118H) resulting in S gene RT-PCR dropout (Leung *et al.*, 2021; Volz *et al.*, 2021). Washington *et al.* (2020) utilized the Helix COVID-19 test, which amplified three viral genes (Orf1ab, N and S) to examine the prevalence of S gene dropout in 2 million samples across USA.

4.3. Antigen Rapid Test (ART)

Point-of-care tests (POCT) have found solid foothold in this COVID-19 pandemic, where long turnaround time has plagued the centralized testing laboratories. As a POCT, lateral flow assays (LFA) are sandwich immunoassays that can detect the presence of a specific viral antigen (antigen rapid test or ART) or antibody of interest (serological LFA). ART tests are for current viral infection, while serological LFA tests are for past viral infection. The basic architecture of the LFA consists of a nitrocellulose matrix strip with immobilized capture agent at one end of the strip, and a conjugate pad containing dried particulate conjugate at the other end (Wong and Tse, 2009). Capillary forces draw the sample through the conjugate pad — where the antigen/antibody (target) present in the sample will bind to the conjugate — towards the immobilized capture agent. The capture agent then binds the antigen/antibody-conjugate, resulting in a colorimetric readout often without the need for a dedicated reader.

In SARS-CoV-2 ART, SARS-CoV-2 nucleocapsid protein (which is the most abundant protein) is usually the target. This test is inexpensive, fast (~15 minutes), and can mostly be used at the point of care, but is less sensitive (~0% to 94%) than nucleic acid test (Blairon *et al.*, 2021; Lambert-Niclot *et al.*, 2020; Mak *et al.*, 2021; Nagura-Ikeda *et al.*, 2020; Porte *et al.*, 2020; Scohy *et al.*, 2020). ARTs are currently authorized to be performed on nasopharyngeal or nasal swab specimens placed directly into the assay extraction buffer or reagent, and the signal is interpreted either by visual read or instrument read. By January 2021, a total of 14 ARTs had obtained EUA by FDA (2021b).

Deployment of SARS-CoV-2 ART is useful for (a) countries or remote areas where access to nucleic acid tests is challenging, and (b) screening testing in high-risk congregational settings, in which repeat testing can quickly identify persons with SARS-CoV-2 infection to prevent transmission. Although SARS-CoV-2 ART has consistently high specificity (>97%), the inconsistency in sensitivity makes data interpretation difficult. ARTs are most likely to perform well in patients with high viral loads (Ct value <25 or >106 genomic copies per mL) which usually appear in the pre-symptomatic (1–3 days before symptom onset) and early symptomatic phases of the illness (within the first 5–7 days of illness) (WHO, 2020a). US CDC has established the antigen test algorithm to interpret SARS-CoV-2 ART results (CDC, 2021a).

4.4. Antibody Detection

Serological testing or antibody detection can provide evidence of the body's immune response to a pathogen. There are many instances where serological testing should be performed in parallel with molecular testing, such as when an individual has cleared the genetic material of the pathogen from their body or when there is a need to investigate apparently unlinked cases retrospectively. In addition, serological testing performed at the population level can provide additional important information. Firstly, it can estimate the true prevalence of an outbreak which can then be used to determine the attack rate (reproduction number). Secondly, it can monitor the longevity of immunity post-infection or post-vaccination. Thirdly, it can map the geographical distribution of epidemics, and identify hotspots and populations at risk. Lastly, pan-species and pan-isotype antibody assays can be used for the surveillance of wildlife and farmed animals, and of residual serum banks that were collected pre-pandemic, in order to trace the origins of the outbreak, identify intermediate animal hosts, and detect spillover/spillback events.

In general, the levels of specific antibodies against SARS-CoV-2 increase over time from the onset of symptoms but will start to wane ~35–40 days after disease resolution. IgM levels can usually be detected earlier in the disease around 12 dpso, peak at 22–24 dpso, and in some patients IgM levels might drop around 35 dpso (Liu *et al.*, 2020; Long *et al.*, 2020; Iyer *et al.*, 2020; Tan *et al.*, 2020b; Whitman *et al.*, 2020). On the other hand, most patients seroconvert for SARS-CoV-2 specific IgG after a median of 19 dpso (Long *et al.*, 2020) and peak at ~30–40 dpso (Young *et al.*, 2021). The longevity of antibody responses varies dramatically depending on symptom severity and individual immune systems. It has recently been reported that IgG can last for at least 8 months pso (Dan *et al.*, 2021). Using a machine learning model based on data from a 9-month longitudinal study, it has been shown that neutralizing antibodies can last from days to decades (Chia *et al.*, 2021). The kinetics of antibody response to SARS-CoV-2 need to be considered when selecting the appropriate serological test to use. Most serological tests can accept plasma or serum interchangeably except for conventional virus neutralization tests or pseudovirus neutralization tests where high levels of anti-clotting agents in plasma samples may be cytotoxic to the cells used in the assay. Some platforms additionally claim that they can detect mucosal antibody responses from saliva samples (Isho *et al.*, 2020; MacMullan *et al.*, 2020) or antibodies in whole blood (in LFA).

There are many serological assays which *in vitro* diagnostics (IVD) companies and academic laboratories have developed for the detection of SARS-CoV-2 infection (https://www.finddx.org/covid-19/tests/). Serological tests can be broadly divided into Enzyme-Linked ImmunoSorbent Assays (ELISA), ChemiLuminescent Immunosorbent Assays (CLIA), Virus Neutralization Tests (VNT), and LFA. They differ in the type of readout (colorimetric, chemiluminescence, measurement of cell cytotoxicity) format (binding or inhibition/neutralization); antigen(s) used (e.g. spike protein and/or nucleocapsid protein); turnaround time (ranging from as short as 10 minutes to days); complexity (can be performed with minimal specialized equipment, containment and personnel — to requiring biosafety level 2 or 3 containment, specialized laboratory equipment and experienced personnel); sensitivity and specificity (Table 4.2). An important consideration in the selection of serology tests involves the choice of target antigen as different antigens provide different information.

Table 4.2. Summary of SARS-CoV-2 serological tests.

	ELISA	CLIA	VNT	LFA
Assay format	Indirect, capture (sandwich), competition formats.	Usually only indirect format where the antigens can be bound to solid phase or onto magnetic microparticles.	cVNT, pVNT, sVNT are all based on inhibition format.	Usually only capture (sandwich) format.
Antigens used	Nucleocapsid and/or Spike antigens.	Nucleocapsid and/or Spike antigens.	Whole virus for cVNT, Spike antigen for pVNT, RBD antigen for sVNT.	Nucleocapsid and/or Spike antigens.
Readout	Colorimetric.	Chemiluminescence.	cVNT — observation of cell death under microscope, pVNT — chemiluminescence or fluorescence, VNT — colorimetric.	Colorimetric.
Equipment and facility requirement	BSL2 and microplate reader with color quantification capability.	BSL2 and most CLIAs require company-specific *in vitro* diagnostics hardware.	cVNT — BSL3 and light microscope, pVNT and sVNT — BSL2 and microplate reader with color, chemiluminescence and fluorescence quantification capabilities.	BSL2 or may be performed without containment environment (i.e. pre-screening for admission to events with large crowds). No specialized equipment needed.

(Continued)

Table 4.2.   (*Continued*)

	ELISA	CLIA	VNT	LFA
Turnaround time	Approximately 4–6 hours.	Approximately 1–2 hours.	cVNT — 4–5 days, pVNT — 1–2 days, sVNT — 1–2 hours.	Approximately 10–30 minutes.
Scalability	High	High	cVNT — low, pVNT — moderate (dependent on cell culture), sVNT — high.	High
What it tells us	Amount of antibodies that bind to antigen-of-interest. May also be able to differentiate between antibody isotypes depending on assay format/ reagents. Generally used for seroprevalence studies. Quantitative readout.	Amount of antibodies that bind to antigen-of-interest. May also be able to differentiate between antibody isotypes depending on kit reagents. Generally used for seroprevalence studies. Quantitative readout.	Amount of antibodies that neutralize the virus entry into cells. Generally used in protective immunity studies.	Amount of antibodies that bind to antigen-of-interest. May also be able to differentiate between antibody isotypes depending on assay format. Generally used for point-of-care diagnostics. Qualitative readout.

Nucleocapsid-based assays are generally more sensitive in detection post infection, as there are many copies of the protein which induces a robust immune response. However, N-based assays may not be as specific as S-based assays, because the N proteins are more conserved among related members of the Coronavirus family. Furthermore, N-antibodies do not last as long as S-antibodies. On the other hand, S-based assays can have good correlation to neutralization and protection from infection. It is important to note that apart from whole inactivated vaccines, more currently approved vaccines are S-based. Hence, S-based antibody tests should be employed to measure vaccine response and longevity. It should be noted that no single test will be suitable for all purposes. The FDA website has a comprehensive list of all commercial assays with FDA certification for EUA (FDA, 2021a). Due to the rapidly evolving developmental landscape of SARS-CoV-2, some of the more notable commercial and non-commercial (academic) assays will be described in this chapter, but it is advisable to also refer to the FDA website for the latest and most comprehensive list.

4.4.1. *ELISA*

ELISA is a plate-based platform for the detection and quantification of soluble substances such as peptides, proteins, antibodies, and hormones. There are generally three different formats — indirect, sandwich and competitive ELISAs used for the detection of antibodies to SARS-CoV-2 (Figure 4.2).

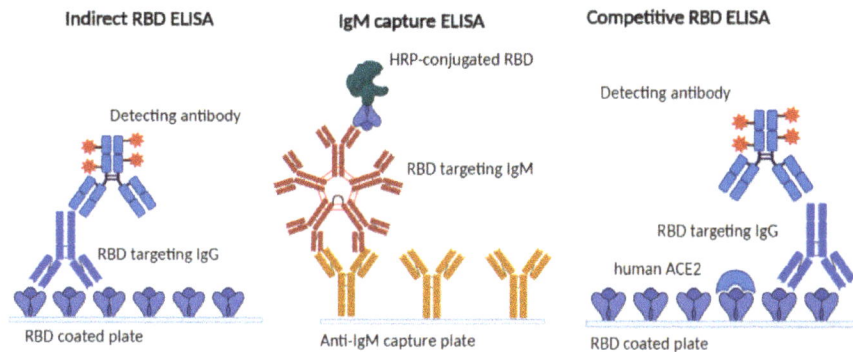

Figure 4.2. Different ELISA formats. Three major formats of ELISA (indirect RBD ELISA, IgM capture ELISA, and competitive RBD ELISA) used in detection of antibodies to SARS-CoV-2.

Indirect ELISA involves the immobilization of the SARS-CoV-2 antigen onto the solid surface of a high-binding microtiter plate by direct adsorption. Free binding sites are blocked with an inert protein buffer. The test sample, which is usually serum or plasma, is diluted with blocking buffer and added to the plate. After washing, the bound specific antibodies are then detected by a secondary antibody that is conjugated to a reporter enzyme such as the anti-human IgG-horseradish peroxidase (HRP) in the presence of the appropriate enzyme substrate (e.g. tetramethylbenzidine or TMB). Several indirect ELISA kits are commercially available with FDA EUA approval (Amanat *et al.*, 2020; Beavis *et al.*, 2020).

In capture (sandwich) ELISA, antibodies specific for certain isotypes of human immunoglobulins (e.g. IgM) are used to coat the microtiter wells. The test serum is next added, and all antibodies of that particular isotype are captured, regardless of their binding specificity. Finally, the antigen-of-interest conjugated to a reporter molecule is added to detect antibodies specific to the antigen. The capture ELISA methodology has been shown to be superior over the indirect ELISA format for the detection of IgM to SARS-CoV-2. This is due to the removal of large amounts of IgG in the serum that interferes with the accessibility of IgM to the antigen, thus improving the assay sensitivity (Chia *et al.*, 2020).

The competitive ELISA format is based on the introduction of an additional binding partner — apart from the S-antibodies in the test sample — that can specifically bind the S protein. During the infection process, the SARS-CoV-2 S protein binds the cell receptor ACE2 to gain cell entry via the specific interaction of the receptor-binding domain (RBD) of the S protein with ACE2. Antibodies that target S (especially RBD) can therefore compete with ACE2 for binding. The procedure for competitive ELISA is generally similar to indirect ELISA, whereby SARS-CoV-2 S (or RBD) is coated onto microtiter wells. A mixture of ACE2 protein and test serum is next added simultaneously to the microtiter well. As the amount of ACE2 protein is fixed in each assay, the level of specific antibodies to S (RBD) in the sample is proportional to colorimetric readout from the secondary anti-IgG-HRP (Isho *et al.*, 2020).

4.4.2. *CLIA and CMIA*

CLIAs are very similar to ELISAs in principle, except that these assays use luminogenic substrates to quantify the readout instead of colorimetric substrates. A subcategory of CLIAs is Chemiluminescent Microparticle Immunosorbent Assays (CMIAs), where the target antigen is not bound to a solid surface in plate wells but instead coated on paramagnetic microparticles. The major advantage for chemiluminescence readout is that the dynamic detection range increases several fold over colorimetric readouts, thus enhancing the sensitivity of the test. Most CLIA/CMIA platforms are developed by IVD companies as part of an enclosed, automated, high-throughput workflow/system for clinical diagnostic labs. The robotics infrastructure is already established in most diagnostic labs as part of the diagnostic capability for other viral infections, such as the quantification of hepatitis B antibodies. For SARS-CoV-2, IVD companies developed specific CLIAs or CMIAs by replacing test antigens (such as N, S, or RBD) using existing hardware. Having a fully enclosed robotics infrastructure means that samples potentially containing the SARS-CoV-2 virus (i.e. collected during the acute phase of disease) can be analyzed in a biosafety level 2 (BSL2) diagnostics lab, and many samples can be processed in a high-throughput manner as the entire workflow is automated.

The most widely adopted CLIA platforms are Abbott Alinity or Architect platforms which can measure either N- or S-specific antibodies, and Roche Elecsys platform which also has kits for measuring N- or S-specific total antibodies (Padoan *et al.*, 2020).

4.4.3. *Virus neutralization test*

VNTs are widely considered as the gold standard for specificity in determining antibody responses to SARS-CoV-2. Conventional VNTs (cVNTs) use live virus and therefore require a biosafety level 3 (BSL3) containment facility, and are conducted in two different formats. In the microneutralization assay, a pre-determined amount of virus is incubated with serially diluted test serum at 37°C for a fixed time. The mixture is next added onto susceptible cells (mostly VeroE6) in microtiter cell culture plates. The cells are incubated with the virus-serum mixture at 37°C for a fixed time before the virus-serum mixture is washed off, and exchanged for fresh culture media. The wells are examined 3–4 days later for cytopathic effects (CPE). The absence of CPE indicates the presence of neutralizing antibodies (NAbs). This method uses endpoint titer quantification, where the well containing the highest serum dilution without CPE is recorded. The second cVNT format is the Plaque Reduction Neutralization Test (PRNT). In PRNT, plaque medium (semi-solid agent such as agarose, methylcellulose, carboxymethylcellulose or Avicel) is added to the cell culture plate after the virus-serum mixture is washed off as for microneutralization test. After incubation for 3–4 days, the plates are then fixed with 4% formaldehyde for 30 minutes, and followed by staining with 0.2% crystal violet. Plaques are visualized by as clear areas surrounded by crystal violet-stained uninfected cells. A reduction in plaque formation with the dilution of serum is used to generate a dose-titration plot. PRNT provides a quantitative percentage inhibition unlike the microneutralization assay which only provides an endpoint titer.

To overcome the limited access to BSL3 containment facilities, multiple groups have developed SARS-CoV-2 S-pseudotyped Virus Neutralization Tests (pVNTs) which can be performed in BSL2 laboratories. The most frequently used pVNTs are based on either vesicular stomatitis virus (VSV) or replication-defective lentivirus backbone carrying a reporter gene such as fluorescence protein or luciferase genes. The ability of S-pseudotyped virus to infect ACE2-expressing cell lines, measured by fluorescence or relative light units, correlates with NAb levels in test sera. The pVNT protocol is similar to cVNT described above — VeroE6 or ACE2-expressing HEK293T cells have been used in pVNT assays. The assay time of 1–2 days for pVNT is shorter than cVNTs.

A third VNT format, a surrogate Virus Neutralization Test (sVNT), was developed based on biochemical simulation of virus-host interaction by establishing a RBD-ACE2 binding assay in an ELISA plate well (Figure 4.3) (Tan *et al.*, 2020a). This totally eliminates the use of any live materials (cells or viruses) or BSL3 containment, and reduces the assay time to 1 hour. Testing serum is pre-incubated with RBD-HRP conjugate for 30 minutes, before the mixture is added to a plate pre-coated with a recombinant soluble ACE2 protein. After incubation for 15 minutes, the unbound RBD-HRP is washed off, and color developed as for standard ELISA assay. The presence of NAbs which block the RBD-ACE2 interaction just as they will in cVNT or pVNT, will lead to lower levels of RBD-HRP, thus giving a weaker colorimetric signal. This assay has been commercialized under the tradename cPass™ by GenScript Biotech, and was the first FDA-approved test to determine NAbs against SARS-CoV-2 (https://www.fda.gov/media/143583/download). The sVNT assay has two

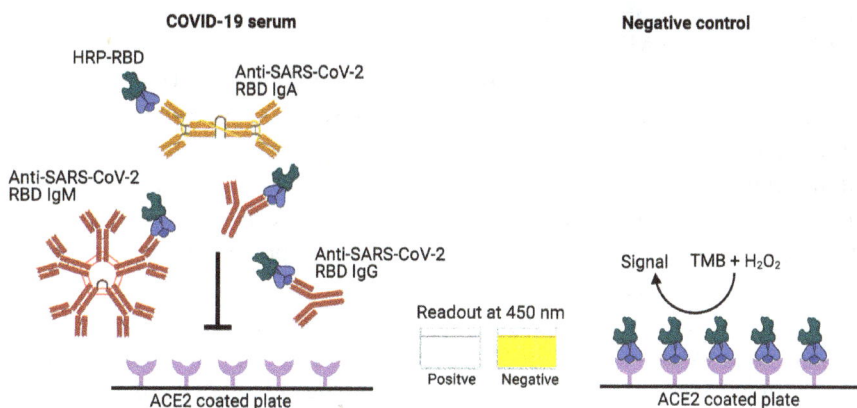

Figure 4.3. Principle of surrogate virus neutralization test (sVNT). Anti-SARS-CoV-2 neutralizing antibodies (Nabs) block HRP-conjugated RBD protein from binding to the hACE2 protein pre-coated on an ELISA plate (on the left), hence reducing the final colorimetric reading. In the absence of NAbs (on the right), the full color change is achieved upon the addition of substrate. The assay detects all RBD-targeting NAbs in a manner independent of antibody isotype (IgG, IgM, IgA, etc.) and host species (human, bat, pangolin, etc.).

key advantages over cVNT or pVNT. Firstly, the manufacture of proteins and kit reagents can be tightly controlled to reduce the inter-day and intra-assay variations, which was the main reason why sVNT is the only FDA-approved NAb test. Secondly, as the readout is unbiased and machine-based, it can be automated as for ELISA, CLIA or CMIA — hence, sVNT can be used for mass screening or testing such as for vaccine efficacy or immunity longevity studies.

4.4.4. *LFA*

Serological LFAs can also be deployed for widespread testing of past infection by SARS-CoV-2 in convalescent patients. The clinical sensitivities of evaluated LFAs can reach up to 100% 2 weeks and beyond after the onset of symptoms (Demey *et al.*, 2020; Whitman *et al.*, 2020). Some LFAs detect total immunoglobulins against SARS-CoV-2 (e.g. Wondfo® SARS-CoV-2 Antibody Test and BioMedomics COVID-19 IgM/IgG

Rapid Test), while others have separate readouts for IgM and IgG (e.g. bioMérieux VIDAS® SARS-CoV-2 Test, Innovita 2019-nCoV Ab Test, and VivaDiag™ SARS-CoV-2 Ag Rapid Test).

The key advantage of LFAs lies in its simplicity. Inexperienced operators in low-resource settings can perform these tests, and obtain interpretable results within 10–30 minutes. The use of capillary action and qualitative colorimetric results eliminate the need for any fluidic equipment or reader system. Reagents coated on the test strip are dried and stored at room temperature, removing the need for dedicated cold chain storage devices. The sample volume required is low (10–20 μL) and is easily obtainable from a finger prick. However, there are multiple hurdles against widespread use of lateral flow tests. Inter-operator variation in assessing colorimetric readouts due to the inherent lack of objective readouts is well-known. The identities of capture antigens coated on the test strip are often protected by the manufacturer as proprietary information and are not readily available. Cross-reactivity against closely related pathogens in LFAs may not be robustly tested. The qualitative nature of the LFAs means that it cannot differentiate high and low titers in convalescent plasma — thus, LFAs cannot be used in certain applications, e.g. to select high-titer plasma for treatment of severe COVID-19 patients.

4.5. T-cell Immunity Assays

T-cells are critical for control and clearance of SARS-CoV-2, and hence reduce disease severity. Early T-cell activation leads to lower viral loads — resulting in earlier disease resolution, and preventing a long disease course where severe COVID-19 complications may manifest (Karlsson *et al.*, 2020). Current literature suggests that male gender, elderly persons, and presence of co-morbidities are risk factors for severe COVID-19 disease — most of these risk factors are directly related to dysfunctional or weaker cellular immune responses. For instance, females appear to mount a stronger T-cell response and in turn experience milder disease (Takahashi *et al.*, 2020), whereas disruption of T-cell and B-cell coordination has been implicated in elderly patients with severe COVID-19 (Rydyznski Moderbacher *et al.*, 2020). A strong T-cell response stems from induction by type I interferons (IFN-I) secreted by innate cells as they initiate antiviral defenses (Murphy and Weaver, 2017). Inborn errors of immunity and auto-antibodies against IFN-I are more commonly detected in severe COVID-19 (Bastard *et al.*, 2020).

T-cell assays usually involve the addition of peripheral blood mononuclear cells (PBMCs) to ELISpot plates coated with capture IFN-γ antibody, stimulating the PBMCs with SARS-CoV-2 peptides to promote IFN-γ secretion, followed by the addition of an anti-IFN-γ antibody conjugated to peroxidase enzyme. Spots can be visualized after the addition of compatible substrate and each spot represents an IFN-γ-secreting T-cell (Le Bert *et al.*, 2020).

Conventionally, T-cell assays are not used as detection or diagnostic tools for SARS-CoV-2 due to two main reasons. Firstly, as high as 20–50% of unexposed SARS-CoV-2 blood donors were found to have pre-existing T-cell immunity to SARS-CoV-2 (Doshi, 2020), possibly attributed to the high amino acid sequence similarity in a number of epitopes between SARS-CoV-2 and seasonal human Coronaviruses. Secondly, T-cell assays are more time-consuming and less suitable for standardization, thus rendering them less adaptable than serology to high-throughput and/or automated assay platforms. At the present time, there is no FDA-approved T-cell immunity test for SARS-CoV-2.

4.6. Other Less Traditional Detection Platforms

Besides the conventional methods of RT-PCR and serology for detecting COVID-19, other platforms have surfaced such as the detection of volatile organic compounds by trained dogs as a surrogate for SARS-CoV-2 infection, and mass spectrometry (MS)-based system with targeted proteomics assay for SARS-CoV-2 nucleoprotein peptides (Table 4.3).

4.6.1. *Dog nose*

In several studies, dogs have been shown to possess an uncanny ability to detect volatile organic compounds unique to different infectious and non-infectious diseases ranging from malaria (Guest *et al.*, 2019) and *Clostridium* infection (Bomers *et al.*, 2014) to colon cancer (Sonoda *et al.*, 2011). Jendrny *et al.* (2020) have shown that trained dogs could also be used for identifying COVID-19 patients, with sensitivity and specificity up to 82.6% and 96.3%, respectively (Jendrny *et al.*, 2020). A similar study showed success rates ranging from 76% to 100% of identifying sweat samples of COVID-19 patients by trained dogs (Grandjean *et al.*, 2020). However, these "proof-of-concept" studies suffer from several

Table 4.3. Summary of other SARS-CoV-2 detection platforms.

Method	Sample Type	Detection Principle	Status/Comment	Limitation	Reference
Graphene-based field-effect transistor (FET) biosensor	Nasal swab	Antibodies against SARS-CoV-2 immobilized on 2D surface of graphene; antigen–antibody binding induces electrical signals read by semiconductor analyzer	Limit of detection down to 242 copies/mL	Sensitivity and specificity not shown	Seo *et al.* (2020)
Dual functional plasmonic photothermal biosensor	Nucleic acid	Complementary nucleic acid strand immobilized on functionalized gold nano-islands binds SARS-CoV-2 RNA sequence; resulting localized surface plasmon resonance measured with spectrophotometer	Tested only on synthetic SARS-CoV-2 RNA strain; limit of detection down to 2.26×10^4 copies	Sensitivity and specificity not shown	Qiu *et al.* (2020)
Trained dogs	Sweat-soaked fabric	Unique volatile organic compound signature emitted from COVID-19 positive patients recognized by trained dogs	Sensitivity and specificity up to 82.6% and 96.3% in one study	Inherent variation in detection accuracy between dogs	Grandjean *et al.* (2020); Jendrny *et al.* (2020)
Mass spectrometry	Nasal swab	Machine learning (ML) algorithm trained with mass spectra from COVID-19 positive swabs	Selected ML model has accuracy up to 93.9%	Viral load decreases over time post-symptom onset	Cardozo *et al.* (2020); Nachtigall *et al.* (2020)
Photonic ring resonance	Whole blood, plasma or serum	Antibodies against SARS-CoV-2 immobilized on silicon-based photonic ring resonator; antigen–antibody binding shifts wavelength of light trapped by resonator	Up to 96.1% sensitivity at 15 days post-symptom onset; FDA EUA	Based on antibody titer, not suitable for early diagnosis	Genalyte (2020)
Multi-analyte profiling (xMAP)	Plasma or serum	Antigen coated on identifiable microsphere binds antibody, secondary antibody labeling detected by microfluidic and optic setup	Up to 98.1% sensitivity at 14 days post-symptom onset; FDA EUA	Based on antibody titer, not suitable for early diagnosis	Dobaño *et al.* (2021); Luminex (2020)

limitations in the authors' claims. Firstly, these studies did not test analytical specificity, i.e. the ability of the trained dogs to differentiate between infections from other respiratory viruses from those of SARS-CoV-2. Secondly, the sensitivities of different dogs within the same study varied widely, raising doubts as to whether sufficient dogs can be trained to scale up for widespread deployment. Many other issues have to be addressed before trained dogs can gain enough credibility for detection of COVID-19 cases in airports, hospitals and other settings (Jendrny *et al.*, 2020).

4.6.2. *Mass spectrometry*

MS has been widely used in clinical microbiology for the identification of bacterial and fungal species (Kostrzewa, 2018), and even antibiotic resistance (Horseman *et al.*, 2020). MS equipment commonly found in clinical laboratories can be utilized for the identification of SARS-CoV-2 in patient samples. In one study, mass spectra of clinical nasal swab samples that were tested by RT-PCR for SARS-CoV-2, were obtained using the matrix-assisted laser desorption/ionization mass spectrometry or MALDI-MS (Nachtigall *et al.*, 2020). Machine learning (ML) algorithms were then used to select characteristic peaks unique to SARS-CoV-2 in these spectra. The selected ML model yielded an accuracy of up to 93.9% in detecting SARS-CoV-2 in nasal swab samples. Cardozo *et al.* (2020) employed another variation of MS, turbulent flow chromatography coupled to tandem mass spectrometry (TFC-MS/MS), to detect SARS-CoV-2 in respiratory tract samples with sensitivity and specificity up to 84% and 97 %, respectively. These studies did not stratify the detection capability of MS based on the days post-symptom onset (Cardozo *et al.*, 2020; Nachtigall *et al.*, 2020; Rocca *et al.*, 2020). Since RT-PCR and MS are designed to detect the presence of SARS-CoV-2 in nasal swabs, both techniques would suffer the same limitation with regards to the limit of detection as the viral load decreases over time post-symptom onset.

4.6.3. *Field-effect transistor*

Another interesting diagnostic method makes use of field-effect transistor (FET) to detect the presence of viral antigen in the transport medium used for nasal swabs (Seo *et al.*, 2020). Briefly, SARS-CoV-2 spike antibody is immobilized on the 2D surface of graphene-based FET. Antigen–Antibody binding induces a change in the conductivity of the FET, which generates an electrical signal. FET boasts an impressive limit of detection of 242 copies/mL (based on RT-PCR quantification), which is comparable to RT-PCR (CDC, 2020a).

4.6.4. *Multiplex assay systems*

A major drawback of ELISA or lateral flow tests in serological testing is the lack of multiplexing in detecting both IgG and IgM against various viral proteins (e.g. nucleocapsid, envelope and spike proteins). Two technologies overcame this disadvantage, and have acquired EUA by the US FDA for use in the COVID-19 pandemic. The first technology makes use of photonic ring resonance phenomena that trap specific wavelengths of light within a circular waveguide (Genalyte, 2020). Antigens bound to the silicon-based photonic ring bind the antibodies present in the sample, and this antigen–antibody interaction changes the wavelength of light trapped in the photonic ring (Mudumba *et al.*, 2017). The presence of the binding activity can then be measured by the shift in the negative peak of the light spectrum that eventually leaves the optical path.

Luminex also developed a multiplex immunoassay for SARS-CoV-2 based on its proprietary Multi-Analyte Profiling (xMAP) technology (Luminex, 2020). Briefly, antigens are coated onto identifiable microspheres and incubated with the sample. After secondary binding with fluorophore-labeled anti-IgG to the microspheres, the latter are passed through a microfluidic setup for the detection of the antibodies and the identification of the unique microspheres. Multiplex immunoassay allows for higher serological throughput and provides a more comprehensive view of the immunogenicity of the virus. The immunoassay is also easily adaptable to include other antigens of interest for a wider panel, and to test specificity of the assay against other respiratory viruses (Dobaño *et al.*, 2021). However, these technologies require dedicated readers (Maverick™ Diagnostic System and MAGPIX® System) that do not have other utilities unlike a thermocycler used for RT-PCR or a plate reader for ELISA.

4.7. Future Challenges and Directions

Since the first report of COVID-19 cases in late 2019, many questions still remain. The two major ones are: (a) Where was SARS-CoV-2 from? and

(b) How can we exit the COVID-19 pandemic eventually? Diagnostic and detection methods described in this chapter can help to address both questions.

In searching for the virus origin, serology has played a pivotal role in identifying the origin of many other bat-borne viruses including Hendra (Young *et al.*, 1996), Nipah (Yob *et al.*, 2001), and SARS-CoV (Li *et al.*, 2005). In the past, serological investigations were facilitated by ELISA, followed by confirmation with other tests including VNT. For SARS-CoV-2, it has been demonstrated that sVNT can combine screening and confirmation into a single test (Wacharapluesadee *et al.*, 2021). The challenge now is to apply the sVNT/cPass assay to as many archived samples (both human and animal origin) in as many geographic locations as possible since the virus can theoretically originate from any part of the world where *Rhinolophus* bats are present, i.e. Australia, Asia, Middle East, Africa, and Europe (Wacharapluesadee *et al.*, 2021).

For exit strategy from the COVID-19 pandemic, it seems unlikely for the world to eradicate the virus, and global herd immunity is thus needed before transmission can be brought under control. With the current speed of vaccine production and administration, it will take years before that can be achieved. It is therefore necessary to consider other exit strategies, at least for certain populations, nations and/or regions. The "immunity passport" (Brown *et al.*, 2021) is the most likely and feasible option. However, with the efficacy varying among different vaccines and the longevity of immunity unclear for the vaccines, relying on vaccine certificates alone may not be sufficient to grant immunity passports. It is also worth noting that binding antibodies, even those targeting RBD, may not correlate with neutralizing antibodies (Muecksch *et al.*, 2021; Tan *et al.*, 2020a). It is therefore important to determine the actual level of neutralizing antibodies, and adopt internationally standardized neutralizing antibody measurement. In this context, it is important to note that WHO and the National Institute of Biological Standards and Control (NIBSC) have established a panel of standard sera with pre-defined international units (IU) of SARS-CoV-2 neutralizing antibodies (WHO, 2020c). All future serological testing should strive to report testing results in IU.

Lastly, the emergence of viral VOCs presents further challenges to develop robust detection methods, both molecular and serological. This will be important not only for epidemiological studies, but also for vaccine efficacy monitoring and for guiding exit strategies. There is already evidence that the current vaccines and serological tests may not be optimal for applications to the Beta (B.1.351) and Delta (B.1.617.2) VOCs

(Chen *et al.*, 2021; Diamond *et al.*, 2021; Mahase, 2021; Planas *et al.*, 2021; Tada *et al.*, 2021). Ongoing and future efforts to develop next-generation vaccines and tests are therefore necessary to address these challenges and new viral variants.

Acknowledgments

COVID-19 and Coronavirus research in our group is supported by grants from the National Medical Research Council (STPRG-FY19-001 and COVID19RF-003), and National Research Foundation (NRF2016NRF-NSFC002-013), Singapore.

Declaration of Interests

Lin-Fa Wang, Chee Wah Tan and Wan Ni Chia are co-inventors on a patent application for the sVNT technology, and a commercial kit, cPass™, is being marketed by GenScript Biotech.

References

Amanat F *et al.* A serological assay to detect SARS-CoV-2 seroconversion in humans. *Nat Med* 2020; 26:1033–1036.

Arizti-Sanz J *et al.* Streamlined inactivation, amplification, and Cas13-based detection of SARS-CoV-2. *Nat Commun* 2020; 11:5921.

Bastard P *et al.* Autoantibodies against type I IFNs in patients with life-threatening COVID-19. *Science* 2020; 370:eabd4585.

Bastos ML *et al.* The sensitivity and costs of testing for SARS-CoV-2 Infection with saliva versus nasopharyngeal swabs: A systematic review and meta-analysis. *Ann Intern Med* 2021; 174:501–510.

Beavis KG *et al.* Evaluation of the EUROIMMUN anti-SARS-CoV-2 ELISA assay for detection of IgA and IgG antibodies. *J Clin Virol* 2020; 129:104468.

Blairon L *et al.* Large-scale, molecular and serological SARS-CoV-2 screening of healthcare workers in a 4-site public hospital in Belgium after COVID-19 outbreak. *J Infect* 2021; 82:159–198.

Bomers MK *et al.* A detection dog to identify patients with *Clostridium difficile* infection during a hospital outbreak. *J Infect* 2014; 69:456–461.

Broughton JP *et al.* CRISPR-Cas12-based detection of SARS-CoV-2. *Nat Biotechnol* 2020; 38:870–874.

Brown RCH *et al*. The scientific and ethical feasibility of immunity passports. *Lancet Infect Dis* 2021; 21:e58–e63.

Cardozo KHM *et al*. Establishing a mass spectrometry-based system for rapid detection of SARS-CoV-2 in large clinical sample cohorts. *Nat Commun* 2020; 11:6201.

Carter LJ *et al*. Assay techniques and test development for COVID-19 diagnosis. *ACS Cent Sci* 2020; 6:591–605.

CDC (Centers for Disease Control and Prevention, USA), 2020a. CDC 2019-Novel Coronavirus (2019-nCov) Real-Time RT-PCR Diagnostic Panel. https://www.fda.gov/media/134922/download (accessed 19 January 2021).

CDC (Centers for Disease Control and Prevention, USA), 2020b. Research Use Only 2019-Novel Coronavirus (2019-nCoV) Real-time RT-PCR Primers and Probes. https://www.cdc.gov/coronavirus/2019-ncov/lab/rt-pcr-panel-primer-probes.html (accessed 6 June 2020).

CDC (Centers for Disease Control and Prevention, USA), 2021a. Interim Guidance for Antigen Testing for SARS-CoV-2. https://www.cdc.gov/coronavirus/2019-ncov/lab/resources/antigen-tests-guidelines.html (accessed 9 September 2021).

CDC (Centers for Disease Control and Prevention, USA), 2021b. Interim Guidelines for Collecting and Handling Clinical Specimens for COVID-19 Testing. https://www.cdc.gov/coronavirus/2019-ncov/lab/guidelines-clini-cal-specimens.html (accessed 31 October 2021).

Chen RE *et al*. Resistance of SARS-CoV-2 Variants to Neutralization by Monoclonal and Serum-derived Polyclonal Antibodies. *Nat Med* 2021; 27:717–726.

Chia WN *et al*. Serological differentiation between COVID-19 and SARS infections. *Emerg Microbes Infect* 2020; 9:1497–1505.

Chia WN *et al*. Dynamics of SARS-CoV-2 neutralising antibody responses and duration of immunity: A longitudinal study. *Lancet Microbe* 2021; 2:e240–e249.

China CDC (Chinese Center for Disease Control and Prevention), 2020. Specific primers and probes for detection of 2019 novel Coronavirus.

Chu DKW *et al*. Molecular diagnosis of a novel Coronavirus (2019-nCoV) causing an outbreak of pneumonia. *Clin Chem* 2020; 66:549–555.

Corman VM *et al*. Detection of 2019 novel Coronavirus (2019-nCoV) by real-time RT-PCR. *Euro Surveill* 2020; 25:2000045.

Dan JM *et al*. Immunological memory to SARS-CoV-2 assessed for up to 8 months after infection. *Science* 2021; 371:eabf4063.

Dao Thi VL *et al*. A colorimetric RT-LAMP assay and LAMP-sequencing for detecting SARS-CoV-2 RNA in clinical samples. *Sci Transl Med* 2020; 12:eabc7075.

Demey B *et al*. Dynamic profile for the detection of anti-SARS-CoV-2 antibodies using four immunochromatographic assays. *J Infect* 2020; 81:e6–e10.

Dobaño C *et al*. Highly sensitive and specific Multiplex antibody assays to quantify immunoglobulins M, A, and G against SARS-CoV-2 antigens. *J Clin Microbiol* 2021; 59:e01731–20.

Doshi P. COVID-19: Do many people have pre-existing immunity? *BMJ* 2020; 370:m3563.

Dudley DM *et al*. Optimizing direct RT-LAMP to detect transmissible SARS-CoV-2 from primary nasopharyngeal swab samples. *PLoS One* 2020; 15:e0244882.

Espy MJ *et al*. Real-time PCR in clinical microbiology: Applications for routine laboratory testing. *Clin Microbiol Rev* 2006; 19:165–256.

Etievant S *et al*. Performance assessment of SARS-CoV-2 PCR assays developed by WHO referral laboratories. *J Clin Med* 2020; 9:1871.

FDA (Food and Drug Administration, USA), 2021a. EUA Authorized Serology Test Performance. https://www.fda.gov/medical-devices/coronavirus-disease-2019-covid-19-emergency-use-authorizations-medical-devices/eua-authorized-serology-test-performance (accessed 28 February 2021).

FDA (Food and Drug Administration, USA), 2021b. *In Vitro* Diagnostics EUAs. https://www.fda.gov/medical-devices/coronavirus-disease-2019-covid-19-emergency-use-authorizations-medical-devices/in-vitro-diagnostics-euas (accessed 28 February 2021).

Genalyte, 2020. Maverick™ SARS-CoV-2 Multi-Antigen Serology Panel v2 0103ART-01. https://www.fda.gov/media/142915/download (accessed 19 January 2021).

Gootenberg JS *et al*. Multiplexed and portable nucleic acid detection platform with Cas13, Cas12a, and Csm6. *Science* 2018; 360:439–444.

Grandjean D *et al*. Can the detection dog alert on COVID-19 positive persons by sniffing axillary sweat samples? A proof-of-concept study. *PLoS One* 2020; 15:e0243122.

Guest C *et al*. Trained dogs identify people with malaria parasites by their odour. *Lancet Infect Dis* 2019; 19:578–580.

Horseman TS *et al*. Rapid qualitative antibiotic resistance characterization using VITEK MS. *Diagn Microbiol Infect Dis* 2020; 97:115093.

Institut Pasteur, 2020. Protocol: Real-time RT-PCR Assays for the Detection of SARS-CoV-2 (WHO). https://www.who.int/docs/default-source/coronaviruse/real-time-rt-pcr-assays-for-the-detection-of-sars-cov-2-institut-pasteur-paris.pdf (accessed 28 February 2021).

Isho B *et al*. Persistence of serum and saliva antibody responses to SARS-CoV-2 spike antigens in COVID-19 patients. *Sci Immunol* 2020; 5:eabe5511.

Iyer AS *et al*. Persistence and decay of human antibody responses to the receptor binding domain of SARS-CoV-2 spike protein in COVID-19 patients. *Sci Immunol* 2020; 5:eabe0367.

Jendrny P *et al.* Scent dog identification of samples from COVID-19 patients — A pilot study. *BMC Infect Dis* 2020; 20:536.

Joung J *et al.* Detection of SARS-CoV-2 with SHERLOCK One-Pot Testing. *N Engl J Med* 2020; 383:1492–1494.

Karlsson AC *et al.* The known unknowns of T cell immunity to COVID-19. *Sci Immunol* 2020; 5:eabe8063.

Kostrzewa M. Application of the MALDI Biotyper to clinical microbiology: Progress and potential. *Expert Rev Proteomics* 2018; 15:193–202.

Lambert-Niclot S *et al.* Evaluation of a rapid diagnostic assay for detection of SARS-CoV-2 antigen in nasopharyngeal swabs. *J Clin Microbiol* 2020; 58:e00977–20.

Le Bert N *et al.* SARS-CoV-2-specific T cell immunity in cases of COVID-19 and SARS, and uninfected controls. *Nature* 2020; 584:457–462.

Leung K *et al.* Early transmissibility assessment of the N501Y mutant strains of SARS-CoV-2 in the United Kingdom, October to November 2020. *Euro Surveill* 2021; 26:2002106.

Li W *et al.* Bats are natural reservoirs of SARS-like Coronaviruses. *Science* 2005; 310:676–679.

Liu W *et al.* Evaluation of nucleocapsid and spike protein-based enzyme-linked immunosorbent assays for detecting antibodies against SARS-CoV-2. *J Clin Microbiol* 2020; 58:e00461–20.

Long QX *et al.* Antibody responses to SARS-CoV-2 in patients with COVID-19. *Nat Med* 2020; 26:845–848.

Luminex, 2020. xMAP® SARS-CoV-2 Multi-Antigen IgG Assay Package Insert. https://www.fda.gov/media/140256/download (accessed 19 January 2021).

Mackay IM *et al.* Real-time PCR in virology. *Nucleic Acids Res* 2002; 30:1292–1305.

MacMullan MA *et al.* ELISA detection of SARS-CoV-2 antibodies in saliva. *Sci Rep* 2020; 10:20818.

Mahase E. COVID-19: Novavax vaccine efficacy is 86% against UK variant and 60% against South African variant. *BMJ* 2021; 372:n296.

Mak GCK *et al.* Evaluation of rapid antigen detection kit from the WHO Emergency Use List for detecting SARS-CoV-2. *J Clin Virol* 2021; 134:104712.

Mautner L *et al.* Rapid point-of-care detection of SARS-CoV-2 using reverse transcription loop-mediated isothermal amplification (RT-LAMP). *Virol J* 2020; 17:160.

Ministry of Public Health, Thailand, 2020. Diagnostic Detection of Novel Coronavirus 2019 by Real-time RT-PCR. https://www.who.int/docs/default-source/coronaviruse/conventional-rt-pcr-followed-by-sequencing-for-detection-of-ncov-rirl-nat-inst-health-t.pdf (accessed 28 February 2021).

Mudumba S *et al*. Photonic ring resonance is a versatile platform for performing multiplex immunoassays in real time. *J Immunol Methods* 2017; 448:34–43.

Muecksch F *et al*. Longitudinal serological analysis and neutralizing antibody levels in Coronavirus disease 2019 convalescent patients. *J Infect Dis* 2021; 223:389–398.

Murphy KM, Weaver C. *Janeway's Immunobiology* (9th edn.). WW Norton, New York, 2017.

Myhrvold C *et al*. Field-deployable viral diagnostics using CRISPR-Cas13. *Science* 2018; 360:444–448.

Nachtigall FM *et al*. Detection of SARS-CoV-2 in nasal swabs using MALDI-MS. *Nat Biotechnol* 2020; 38:1168–1173.

Nagura-Ikeda M *et al*. Clinical evaluation of self-collected saliva by quantitative reverse transcription-PCR (RT-qPCR), direct RT-qPCR, reverse transcription-loop-mediated isothermal amplification, and a rapid antigen test to diagnose COVID-19. *J Clin Microbiol* 2020; 58:e01438–20.

Notomi T *et al*. Loop-mediated isothermal amplification of DNA. *Nucleic Acids Res* 2000; 28:E63.

Padoan A *et al*. Analytical and clinical performances of five immunoassays for the detection of SARS-CoV-2 antibodies in comparison with neutralization activity. *EBioMedicine* 2020; 62:103101.

Pan Y *et al*. Viral load of SARS-CoV-2 in clinical samples. *Lancet Infect Dis* 2020; 20:411–412.

Patchsung M *et al*. Clinical validation of a Cas13-based assay for the detection of SARS-CoV-2 RNA. *Nat Biomed Eng* 2020; 4:1140–1149.

Planas D *et al*. Reduced sensitivity of SARS-CoV-2 variant delta to antibody neutralization. *Nature* 2021; 596:276–280.

Porte L *et al*. Evaluation of a novel antigen-based rapid detection test for the diagnosis of SARS-CoV-2 in respiratory samples. *Int J Infect Dis* 2020; 99:328–333.

Qiu G *et al*. Dual-functional plasmonic photothermal biosensors for highly accurate severe acute respiratory syndrome Coronavirus 2 detection. *ACS Nano* 2020; 14:5268–5277.

Rabe BA, Cepko C. SARS-CoV-2 detection using isothermal amplification and a rapid, inexpensive protocol for sample inactivation and purification. *Proc Natl Acad Sci USA* 2020; 117:24450–24458.

Rocca MF *et al*. A combined approach of MALDI-TOF mass spectrometry and multivariate analysis as a potential tool for the detection of SARS-CoV-2 virus in nasopharyngeal swabs. *J Virol Methods* 2020; 286:113991.

Rydyznski Moderbacher C *et al*. Antigen-specific adaptive immunity to SARS-CoV-2 in acute COVID-19 and associations with age and disease severity. *Cell* 2020; 183:996–1012.e19.

Scohy A *et al*. Low performance of rapid antigen detection test as frontline testing for COVID-19 diagnosis. *J Clin Virol* 2020; 129:104455.

Seo G *et al*. Rapid detection of COVID-19 causative virus (SARS-CoV-2) in human nasopharyngeal swab specimens using field-effect transistor-based biosensor. *ACS Nano* 2020; 14:5135–5142.

Sethuraman N *et al*. Interpreting diagnostic tests for SARS-CoV-2. *JAMA* 2020; 323:2249–2251.

Shirato K *et al*. Development of genetic diagnostic methods for detection for novel Coronavirus 2019(nCoV-2019) in Japan. *Jpn J Infect Dis* 2020; 73:304–307.

Sonoda H *et al*. Colorectal cancer screening with odour material by canine scent detection. *Gut* 2011; 60:814–819.

Tada T *et al*. Convalescent-phase sera and vaccine-elicited antibodies largely maintain neutralizing titer against global SARS-CoV-2 variant spikes. *mBio* 2021; 12:e0069621.

Takahashi T *et al*. Sex differences in immune responses that underlie COVID-19 disease outcomes. *Nature* 2020; 588:315–320.

Tan CW *et al*. A SARS-CoV-2 surrogate virus neutralization test based on antibody-mediated blockage of ACE2-spike protein-protein interaction. *Nat Biotechnol* 2020a; 38:1073–1078.

Tan W *et al*. Viral kinetics and antibody responses in patients with COVID-19. *medRxiv* 2020b; 2020.03.24.20042382.

Vogels CBF *et al*. Analytical sensitivity and efficiency comparisons of SARS-CoV-2 RT-qPCR primer-probe sets. *Nat Microbiol* 2020; 5:1299–1305.

Volz E *et al*. Assessing transmissibility of SARS-CoV-2 lineage B.1.1.7 in England. *Nature* 2021; 593:266–269.

Wacharapluesadee S *et al*. Evidence for SARS-CoV-2 related Coronaviruses circulating in bats and pangolins in Southeast Asia. *Nat Commun* 2021; 12:972.

Wang C *et al*. A novel Coronavirus outbreak of global health concern. *Lancet* 2020a; 395:470–473.

Wang LF *et al*. From Hendra to Wuhan: What has been learned in responding to emerging zoonotic viruses. *Lancet* 2020b; 395:e33–e34.

Wang W *et al*. Detection of SARS-CoV-2 in different types of clinical specimens. *JAMA* 2020c; 323:1843–1844.

Washington NL *et al*. S gene dropout patterns in SARS-CoV-2 tests suggest spread of the H69del/V70del mutation in the US. *medRxiv* 2020; 2020.12.24.20248814.

Whitman JD *et al*. Evaluation of SARS-CoV-2 serology assays reveals a range of test performance. *Nat Biotechnol* 2020; 38:1174–1183.

WHO (World Health Organization), 2020a. Antigen-detection in the Diagnosis of SARS-CoV-2 Infection Using Rapid Immunoassays. https://apps.who.int/iris/bitstream/handle/10665/334253/WHO-2019-nCoV-Antigen_Detection-2020.1-eng.pdf (accessed 28 Feburary 2021).

WHO (World Health Organization), 2020b. COVID-19 Status Report. https://www.who.int/emergencies/diseases/novel-coronavirus-2019/situation-reports (accessed 28 Feburary 2021).

WHO (World Health Organization), 2020c. Establishment of the WHO International Standard and Reference Panel for Anti-SARS-CoV-2 Antibody. https://www.who.int/publications/m/item/WHO-BS-2020.2403 (accessed 28 Feburary 2021).

Wong R, Tse H. *Lateral Flow Immunoassay*. Humana Press, Totowa, 2009.

Yob JM *et al*. Nipah virus infection in bats (order Chiroptera) in peninsular Malaysia. *Emerg Infect Dis* 2001; 7:439–441.

Young BE *et al*. Viral dynamics and immune correlates of Coronavirus disease 2019 (COVID-19) severity. *Clin Infect Dis* 2021; 73:e2932–e2942.

Young PL *et al*. Serologic evidence for the presence in Pteropus bats of a paramyxovirus related to equine morbillivirus. *Emerg Infect Dis* 1996; 2:239–240.

Zhou P *et al*. A pneumonia outbreak associated with a new Coronavirus of probable bat origin. *Nature* 2020; 579:270–273.

Chapter 5

Aerosol Transmission and Control of SARS-CoV-2

Julian W. Tang[*,‡] **and Nan Zhang**[†,¶]

Department of Respiratory Sciences, University of Leicester, Leicester, United Kingdom

†*Beijing Key Laboratory of Green Built Environment and Energy Efficient Technology, Beijing University of Technology, Beijing, China*

‡*julian.tang@uhl-tr.nhs.uk*
‡*jwtang49@hotmail.com*
¶*zhangn@bjut.edu.cn*

Abstract

One fundamental question about any novel pathogen is: how does it transmit? Answering this question will help to protect ourselves from the agent, at least until effective vaccines and antiviral therapies can be developed, especially if it is an agent of moderate to high lethality. Initially, at the start of the Coronavirus disease 2019 (COVID-19) pandemic, more emphasis was placed on handwashing rather than on droplet and aerosol transmission. Although severe acute respiratory syndrome Coronavirus 2 (SARS-CoV-2)-infected secretions such as saliva can spread the virus to hands, it became increasing evident that the virus mostly transmitted through close contact (though not necessarily touching), whilst people were breathing, talking, laughing, singing, coughing and sneezing near one another. During such respiratory activities, droplets and aerosols are produced together, and the amount of transmission due to these different-sized liquid particles will likely vary between individuals at different stages of their infection and illness. This question became even more complex as it emerged that viral transmission can occur for several days before symptom onset, and that asymptomatic cases can also shed just as much virus and potentially transmit it just as well as symptomatic cases. This chapter summarizes our understanding of how SARS-CoV-2 transmits and the infection control precautions to reduce this.

Keywords: COVID-19; SARS-CoV-2; transmission; epidemiology; infection control; outbreak; contact; fomite; droplet; aerosol; prevention; personal protective equipment; social distancing; handwashing; mask; gloves; gown; face shield visor; breathing; talking; laughing; singing; coughing; sneezing

5.1. Introduction: How Did It Start?

Reports from China during December 2019 to January 2020 described an outbreak of a novel Coronavirus causing respiratory illness concentrated in the city of Wuhan (Tang *et al.*, 2020). This appeared to be spreading amongst customers and workers with some efficiency, and soon spread beyond China to other countries (Wu *et al.*, 2020), triggering the declaration of a Public Health Emergency of International Concern (PHEIC) by the World Health Organization (WHO) soon afterwards on 30 January 2020 (WHO, 2020a). Within a few weeks of this, and due to the increasing spread of the disease to other countries, the WHO declared a pandemic, renaming the virus as severe acute respiratory syndrome Coronavirus 2 (SARS-CoV-2) and the disease that it causes as Coronavirus disease 2019 (COVID-19) (WHO, 2020a).

Other countries that reported imported cases of COVID-19 very early in January 2020 included France, Italy, Spain, UK, USA, Canada, and Australia (Caly *et al.*, 2020; Holshue *et al.*, 2020; Lillie *et al.*, 2020; Silverstein *et al.*, 2020; Spiteri *et al.*, 2020).

Although most of the national guidance of these affected countries initially emphasized hand-washing without masking to control this virus, it became apparent very quickly that the virus was spreading further and more widely than if contact transmission alone was responsible for most of the transmission. Soon after, the wearing of masks was initially recommended and then mandated, first in hospitals and other clinical areas, and then on public transport and in shared public areas such as shops, hairdressers, cinemas (Han *et al.*, 2020). Masking in bars and restaurants was not possible with eating and drinking, but engineering regulations were also updated to recommend more ventilation in indoor areas to reduce aerosol transmission of SARS-CoV-2 (ASHRAE, 2020; REHVA, 2020a, 2020b).

Despite this, there has been ongoing debate about the "main" mode of transmission of SARS-CoV-2, i.e. whether via contact or fomite, droplet or aerosol routes, and in what situations which of these routes is more important. This is a very difficult question to answer for every situation, though increasingly, opinions and evidence are against contact or fomite routes being the main way that this virus transmits (CDC, 2020a; UK Government, 2020; UK SAGE, 2020). In fact, a global analysis ranking the effectiveness of different infection control measures ranked various social distancing measures and use of mask and other personal protective equipment (PPE) the most effective, and environmental cleaning, enhanced testing, tracking and tracing the least effective (Haug *et al.*, 2020).

5.2. Useful Selected Facts About SARS-CoV-2 and COVID-19

Taxonomy: Strain: Severe acute respiratory syndrome coronavirus 2;
Species: Severe acute respiratory syndrome coronavirus;
Subgenus: *Sarbecovirus*;
Genus: *Betacoronavirus*;
Family: *Coronaviridae* (ICTV, 2020).

Structure: Enveloped, single-stranded, positive-sense RNA genome (size ~30,000 bases).

Reservoir: Bats, pangolins, others? (Boni *et al.*, 2020; Lam *et al.*, 2020).

Incubation period (humans): 5–6 days (range 2–14 days) (CDC, 2020b; Cevik *et al.*, 2020).

Cellular receptor: Angiotensin-converting enzyme 2 (ACE2) with priming by TMPRSS2 (transmembrane protease serine 2) (Lukassen *et al.*, 2020). ACE2 distribution is ubiquitous in cardiovascular, respiratory, gastrointestinal and urinary systems; but most concentrated in the small intestine, kidneys and heart; moderately concentrated in the lungs, colon, liver and bladder; and least concentrated in the spleen, blood (including bone marrow and blood vessels), brain and muscle (Dai *et al.*, 2020; Li *et al.*, 2020).

Infectious dose (*humans*): Unknown, but likely to differ between individuals. One estimate for SARS-CoV based on animal studies is about 200–300 viruses (similar to estimates for influenza) (Fang *et al.*, 2021), but this may be different for SARS-CoV-2.

5.3. Different Routes of SARS-CoV-2 Transmission and the Evidence for Them

There is a general consensus that SARS-CoV-2 can transmit by direct contact (via contaminated hands to eyes, nose, mouth) or indirect contact (via contaminated fomites to hands to eyes, nose, mouth), droplets (over short-range, conversational distances, <1 m), and aerosols (over both short-range conversational distance and longer range airborne spread >2 m). The numbers and sizes of droplets and aerosols transported over these distances may vary between individuals, depending on whether they are talking, breathing, laughing, singing, coughing, or sneezing (Bourouiba *et al.*, 2020; Chen *et al.*, 2020; Gao *et al.*, 2021; Xie *et al.*, 2007), with aerosols assumed to move with (and therefore carry viruses) with the airstreams produced (Tang *et al.*, 2011, 2012, 2013). In laboratory studies, SARS-CoV-2 has been shown to survive for hours to days in aerosols and various surfaces (Chin *et al.*, 2020; van Doremalen *et al.*, 2020).

It is also understood is that the comparative importance and contribution of each of these transmission routes may differ in different situations (Chen *et al.*, 2020; Gao *et al.*, 2021).

Evidence for the transmission of a novel pathogen can take several forms: (a) the epidemiology of real-life outbreak studies — particularly at the beginning of an epidemic in a population, as this limits the number of alternative sources for the pathogen; (b) laboratory studies, usually with either human volunteers or suitable animal models, where contact, short-range and long-range droplet and aerosol transmission can be investigated; (c) mathematical modelling studies where different modes of transmission are inferred from epidemiological and laboratory input data

(Tang *et al.*, 2022). The scope, interpretation and overall quality of these SARS-CoV-2 studies has varied enormously.

5.4. Real-Life Examples of Likely Airborne Spread of SARS-CoV-2

Various examples have been published of SARS-CoV-2 spread in restaurants (Lu *et al.*, 2020), public transport (Shen *et al.*, 2020), choirs (Hamner *et al.*, 2020; Miller *et al.*, 2021), call-centers (Park *et al.*, 2020), and other recreational events (Qian *et al.*, 2021) — that strongly indicate a predominance of airborne transmission. This does not mean that contact, fomite or shorter-range droplet transmission does not occur or contribute — rather that most of the cases in these outbreaks were more likely acquired via inhalation of airborne virus in aerosols.

Indeed, the UK government advisory body (Scientific Advisory Group for Emergencies, SAGE) has also published a mini-review concluding that for respiratory viruses, the contact/fomite route appears to account for only about 20% of all transmission (UK SAGE, 2020), implying that the majority of transmission for such viruses is via droplets and aerosols.

Another independent, global analysis also concluded that environmental cleaning (of surfaces) was also almost completely ineffective in controlling the spread of the virus (Haug *et al.*, 2020). This fits with the evidence that is accumulating so far with SARS-CoV-2. The WHO has admitted that there is no evidence of contact/fomite transmission for SARS-CoV-2 (WHO, 2020b), but stated that they believe this transmission route exists, based on the behavior of other respiratory viruses. However, if this is true for SAR-CoV-2, this would only account for up to 20% of all transmission — as the UK SAGE review found (UK SAGE, 2020).

There is also ample evidence that there are naturally occurring antiviral and antibacterial components in human saliva (e.g. salivary glycoprotein gp340, human defensins) (Malamud *et al.*, 2011; White *et al.*, 2009); sweat (e.g. human cathelicidin, human β-defensins) (Chessa *et al.*, 2020); and tears (e.g. rapidly appearing antiviral antibodies, lactoferrin, lysozymes) (Berlutti *et al.*, 2011; Hanstock *et al.*, 2019; Langford *et al.*, 1979) — which all make direct inoculation of live virus through casual contact relatively difficult to cause infection.

For droplets and aerosols, it is difficult to separate the two, as they are both produced by human respiratory activities (breathing, talking,

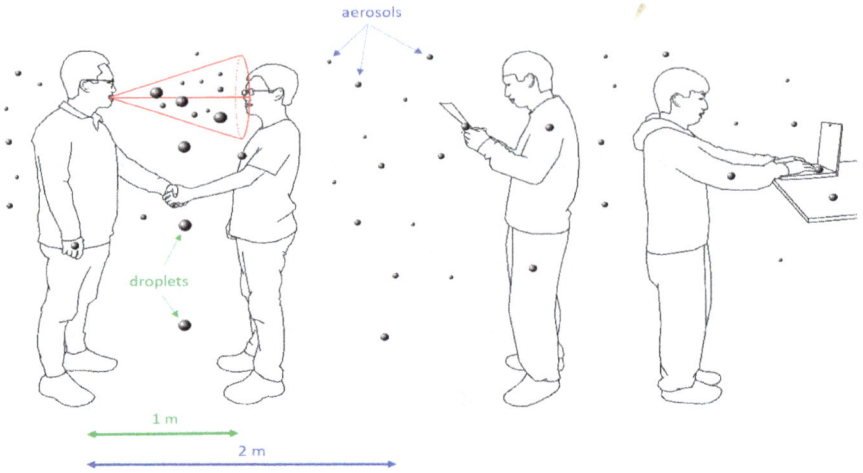

Figure 5.1. Droplets and aerosols distinguished by relative sizes and/or distances traveled.

laughing, singing, coughing, sneezing, etc.), and they exist on the same sliding scale of particle size and behavior (Asadi *et al.*, 2019; Miller *et al.*, 2021; Stadnytskyi *et al.*, 2020; Stelzer-Braid *et al.*, 2009). Furthermore, aside from modelling studies, it is difficult to separate short-range aerosol transmission occurring over typical conversational distances (<1 m) from long-range aerosol transmission when airborne virus is present in the air and can travel >2 m to infect another person (Figure 5.1).

No studies on influenza and other respiratory viruses have claimed to have successfully done this, but there are now multiple studies showing the exhalation of live influenza and SARS-CoV-2 from infected patients (Ma *et al.*, 2021; Milton *et al.*, 2013; Yan *et al.*, 2018; Zhou *et al.*, 2021; Coleman *et al.*, 2021; Adenaiye *et al.*, 2021). In addition, the presence of live virus collected in air samples has been reported for influenza and other respiratory viruses such as respiratory syncytial virus (RSV) (Kulkarni *et al.*, 2016) and Middle East respiratory syndrome Coronavirus (MERS-CoV) (Kim *et al.*, 2016).

5.5. Infectious Dose of SARS-CoV-2?

The missing link for all of these air-sampling studies is the demonstration of susceptible persons actually inhaling the virus from the air and developing infection and disease from that particular inhalation event (i.e. to the exclusion of all other sources of the virus). This is very difficult to do even with well-known pathogens like influenza. Where this has been tried with influenza, using a laboratory strain of the virus in a well-controlled and isolated environment, the study failed to show any transmission at all in the test group (Nguyen-Van-Tam *et al.*, 2020).

Yet, this also raises the interesting (and often asked) question of the actual infectious dose of airborne and inhaled SARS-CoV-2. Such estimates are available for influenza (Nikitin *et al.*, 2014) and SARS-CoV-1 (Fang *et al.*, 2021; Schroder, 2020; Watanabe *et al.*, 2010), and these may be similar amongst respiratory viruses for immunologically naïve (i.e. fully susceptible) individuals (including SARS-CoV-2). So, this might be around 10–1000 viruses inhaled within a few breaths (i.e. with a single high intensity exposure), depending on the rapidity of the host innate immune response to clear the virus before any can find and bind successfully to a permissive host cell.

5.6. The Important Concept of Short-Range Aerosol Transmission

The generally-accepted short-range aerosol transmission mode includes two routes: short-range airborne and large droplet transmission. As shown in Figure 5.2(a), small particles (<5–10 μm) generated by respiratory activities (e.g. breathing, talking, laughing, singing, coughing, sneezing) can easily follow the airstreams and are potentially capable of short-range transmission by inhalation. Small particles (<5 μm) readily penetrate the airways all the way down to the alveolar space, whereas larger particles (<10 μm) readily penetrate below the glottis (Tellier *et al.*, 2019). The short-range exposure can be affected by body micro-environment, such as thermal body plumes (Licina *et al.*, 2015). Possibly the first study (Lewis *et al.*, 1969) of the near-body environment showed that the near-body microenvironment contains 30–400% more microorganisms than the ambient environment, and this work was followed by studies on near-body flows, respiration and thermal body plumes (Murakami *et al.*, 2000).

Large droplets (>10 μm), a concept originating from Flügge (1897), are too large to follow inhalation airflows. They are too big to be deposited in the lower respiratory tract or even be inhaled, but they can deposit directly on the mucous membranes of the eyelids, nostrils, and lips

(Liu *et al.*, 2017). Such large droplets are less likely to develop into airborne droplet nuclei that then stay suspended in air in the room (Eames *et al.*, 2009). The large droplet route has been considered a primary transmission route for some respiratory infectious diseases such as influenza, SARS, and MERS (Brankston *et al.*, 2007; Christian *et al.*, 2004; Mackay and Arden, 2015). However, there is no direct evidence for this belief. Both short-range airborne and large droplet routes may be affected to different degrees by the local ventilation system.

Exactly what range is short-range? According to the currently available evidence, WHO (2020c) considered the threshold range to be ~1 m, while the US CDC suggested a value of 6 feet (1.8 m) (CDC, 2020c). Flügge (1897) first suggested the large droplet route, and found that respiratory activities release droplets, and that the exhaled organisms could not be recovered when the sampling plates were exposed at distances beyond 1–2 m from the infectious person releasing the droplets. Recent mechanistic studies showed that the threshold horizontal interpersonal distance can be more than 2 m (Chen *et al.*, 2020).

The relative importance of short-range airborne and large droplet route depends on the virus concentration in particles of different sizes. Using influenza A, for example, 64% of the viral genome copies were associated with fine particles smaller than 2.5 μm (Yang *et al.*, 2011). Milton *et al.* (2013) also found that fine particles contained 8.8-fold more viral copies than did coarse particles (95% CI: 4.1–19). However, in contrast, some research showed that the number of RNA copies was thousands of times higher in larger particles of 10 μm diameter compared to smaller particles of 1 μm (Alonso *et al.*, 2015). If we consider that virus concentration is uniform in all sizes of particles, within 2 m, the short-range airborne route is mechanistically found to dominate at most distances during both talking and coughing (Chen *et al.*, 2020).

The vulnerable surface area of mucous membranes that may allow entry of infection is less than 10% of the area of the face (Chen *et al.*, 2020). More than 97% of large droplets landing on the facial skin will therefore settle on non-mucous areas of the face. Humans touch their face and mucous membranes more than 40 and 30 times per hour, respectively, potentially exposing these surfaces to virus entry (Figure 5.2(b)) — known as the immediate surface route of transmission (Zhang *et al.*, 2020). However, in reality, very little support is found for this mode of transmission, both for other respiratory viruses (UK SAGE, 2020), and for

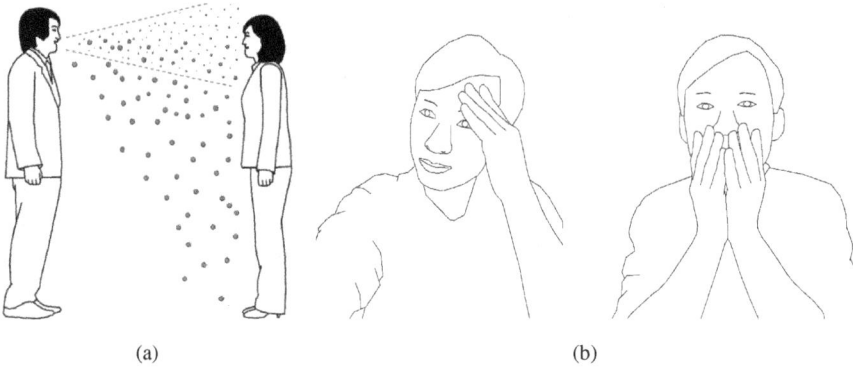

Figure 5.2.   Short-range aerosol transmission. (a) Short-range airborne and large droplet routes. (b) Immediate surface route.

SARS-CoV-2 (Haug *et al.*, 2020), and this is currently not thought to be the main way that this virus is spread (CDC, 2020a).

Thus, the short-range aerosol transmission may be the most important route in many respiratory infectious disease transmissions, as some studies have already suggested (Asadi *et al.*, 2019; Ma *et al.*, 2021; Milton *et al.*, 2013; Stadnytskyi *et al.*, 2020; Yan *et al.*, 2018; Zhou *et al.*, 2021).

5.7.   Related Infection Control Precautions and Interventions

All countries affected by the COVID-19 pandemic have applied various combinations of non-pharmaceutical, physical measures of social distancing to reduce the spread of SARS-CoV-2, including: border and travel restrictions, the cancellation of small and large gatherings, a 1–2 m distancing rule between people in public areas, restricting the mixing of households, curfews and stay-at-home orders as part of local or national lockdown measures. These have been compared and analyzed by several studies and ranked (Han *et al.* 2020; Haug *et al.* 2020). These measures have been followed to greater or lesser extents by various populations, but perhaps the most controversial intervention has been the use of masks.

Despite earlier guidance from multiple countries in the West initially stating that masking was not useful and not to buy masks (even though they were accepted to be useful on hospital wards) (Huang, 2020; Molteni and Rogers, 2020) — this has now been reversed globally. Masking in healthcare facilities and potentially crowded indoor public areas (including public transport) with poor ventilation, is now mandated in most countries (Han *et al.*, 2020; Haug *et al.*, 2020).

Despite earlier debates in the media and at government level about the lack of evidence for the effectiveness of masks, there is in fact a lot of published evidence already. Studies have already shown that surgical masks can contain and therefore reduce the dissemination of viruses in droplets and aerosols by up to 2–4-fold (i.e. ~67–75%) when worn by an infected person to protect others (Leung *et al.*, 2020; Milton *et al.*, 2013). Surgical masks can also protect the wearer to some degree by reducing exposure to incoming droplets and aerosols by up to 6-fold (i.e. ~83%), from others who are infected (HSE, 2008; Makison Booth *et al.*, 2013). Similarly, one study showed that homemade cloth masks (made from a tea towel) can reduce the exposure from incoming aerosols by up to 2–4-fold (i.e. ~50–75%) (van der Sande, 2008). The effectiveness of such homemade masks may vary considerably, but will ultimately depend on the material and the number of layers, as well as the tightness of fit to the facial skin.

One intuitive way to understand these various mask protection factors more clearly is to consider the impact of wearing the mask if 1000 viruses are coming towards you in droplet and/or aerosol form. Hence, a 6-fold reduction indicates that you will only be exposed to one-sixth of these viruses (i.e. $1000/6 = 167$ viruses); a 2–4-fold reduction would indicate that only half (i.e. 500 viruses) to one-quarter (i.e. 250 viruses) of these viruses would reach you. Similarly, if wearing a mask contains and reduces the amount of virus that you are spreading to others by 3–4-fold, this effectively reduces these 1000 viruses to just 333 or 250 viruses.

So, in combination, where two persons are both wearing masks that can each reduce the outgoing and incoming viral aerosols by 4-fold, then any exposure between the two of them could theoretically be reduced to around 62 virus particles, i.e. $\frac{1}{4} \times \frac{1}{4} = 16$-fold reduction of the initial exhaled 1000 viruses (Figure 5.3).

Regarding face shields (or visors), one review article suggested a protection efficacy slightly higher than surgical masks initially from immediate (droplet) exposures, but the protectiveness over a longer period will be lower as aerosols start to be inhaled underneath or from around the sides of the visor (Roberge, 2016). Thus, to optimize the protection of face shields, they should curve round the sides of the face as far as the ears,

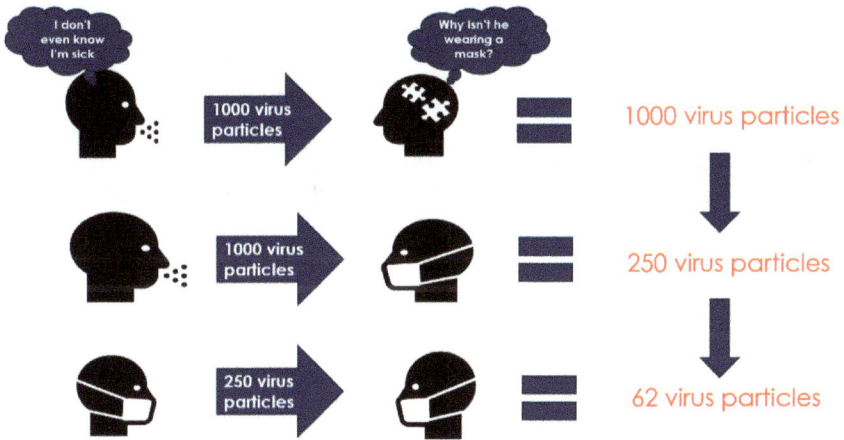

Courtesy of Mark Copeland, 3T Medical Systems, Inc., Canton, MI, USA

Figure 5.3. Theoretical effectiveness of masks to contain aerosols and/or to protect against incoming aerosols. The exact reduction factors will vary between masks. The diagram makes the simplifying assumption that the mask can reduce the outward viral load to 25% (i.e. a 4-fold reduction), and can also decrease the incoming aerosol viral load to 25% (i.e. a 4-fold reduction), thereby reducing the overall exposure to about 6% (i.e. a 16-fold reduction).

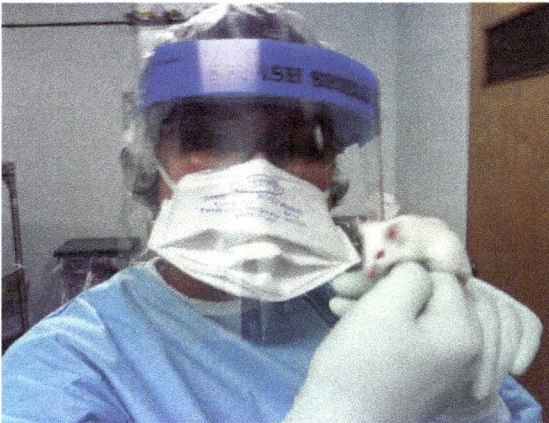

Figure 5.4. Example of face shield or visor, worn together with a face mask. From US CDC Public Image Library (https://phil.cdc.gov/Details.aspx?pid=16422).

and extend far down in front of the face, to minimize such aerosol entry as much as possible. Face shields or visors also offer eye protection, which surgical masks alone do not. They are also washable and readily reusable and are generally less claustrophobic than masks. They also allow more normal communication compared to masks which can muffle the voice. For increased protection, face shield can be worn with a mask for added protection (Figure 5.4).

5.8. Conclusions

In summary, there are already numerous examples of real-life SARS-CoV-2 outbreaks in crowded, poorly ventilated indoor settings that can easily be explained by short-range aerosol transmission (Qian and Zheng, 2018; Somsen *et al.*, 2020). However, without the ability to characterize these exposure events in detail in real-time as they unfold, this will always be difficult to prove conclusively (Qian *et al.*, 2021).

Nonetheless, there is sufficient evidence of aerosol transmission of SARS-CoV-2 to make new recommendations to reduce this route of spread — including improved ventilation without recirculation, the use of air-cleansing technologies, and reducing crowding in poorly-ventilated indoor spaces (Morawska *et al.*, 2020; Morawska and Milton, 2020) — which have already been adopted in updated engineering guidance (ASHRAE, 2020; REHVA, 2020a, 2020b).

The US Centers for Disease Control and Prevention, UK Public Health England, and the WHO have all updated their guidance to recognize the role of aerosols in transmitting SARS-CoV-2 (outside of aerosol-generating procedures) in the transmission of SARS-CoV-2, particularly in crowded, poorly ventilated indoor spaces (UK Government, 2020; CDC, 2020a; WHO, 2020b).

References

Adenaiye OO, *et al.* Infectious SARS-CoV-2 in exhaled aerosols and efficacy of masks during early mild infection. *Clin Infect Dis* 2021; ciab797.

Alonso C, *et al.* Concentration, size distribution, and infectivity of airborne particles carrying swine viruses. *PLoS One* 2015; 10:e0135675.

Asadi S, *et al.* Aerosol emission and superemission during human speech increase with voice loudness. *Sci Rep* 2019; 9:2348.

ASHRAE (American Society for Heating, Refrigeration and Air-Conditioning Engineers), 20 April 2020. https://www.ashrae.org/about/news/2020/ashrae-issues-statements-on-relationship-between-covid-19-and-hvac-in-buildings (accessed 1 December 2020).

Berlutti F, *et al*. Antiviral properties of lactoferrin — A natural immunity molecule. *Molecules* 2011; 16:6992–7018.

Boni MF, *et al*. Evolutionary origins of the SARS-CoV-2 sarbecovirus lineage responsible for the COVID-19 pandemic. *Nat Microbiol* 2020; 5:1408–1417.

Bourouiba L. Turbulent gas clouds and respiratory pathogen emissions: Potential implications for reducing transmission of COVID-19. *JAMA* 2020; 323: 1837–1838.

Brankston G, *et al*. Transmission of influenza A in human beings. *Lancet Infect Dis* 2007; 7:257–265.

Caly L, *et al*. Isolation and rapid sharing of the 2019 novel coronavirus (SARS-CoV-2) from the first patient diagnosed with COVID-19 in Australia. *Med J Aust* 2020; 212:459–462.

CDC (US Centers for Disease Prevention and Control), 2020a. How COVID-19 Spreads. Updated 28 October 2020. https://www.cdc.gov/Coronavirus/2019-ncov/prevent-getting-sick/how-covid-spreads.html (accessed 1 December 2020).

CDC (US Centers for Disease Control and Prevention), 2020b. Interim Clinical Guidance for Management of Patients with Confirmed Coronavirus Disease (COVID-19). https://www.cdc.gov/Coronavirus/2019-ncov/hcp/clinical-guidance-management-patients.html (accessed 1 December 2020).

CDC (Centers for Disease Control and Prevention, USA), 2020c. Social Distancing. 15 July 2020. https://www.cdc.gov/Coronavirus/2019-ncov/prevent-getting-sick/social-distancing.html (accessed 5 December 2020).

Cevik M, *et al*. Virology, transmission, and pathogenesis of SARS-CoV-2. *BMJ* 2020; 371:m3862.

Chen W, *et al*. Short-range airborne route dominates exposure of respiratory infection during close contact. *Build Environ* 2020; 176:106859.

Chessa C, *et al*. Antiviral and immunomodulatory properties of antimicrobial peptides produced by human keratinocytes. *Front Microbiol* 2020; 11: 1155.

Chin AWH, *et al*. Stability of SARS-CoV-2 in different environmental conditions. *Lancet Microbe* 2020; 1:e10.

Christian MD, *et al*. Possible SARS coronavirus transmission during cardiopulmonary resuscitation. *Emerg Infect Dis* 2004; 10:287–293.

Coleman KK, *et al*. Viral load of SARS-CoV-2 in respiratory aerosols emitted by COVID-19 patients while breathing, talking, and singing. *Clin Infect Dis* 2021; ciab691.

Dai YJ, *et al.* A profiling analysis on the receptor ACE2 expression reveals the potential risk of different type of cancers vulnerable to SARS-CoV-2 infection. *Ann Transl Med* 2020; 8:481.

Eames I, *et al.* Airborne transmission of disease in hospitals. *J R Soc Interface* 2009; 6(Suppl 6):S697–S702.

Fang FC, *et al.* COVID-19 — Lessons learned and questions remaining. *Clin Infect Dis* 2021; 72:2225–2240.

Flügge C. Uber luftinfection. *Z Hyg Infektionskr* 1897; 25:179–224.

Gao CX, *et al.* Multi-route respiratory infection: When a transmission route may dominate. *Sci Total Environ* 2021; 752:141856.

Hamner L, *et al.* High SARS-CoV-2 attack rate following exposure at a choir practice — Skagit County, Washington, March 2020. *MMWR — Morb Mortal Wkly Rep* 2020; 69:606–610.

Han E, *et al.* Lessons learnt from easing COVID-19 restrictions: An analysis of countries and regions in Asia Pacific and Europe. *Lancet* 2020; 396: 1525–1534.

Hanstock HG, *et al.* Tear lactoferrin and lysozyme as clinically relevant biomarkers of mucosal immune competence. *Front Immunol* 2019; 10:1178.

Haug N, *et al.* Ranking the effectiveness of worldwide COVID-19 government interventions. *Nat Hum Behav* 2020; 4:1303–1312.

Holshue ML, *et al.* First case of 2019 novel Coronavirus in the United States. *N Engl J Med* 2020; 382:929–936.

HSE (Health and Safety Executive UK), 2008. RR619 Evaluating the Protection Afforded by Surgical Masks Against Influenza Bioaerosols. https://www.hse. gov.uk/research/rrhtm/rr619.htm (accessed 13 July 2020).

ICTV (Coronaviridae Study Group of the International Committee on Taxonomy of Viruses). The species severe acute respiratory syndrome-related Coronavirus: Classifying 2019-nCoV and naming it SARS-CoV-2. *Nat Microbiol* 2020; 5:536–544.

Kim SH, *et al.* Extensive viable Middle East respiratory syndrome (MERS) Coronavirus contamination in air and surrounding environment in MERS isolation wards. *Clin Infect Dis* 2016; 63:363–369.

Kulkarni H, *et al.* Evidence of respiratory syncytial virus spread by aerosol. Time to revisit infection control strategies? *Am J Respir Crit Care Med* 2016; 194:308–316.

Lam TT, *et al.* Identifying SARS-CoV-2-related Coronaviruses in *Malayan pangolins. Nature* 2020; 583:282–285.

Langford MP, *et al.* Early-appearing antiviral activity in human tears during a case of picornavirus epidemic conjunctivitis. *J Infect Dis* 1979; 139: 653–658.

Leung NHL, *et al.* Respiratory virus shedding in exhaled breath and efficacy of face masks. *Nat Med* 2020; 26:676–680.

Lewis HE, *et al*. Aerodynamics of the human microenvironment. *Lancet* 1969; 293:1273–1277.

Li MY, *et al*. Expression of the SARS-CoV-2 cell receptor gene ACE2 in a wide variety of human tissues. *Infect Dis Poverty* 2020; 9:45.

Licina D, *et al*. Human convective boundary layer and its interaction with room ventilation flow. Indoor Air 2015; 25:21–35.

Lillie PJ, *et al*. Novel Coronavirus disease (COVID-19): The first two patients in the UK with person to person transmission. *J Infect* 2020; 80:578–606.

Liu L, *et al*. Short-range airborne transmission of expiratory droplets between two people. *Indoor Air* 2017; 27:452–462.

Lu J, *et al*. COVID-19 outbreak associated with air conditioning in restaurant, Guangzhou, China, 2020. *Emerg Infect Dis* 2020; 26:1628–1631.

Lukassen S, *et al*. SARS-CoV-2 receptor ACE2 and TMPRSS2 are primarily expressed in bronchial transient secretory cells. *EMBO J.* 2020; 39:e105114.

Ma J, *et al*. Coronavirus disease 2019 patients in earlier stages exhaled millions of severe acute respiratory syndrome Coronavirus 2 per hour. *Clin Infect Dis* 2021; 72:e652–e654.

Mackay IM, Arden KE. MERS Coronavirus: Diagnostics, epidemiology and transmission. *Virol J* 2015; 12:222.

Makison Booth C, *et al*. Effectiveness of surgical masks against influenza bio-aerosols. *J Hosp Infect* 2013; 84:22–26.

Malamud D, *et al*. Antiviral activities in human saliva. *Adv Dent Res* 2011; 23:34–37.

Miller SL, *et al*. Transmission of SARS-CoV-2 by inhalation of respiratory aerosol in the Skagit Valley Chorale superspreading event. *Indoor Air* 2021; 31:314–323.

Milton DK, *et al*. Influenza virus aerosols in human exhaled breath: Particle size, culturability, and effect of surgical masks. *PLoS Pathog* 2013; 9:e1003205.

Molteni M, Rogers A, 2020. WIRED. How Masks Went From Don't-Wear to Must-Have. https://www.wired.com/story/how-masks-went-from-dont-wear-to-must-have/ (accessed 2 July 2020).

Morawska L, Milton DK. It is time to address airborne transmission of Coronavirus disease 2019 (COVID-19). *Clin Infect Dis* 2020; 71: 2311–2313.

Morawska L, *et al*. How can airborne transmission of COVID-19 indoors be minimised? *Environ Int* 2020; 142:105832.

Murakami S, *et al*. Combined simulation of airflow, radiation and moisture transport for heat release from a human body. *Build Environ* 2000; 35: 489–500.

Nguyen-Van-Tam JS, *et al*. Minimal transmission in an influenza A (H3N2) human challenge-transmission model within a controlled exposure environment. *PLoS Pathog* 2020; 16:e1008704.

Nikitin N, *et al*. Influenza virus aerosols in the air and their infectiousness. *Adv Virol* 2014; 2014:859090.

Park SY, *et al*. Coronavirus disease outbreak in call center, South Korea. *Emerg Infect Dis* 2020; 26:1666–1670.

Qian H, Zheng X. Ventilation control for airborne transmission of human exhaled bio-aerosols in buildings. *J Thorac Dis* 2018; 10(Suppl 19): S2295–S2304.

Qian H, *et al*. Indoor transmission of SARS-CoV-2. *Indoor Air* 2021; 31:639–645.

REHVA (Federation of European Heating, Ventilation and Air Conditioning Associations), 2020a. COVID-19 Guidance Document. https://www.rehva. eu/fileadmin/user_upload/REHVA_COVID-19_guidance_document_ V3_03082020.pdf (accessed 3 August 2020).

REHVA (Federation of European Heating, Ventilation and Air Conditioning Associations), 2020b. Guidance for Schools. https://www.rehva.eu/ fileadmin/user_upload/REHVA_COVID-19_Guidance_School_Buildings. pdf (accessed 1 December 2020).

Roberge RJ. Face shields for infection control: A review. *J Occup Environ Hyg* 2016; 13:235–242.

Schroder I. COVID-19: A risk assessment perspective. *ACS Chem Health Saf* 2020; 27:160–169.

Shen Y, *et al*. Community outbreak investigation of SARS-CoV-2 transmission among bus riders in eastern China. *JAMA Intern Med* 2020; 180:1665–1671.

Silverstein WK, *et al*. First imported case of 2019 novel Coronavirus in Canada, presenting as mild pneumonia. *Lancet* 2020; 395:734.

Somsen GA, *et al*. Small droplet aerosols in poorly ventilated spaces and SARS-CoV-2 transmission. *Lancet Respir Med* 2020; 8:658–659.

Spiteri G, *et al*. First cases of Coronavirus disease 2019 (COVID-19) in the WHO European Region, 24 January to 21 February 2020. *Euro Surveill* 2020; 25:2000178.

Stadnytskyi V, *et al*. The airborne lifetime of small speech droplets and their potential importance in SARS-CoV-2 transmission. *Proc Natl Acad Sci USA* 2020; 117:11875–11877.

Stelzer-Braid S, *et al*. Exhalation of respiratory viruses by breathing, coughing, and talking. *J Med Virol* 2009; 81:1674–1679.

Tang JW, *et al*. Hypothesis: All respiratory viruses (including SARS-CoV-2) are aerosol-transmitted. *Indoor Air* 2022; 32:e12937.

Tang JW, *et al*. Qualitative real-time schlieren and shadowgraph imaging of human exhaled airflows: An aid to aerosol infection control. *PLoS One* 2011; 6:e21392.

Tang JW, *et al*. Airflow dynamics of coughing in healthy human volunteers by shadowgraph imaging: An aid to aerosol infection control. *PLoS One* 2012; 7:e34818.

Tang JW, Tellier R, Li Y. Hypothesis: All respiratory viruses (including SARS-CoV-2) are aerosol-transmitted. *Indoor Air* 2022; 32:e12937.

Tang JW, *et al.* Airflow dynamics of human jets: Sneezing and breathing — Potential sources of infectious aerosols. *PLoS One* 2013; 8:e59970.

Tang JW, *et al.* Emergence of a novel Coronavirus causing respiratory illness from Wuhan, *China. J Infect* 2020; 80:350–371.

Tellier R, *et al.* Recognition of aerosol transmission of infectious agents: A commentary. *BMC Infect Dis* 2019; 19:101.

UK Government, 2020. Review of Two Metre Social Distancing Guidance. https://www.gov.uk/government/publications/review-of-two-metre-social-distancing-guidance/review-of-two-metre-social-distancing-guidance (accessed 26 June 2020).

UK SAGE, 2020. What is the Evidence for the Effectiveness of Hand Hygiene in Preventing the Transmission of Respiratory Viruses? https://assets.publishing.service.gov.uk/government/uploads/system/uploads/attachment_data/file/897598/S0574_NERVTAG-EMG_paper_-_hand_hygiene_010720_Redacted.pdf (accessed 1 December 2020).

van der Sande M, *et al.* Professional and home-made face masks reduce exposure to respiratory infections among the general population. *PLoS One* 2008; 3:e2618.

van Doremalen N, *et al.* Aerosol and surface stability of SARS-CoV-2 as compared with SARS-CoV-1. *N Engl J Med* 2020; 382:1564–1567.

Watanabe T, *et al.* Development of a dose-response model for SARS Coronavirus. *Risk Anal* 2010; 30:1129–1138.

White MR, *et al.* Multiple components contribute to ability of saliva to inhibit influenza viruses. *Oral Microbiol Immunol* 2009; 24:18–24.

WHO (World Health Organization), 2020a. Timeline of WHO's Response to COVID-19. Updated 9 September 2020. https://www.who.int/news/item/29-06-2020-covidtimeline (accessed 1 December 2020).

WHO (World Health Organization), 2020b. Transmission of SARS-CoV-2: Implications for Infection Prevention Precautions. https://www.who.int/news-room/commentaries/detail/transmission-of-sars-cov-2-implications-for-infection-prevention-precautions (accessed 9 July 2020).

WHO (World Health Organization), 2020c. Coronavirus Disease 2019 (COVID-19) Situation Report — 66. https://www.who.int/docs/default-source/Coronaviruse/situation-reports/20200326-sitrep-66-covid-19.pdf (accessed 26 March 2020).

Wu P, *et al.* Real-time tentative assessment of the epidemiological characteristics of novel Coronavirus infections in Wuhan, China, as at 22 January 2020. *Euro Surveill* 2020; 25:2000044.

Xie X, *et al.* How far droplets can move in indoor environments — Revisiting the Wells evaporation-falling curve. *Indoor Air* 2007; 17:211–225.

Yan J, *et al*. Infectious virus in exhaled breath of symptomatic seasonal influenza cases from a college community. *Proc Natl Acad Sci USA* 2018; 115: 1081–1086.

Yang W, *et al*. Concentrations and size distributions of airborne influenza A viruses measured indoors at a health centre, a day-care centre and on aeroplanes. *J R Soc Interface* 2011; 8:1176–1184.

Zhang N, *et al*. Close contact behavior in indoor environment and transmission of respiratory infection. *Indoor Air* 2020; 30:645–661.

Zhou L, *et al*. Breath-, air- and surface-borne SARS-CoV-2 in hospitals. *J Aerosol Sci* 2021; 152:105693.

Chapter 6

COVID-19 Containment Measures

Jacinta I-Pei Chen[*], **Li Yang Hsu**[†], **Alex R. Cook**[‡],
and Jason Chin-Huat Yap[§]

Saw Swee Hock School of Public Health,
National University Health System,
National University of Singapore,
Kent Ridge, Singapore

[*]*ephcij@nus.edu.sg*
[†]*mdchly@nus.edu.sg*
[‡]*ephcar@nus.edu.sg*
[§]*jasonyap@nus.edu.sg*

Abstract

As medical countermeasures are usually not immediately available during pandemics, non-pharmaceutical measures are important and often the only options available to governments before the arrival of pharmaceutical interventions. This chapter provides an overview of containment measures historically and typically used in pandemic outbreak of respiratory diseases and in the context of Coronavirus disease 2019 (COVID-19) up until August 2021, summarizes the evidence on their effectiveness and efficiency, and considerations and impact from their deployment.

Keywords: Containment measures; non-pharmaceutical interventions; border control; travel restrictions; isolation; quarantine; detection; community hygiene measures; physical distancing; social distancing

6.1. Introduction

As we have re-learned since the onset of the Coronavirus disease 2019 (COVID-19) pandemic, pharmaceutical countermeasures during pandemics may not be immediately available. For novel diseases, the delivery of vaccines and therapeutics is dependent on the discovery and development pipelines, with potential bottlenecks at various stages including clinical trials, regulatory hurdles, and ramping-up of production, all of which normally take years to be passed (WHO, 2020b). Although the speed at which vaccines have reached the market during the COVID-19 pandemic shows the feasibility of shortening the process, several waves of the pandemic had passed by the time emergency use approval was obtained. Therefore, non-pharmaceutical interventions (NPIs) will always be important and are often the main options available to governments to contain a major outbreak. However, the evidence to support their use and to decide which NPIs have acceptable benefit-to-cost ratios has mostly been lacking until COVID-19 (Aldedort *et al.*, 2007; Fong *et al.*, 2020; Xiao *et al.*, 2020).

Governments have traditionally adopted a wide range of NPIs to contain or mitigate the spread of a virus at varying levels, drawing from pandemic preparedness plans that have been promoted by the World Health Organization (WHO) since the years after severe acute respiratory syndrome (SARS) and fears of avian influenza giving rise to an influenza pandemic. This chapter provides an overview of these containment measures, the scientific evidence and insights surrounding them up until August 2021, and guiding principles on how they are deployed. For a systematic discussion, a framework categorizing the measures into varying levels of containment is applied.

6.2. Factors Determining Transmission of SARS-CoV-2

Factors influencing transmission rates are important considerations when formulating and implementing NPIs (Frieden and Lee, 2020; NUS Saw Swee Hock School of Public Health, 2020e). For SARS Coronavirus-2 (SARS-CoV-2) and COVID-19, these include:

(a) **Pathogen-specific factors:** Current evidence points to key transmission via respiratory droplets, transmission via aerosols under limited circumstances (Bourouiba, 2020; Liu *et al.*, 2020c), possible fecal transmission (Amirian, 2020; Tian *et al.*, 2020b; Zhou *et al.*, 2020), and possible transmission via surfaces with potential viral viability up to 72 hours on certain surfaces (Biryukov *et al.*, 2020; Chin *et al.*, 2020a; Guo, 2020; Ong *et al.*, 2020; Rawlinson *et al.*, 2020; van Doremalen *et al.*, 2020). As the pandemic evolved, variants of interest with genetic changes that affect virus characteristics have indicated likely increase in aerosol transmission potential (Port *et al.*, 2021).

(b) **Host factors:** The median incubation period is ~5–6 days (Backer *et al.*, 2020; Linton *et al.*, 2020; NUS Saw Swee Hock School of Public Health, 2020b; Park *et al.*, 2020), with strong evidence that asymptomatic or presymptomatic transmission plays a significant role in epidemic spread (Arons, 2020; Ferretti *et al.*, 2020; Gandhi *et al.*, 2020; He *et al.*, 2020; Huang *et al.*, 2020a; Moghadas *et al.*, 2020; Qian *et al.*, 2020; Tindale *et al.*, 2020; Wei *et al.*, 2020; Zhu *et al.*, 2020). Preliminary studies have suggested shorter incubation periods for some variants of interests (such as the Delta variant), with viral loads reaching higher and detectable levels more quickly from time of exposure (Li *et al.*, 2021; Reardon, 2021).

(c) **Environmental factors:** Population density (Frieden and Lee, 2020; Kucharski *et al.*, 2020; Korevaar *et al.*, 2020; Rubin *et al.*, 2020; Summan and Nandi, 2021), sanitary conditions (Caruso and Freeman, 2020; UNICEF, 2020), and weather conditions influence transmission. Emerging data suggest that cold and dry conditions aid the spread of SARS-CoV-2 (Benedetti *et al.*, 2020; Biryukov *et al.*, 2020; CEBM, 2020a, 2020b).

(d) **Behavioral factors:** These include personal hygiene, health-seeking behavior, sociability, compliance to government, and personality traits such as individualism and being prosocial, among others (Aschwanden *et al.*, 2020).

6.3. Conceptual Overview of Levels of Containment

In a pandemic, the causative virus can be imported into a country, give rise to autochthonous infections, which in turn beget new clusters which can lead to initial exponential growth. Non-pharmaceutical containment and mitigating measures are usually built around key points in the virus transmission pathways, forming three key layers of defense and protection against spread of the disease (Table 6.1).

Table 6.1. Framework of measures by varying levels of containment.

Measures			Examples
Border controls	Directly from the source area to one's country, which may be extended over time		From Wuhan, then Hubei, to Singapore
	Indirectly from the source country by persons travelling from the source areas to a transit point outside and then to one's country		From elsewhere in China
	From other countries or areas from which there have been subsequent incidences of infections		
Active measures	Detection of potential cases	Imported cases	Through screening at healthcare and other facilities
		Unlinked cases	
		Contacts of confirmed cases	By contact tracing
	Isolation or quarantine	In healthcare facilities	Hospital infection control, protection of healthcare personnel
		In homes	"Stay Home Notices"
		In quarantine facilities	Hotels, purpose-built
	Treatment of diagnosed cases, including financial support for treatment costs and loss of income		Hospital clinical facilities Support programs
	Release of cases when safe		Testing for infectiousness Durations of quarantines
General measures (community measures, mitigating measures, etc.)	Measures to reduce contact within the community		Reducing public gatherings, school closures
	Public communications		Community sanitation and hygiene, mask use, self-isolation if unwell
	Provision of necessities and other supplies		Masks, medical and food supplies
	Environmental measures		Environmental cleansing, etc.
	Socioeconomic measures		Business continuity, disaster recovery, etc.

6.4. Border Controls

Border controls and travel restrictions are common first-response measures governments implement at the onset of a pandemic (US Department of Health and Human Services, 2017). They seek to prevent importation of a disease into the country, and include entry or exit screening, travel advisories/restrictions, border quarantine and border closures (Cochrane, 2020). Early months of the COVID-19 outbreak in 2020 saw several countries across the world implementing screening and restriction of travelers to or from Wuhan (Chinazzi *et al.*, 2020), and then extending to closure of borders to mainland China and selected countries, and then globally, as the epicenter expanded beyond Wuhan and new foci became established in Europe and the Americas (Russell *et al.*, 2021).

6.4.1. *Effectiveness and influencing factors*

Border controls may delay the spread of an epidemic and reduce the impact from imported cases on the population of the destination country (Cochrane, 2020). Modeling to quantify the effects of this have shown that it can be substantial (Adekunle *et al.*, 2020; Costantino *et al.*, 2020; Dickens *et al.*, 2020a; Ryu *et al.*, 2020; Wells *et al.*, 2020). However, the effectiveness of border controls is highly dependent on the virus transmissibility, natural history, and symptom presentation (which may be uncertain for novel infections), and the timing of implementation. High transmissibility necessitates quicker action, within days for SARS-CoV-2's basic reproduction number (R0), which has been estimated to range between 2 and 4.5 (Billah *et al.*, 2020; Katul *et al.*, 2020; Rahman *et al.*, 2020; Wang *et al.*, 2020c) and even higher for variants of interest, such as the Alpha and Delta variants (Alizon *et al.*, 2021; Hagen, 2021; Liu and Rocklov, 2021). Prior to importation and sustained transmission of the virus in a country, effecting the controls early (in terms of weeks and before there are thousands of cases at the source epidemic) would reduce peak magnitude of the outbreak in the seeded country (Hollingsworth *et al.*, 2006; Wells *et al.*, 2020).

Pre-COVID studies have indicated longer periods of delay in epidemic spread (of the order of weeks) for islands and remote communities where alternatives to aircraft travel are difficult (Boyd *et al.*, 2017; Gostin, 2007; Nishiura *et al.*, 2009). Simulations of the benefits of targeted air travel control strategies showed that allocating screening resources and restrictions to the most connected airports and those with shortest path distances from the epidemic source is more effective from a cost-benefit analysis standpoint than a blanket reduction in global air travel. However, such circumstances and strategies make a difference only when global case numbers are low at the very early onset of an epidemic (Hollingsworth *et al.*, 2006; Zlojutro *et al.*, 2019).

At the start of an evolving pandemic, there is a critically short time-line during which border controls may make a major difference, after which local control will play a more central role in suppressing local community transmissions. Implementing timely border controls is challenged by delays in recognizing that a pandemic has begun, by which time further loci of infection may have already seeded far from the initial epicenter. This is why travel restrictions usually and eventually have limited effect on preventing the advent of global pandemics (Carter, 2016). With COVID-19, multiple border closures across countries worldwide over the months of February to May 2020 failed to prevent the pandemic being established — as by the time awareness of an international epidemic had set in, cases had been seeded in enough countries to sustain transmission within national borders and to serve as additional sources for global transmission.

Other influencing factors include population density and traveler traffic, with delays to epidemic spread brought about by travel restrictions being shorter for cities with larger populations and traveler volumes from the source region during the COVID-19 pandemic (Chinazzi *et al.*, 2020; Liebig *et al.*, 2020; Tian *et al.*, 2020a). However, the number of travelers continuing to travel despite border restrictions may not be easy to predict based on regular travel patterns.

6.4.2. *Quarantine of ships*

The practice of quarantine began in the Middle Ages in an effort to protect coastal cities from plague epidemics, where ships arriving in Venice from infected ports were required to sit at anchor for a period of 40 days. In fact, the term "quarantine" originated from the Italian words "*quaranta giorni*" which mean 40 days (CDC, 2020).

The quarantine of ships also generated substantial academic research and reflection following high profile outbreaks on board cruise ships during the COVID-19 pandemic (Liu and Chang, 2020; Moriarty *et al.*,

2020) — as significantly higher risks of transmission for those on board must be considered against implications of disease spread to the larger shore-based population. While on-ship quarantine of all occupants, and containment of spread with segregation of suspect cases from unexposed groups, have been shown to have helped reduce disease spread within ships, the general consensus is to evacuate all occupants when the virus is airborne and the ship has closed air-conditioning without HEPA filters (Liu *et al.*, 2020a; Liu and Chang, 2020; Moriarty *et al.*, 2020; Rocklöv *et al.*, 2020; Sawano *et al.*, 2020; Sekizuka *et al.*, 2020; Vera *et al.*, 2014).

6.4.3. *Preventing the second and subsequent waves*

As the pandemic continued, the outbreak from the first wave of infection was brought under control within many countries, but second and subsequent waves of infection rage on in others. In an ongoing pandemic, border controls continue to play an important part in preventing importation and another outbreak for some local communities. The porous borders between countries in Europe since the post-lockdown period from May 2020 to Jan 2021 resulted in spikes in Coronavirus cases and prompted the progressive national lockdowns of countries such as France, Germany, and UK again from October 2020. The unpredictable emergence of viral variants with varying transmission dynamics adds complexity and challenges to border control policies. For example, the more transmissible Delta variant originating from India has sparked off large subsequent waves of infection in Southeast Asia in 2021. Singapore has been practicing a variegated border control policy approach with travelers from different countries fulfilling quarantine-test protocols of varying duration and intensity depending on their departing countries' relative importation risk. The country saw the imported variant sparking off two of the largest community clusters in May 2021 (Tan, 2021), prompting Singapore to shift into a phase of tightened containment measures.

In a continuing pandemic, countries need to maintain a constantly vigilant border control approach. This can be challenging for larger countries with less well-defined borders, inter-state travel, and multiple points of entry for travelers via air, sea and land — which will face the added complexity of policy formulation and implementation across states, provinces, and different points of entry and modes of travel. Even Singapore, an island nation with well-defined borders and limited points of entry, experienced one of her largest community clusters likely seeded by fishing boats into one of her fishery ports (Ang, 2021), two months after the Delta variant sparked off a large cluster from her airport (Sim and Kok, 2021).

6.4.4. *Economic impact and transboundary considerations*

The COVID-19 pandemic has brought about unprecedented impact on global air connectivity and the international movement of people and goods, and has affected the livelihood of hundreds of millions of people worldwide who have made this connectivity possible. As at November 2020, the world has recorded 300 million fewer tourists globally and some 320 billion USD in lost revenue (Nortajuddin, 2020; UNWTO, 2020).

Given the transboundary nature and economic impact of travel advisories and border closures, solidarity among nations and collaborative approaches that are balanced against traditional values of self-interest and territoriality are required during pandemics. In shaping opportunities to mitigate the economic impact from travel restrictions, responsibilities are shared by individual countries — in communicating relevant information with regards to intra-country epidemiological spread — as well as international coordinating organizations (Gostin and Berkman, 2007; WHO, 2018a).

Bilateral or bloc arrangements among countries can be established to support continuing export and import activities, as seen with some countries during the early lockdown period in the first half of 2020 (Boyd *et al.*, 2017). After Malaysia announced its border lockdown on 16 March 2020, the Singapore government worked with companies and provided subsidies for the arrangement of accommodation to Malaysian workers who used to commute daily by land to and from Johor to Singapore. An in-principle agreement was worked out between Singapore and Malaysia on the continuation of smooth transporting of necessities such as food across both countries' land checkpoints. These helped to prevent disruption to essential services and supplies in Singapore while safeguarding the livelihoods of Malaysian workers (*The Straits Times*, 2020; *Today*, 2020).

The increasing cooperation among civil aviation authorities, cruise operators, and public health authorities in countries has also brought about the emergence of common preventive public health guidelines for operating air travel and cruises in the pandemic situation, and limited resumption of such operations in and between some regions (Royal Caribbean

International, 2020; The Royal Caribbean and Norwegian Cruise Line, 2020). Common frameworks of reporting coordinated by international coordinating organizations can provide information on countries' and operators' compliance with the guidelines and countries' situation of epidemiological spread, public health structures, and health system capacity. This can help individual countries to assess the relative importation risk from and to different destinations and make decisions on air travel or cruising arrangements in relation to what is tolerable for their own response capacity. Emerging research on the relative effectiveness of different combinations of pre-departure and post-arrival testing with varying quarantine periods can help guide these decisions (Dickens *et al.*, 2020a; ICAO, 2020).

6.5. Active Measures

Active measures are deployed when imported cases have been seeded within national borders. They are aimed at preventing disease spread from infected people into the community.

6.5.1. *Detection*

Accurate identification of infected and potentially infected persons is necessary to separate them promptly from the non-exposed population, if isolation of cases is politically achievable. Identification of cases also allows the government to monitor the degree of autochthonous transmission. Governments typically set out suspect case criteria — clinical symptoms, travel history, close contact with infected cases, etc. — and referral protocols to which screening points and clinics can use to refer cases for diagnostic testing. Such criteria are revised according to new information about the virus and developments in its epidemic spread (CDC, 2020c; China National Health Commission, 2020a; Ministry of Health, Singapore, 2020b).

Polymerase chain reaction (PCR) tests, also known as nucleic acid tests, using nasopharyngeal swabs to detect the virus are currently the most reported technique (Giri *et al.*, 2021). Limitations of the test and other disease characteristics have increased the complexity of the testing process. The limited sensitivity of nasal swabs and wide ranging incubation period — typically 4–6.4 days but possibly up to 38 days (Backer *et al.*, 2020; Baettig *et al.*, 2021; Guan *et al.*, 2020; Jiang *et al.*, 2020;

Linton *et al.*, 2020; Liu and Chang, 2020; NUS Saw Swee Hock School of Public Health, 2020b, 2020d; Wallace *et al.*, 2020) — means possible false negative results, and someone who has tested negative may become a positive case even shortly after an earlier test. Serial testing can improve test accuracy (Baettig *et al.*, 2021; Crotty *et al.*, 2020; Farrell *et al.*, 2013; Hastings *et al.*, 2015; Liu and Chang, 2020; Miyamae *et al.*, 2020; Njuguna *et al.*, 2020). There has been rapid development of other testing methods that can be potentially more cost-effective, accurate, rapid and scalable, including saliva testing, serological tests, multi-stage pooled testing, and use of multiple methods in combination. For example, a combination of different or symptom-oriented swab location may improve test accuracy, since sites of biological sampling affect the sensitivity of PCR tests (Anderson *et al.*, 2020; Baettig *et al.*, 2021; Eberhardt *et al.*, 2020; NUS Saw Swee Hock School of Public Health, 2020d; Pulia *et al.*, 2020; Yang *et al.*, 2021). Some countries have also explored use of serological tests to confirm historical infections and appreciate the true extent of spread (Hafstad, 2020; Hoang, 2020; Ministry of Health, Singapore, 2020c; Peeling *et al.*, 2020).

Targeted broad-based testing of suspected clusters or higher risk population groups can also facilitate rapid identification of infected persons. Examples include South Korea's outreach to test all 200,000 members of the Shincheonji Church of Jesus linked to a COVID-19 cluster in February 2020 (Business Insider, 2020), and Singapore's universal testing of nursing home staff (Crotty *et al.*, 2020) and rostered routine testing of certain migrant worker groups (Ministry of Manpower, Singapore, 2020). The development of new methods such as wastewater and environmental surface testing can further support and improve surveillance testing efforts in the future (Ahmed *et al.*, 2020; Marshall *et al.*, 2020).

The detection capacity of a country or region is defined by how developed is its testing capacity and expertise, how swiftly its suspect case criteria is aligned to epidemic developments, and how well testing strategies and protocols are executed. This explains the variability in detection capacity across countries observed in a few early COVID-19 studies (De Salazar *et al.*, 2020; Ng *et al.*, 2020; Niehus *et al.*, 2020). Detection capacity impacts mortality, with some studies revealing negative association between COVID-19 mortality rate and test rate — a likely result of its facilitation of early detection, treatment and tackling of transmission via presymptomatic and never-symptomatic patients (Kenyon, 2020; Leffler *et al.*, 2020).

6.5.2. *Contact tracing*

It is important to combine isolation of symptomatic cases with rapid contact tracing to identify and quarantine presymptomatic and asymptomatic individuals prior to their infectious period (James *et al.*, 2021; Moghadas *et al.*, 2020).

Contact tracing and testing strategies can be mutually reinforcing. Decreasing time to test and quarantine by a matter of days can improve the detection ratio by as much as 40% (Yuan *et al.*, 2020). Conversely, poor testing efficacy can undermine contact tracing with the possible release of false negative cases from quarantine; incorporating additional days of quarantine for negative cases can reduce such risk (Davis *et al.*, 2020; Fiore *et al.*, 2021; Kucharski *et al.*, 2020). In view of the substantial demands contact tracing places on public health authorities, applying a less strict definition of "close contact" for suspect cases can potentially reduce administrative burden without impacting efficacy significantly (Keeling *et al.*, 2020).

Governments can consider varying combinations of testing methods and strategies, contact tracing speed, and quarantine/isolation duration to achieve maximal possible efficiency in these areas, bearing in mind national considerations of testing capacity, administrative burden, and manpower or infrastructural availability.

Digital contact tracing can improve contact tracing speed and several countries have adopted mobile phone applications to location trace and notify "close contacts" of diagnosed COVID-19 cases (Cencetti *et al.*, 2021; Currie *et al.*, 2020; Ekong *et al.*, 2020; Ferretti *et al.*, 2020). However, digital contact tracing is limited by and dependent on mobile app adoption and self-reporting by individuals. Most modeling studies project an uptake of at least 60% to suppress the epidemic (Cencetti *et al.*, 2021; Currie *et al.*, 2020; Hinch *et al.*, 2020). Digital tracing should therefore be an adjunct to traditional manual tracing and accompanying testing efforts.

6.5.3. *Quarantine and isolation*

Quarantine is the restriction of the activities of asymptomatic persons who have been exposed to a communicable disease to prevent disease transmission should they transpire to be infected. In contrast, isolation is the separation of known infected persons. Both approaches have the goal of preventing subsequent transmission of the disease. Quarantine and isolation can be done by various means, including confining people to their own homes, restricting travel out of an affected area, and keeping people in a designated facility (Gostin and Berkman, 2007). It has been argued that home-based isolation of milder cases of COVID-19 severely hampers epidemic control (Dickens *et al.*, 2020b), and countries that adopt institutional isolation of cases are also those with better controlled outbreaks (Cook *et al.*, 2021). Use of quarantine zones, where possibly infected persons are confined to designated areas, may be limited for smaller nations which do not have the benefit of space.

Both quarantine and isolation have public health ethical considerations as they restrict the freedoms of an individual to protect the health of the community. Quarantine is comparatively more controversial as it involves restricting the liberty of individuals who *might* pose a danger to public health in contrast to known infected individuals who *do* pose a danger.

6.5.3.1. *Effectiveness*

Prior to COVID-19, modeling studies have already attempted to examine the extent to which quarantine contributes to the control of infectious disease spread. These generally conclude that quarantine (accompanied with effective isolation) is likely to be effective if the asymptomatic transmission period is not too short such that the probability of an infectious person getting quarantined before symptoms emerge is low, and not too long such that it becomes extremely difficult to identify possibly infected individuals. In other words, quarantine is effective for diseases with a high proportion of identifiable asymptomatic infections (Day *et al.*, 2006; Fraser *et al.*, 2004). While the relevance of quarantine was questionable for SARS (Annas, 2007; Hsieh *et al.*, 2007; Mubayi *et al.*, 2010), which was likely contagious upon symptom onset, evidence of asymptomatic transmission for COVID-19 within a reasonably identifiable transmission period meets the qualifying conditions for effective use of quarantine (Anderson *et al.*, 2020; Peak *et al.*, 2020; The Novel Coronavirus Pneumonia Emergency Response Epidemiology Team, 2020; Xia *et al.*, 2020; Yang *et al.*, 2020; Zou *et al.*, 2020a). Testing and contact tracing strategies can further improve the identification rate of possibly infected individuals and achieve higher intervention performance.

However, quarantine operations are resource heavy, and as an outbreak spreads, maintaining good intervention performance may become unrealistic. In such circumstances, resources can be prioritized for scalable interventions such as social distancing, active monitoring, and more selective individual quarantine (e.g. the family or household members of patients) (Peak *et al.*, 2020).

6.5.3.2. *Influencing factors and considerations*

A review found that adherence to quarantine ranged from as low as 0% up to 92.8% (Webster *et al.*, 2020). Main factors influencing compliance were people's knowledge about the disease and quarantine procedure, whether it is home or facility-based quarantine, social norms, perceived benefits of quarantine and perceived risk of disease, and practical issues such as accessibility to necessities or consequences of absence from work (Webster *et al.*, 2020).

Variation in acceptability of restrictive measures was observed across cultures and countries during the COVID-19 pandemic. China's quarantine operations, described by some literature as the "largest and most draconian quarantine in history", and Singapore's "strict hospital and home quarantine regimen", helped contain spread but may not be replicable in other cultures and parts of the world. In the US, for example, concerns were raised about quarantine measures being excessive and infringing on individual liberties (*Channel News Asia*, 2020b; Gostin and Hodge, 2020; Heijmans and Bloomberg, 2020; *The Economist*, 2020).

The provision of regular and timely information by the government can help build societal understanding of the risk of the disease and improve community cooperation (Webster *et al.*, 2020).

The psychological impact from quarantine can also be wide-ranging and substantial, and longer quarantine durations are associated with poorer mental health outcomes. Restricting the length of quarantine to the minimum necessary and provision of forms of support — access to social networks, social media, psychological advice and so on — and financial compensation can make the experience more tolerable (Blendon *et al.*, 2006; Brooks *et al.*, 2020).

Internet connectivity and e-commerce services can facilitate ordering and delivery of necessities and good contact with the workplace, family and friends for persons under quarantine, making the experience less inconvenient and resource-intensive. For example, Singapore benefits from its compactness and relative maturity of e-commerce services, where it is relatively easy and inexpensive to order cooked food and other items online (Lim, 2020a).

6.5.3.3. *Guiding principles and general consensus*

Techniques for quarantine and isolation can vary, but it is important to treat symptomatic, potentially infected, and non-exposed populations differently (Gostin and Berkman, 2007). Decisions on restrictive measures should also be scientifically based, made in an open and fair manner (Heyman, 2005; Markovits, 2005), and bear in mind cultural norms and contexts. Considering the various influencing factors and considerations, WHO has developed guidelines for the quarantine of individuals in the context of COVID-19, addressing issues such as appropriateness of quarantine facilities, necessary provision of necessities and information, and minimum infection prevention and control measures (WHO, 2020c).

6.5.4. *Release after treatment or from quarantine*

The quarantine period should be based on incubation period of the disease. In the case of COVID-19, WHO and other international/authoritative bodies generally recommend a 14-day period (CDC, 2020a; WHO, 2020c).

In earlier months of the COVID-19 outbreak, release from isolation for infected persons was based on resolution of fever and respiratory symptoms, or serial negative swab tests, or both, with variations noted across countries. As the epidemic evolved, instances of patients continuing to test positive for more than 14 days (up to 36 days) and evidence that the virus is likely no longer viable after 14 days has caused countries (including South Korea, UK, US and Singapore) as well as WHO, to adopt or recommend a time-based discharge criterion rather than a test-based one (Korea Centers for Disease Control and Prevention, 2020; Marchand-Senecal *et al.*, 2020; Ministry of Health, Singapore, 2020a; NCID, Academy of Medicine Singapore, Chapter of Infectious Disease Physicians, 2020; Public Health England, 2016).

The phenomenon of patients with mild symptomatology and scientific observation of their stable disease course have also led to management of such cases outside of acute hospital settings, in field hospitals or isolation facilities converted from exhibition centers or hotels (Dezan Shira & Associates Staff in Vietnam, 2020; Kmar *et al.*, 2020; Mangosing, 2020; Marchand-Senecal *et al.*, 2020; Wölfel *et al.*, 2020). In the case of limited hospital bed capacity, the strategy of early discharge with ensuing home isolation after a 10-day period when residual risk of infectivity is low was recommended by some studies (Marchand-Senecal *et al.*, 2020; Wölfel *et al.*, 2020).

6.5.4.1. *Alignment to national guidelines*

Healthcare and screening providers should align with government guidelines in terms of diagnostic and isolation discharge criteria. A stricter approach than what is proposed by national guidelines can undermine the national position, change the pick-up specificity, and create a culture of mistrust in the government.

6.5.5. *Infection control in hospitals and clinics*

Active measures to identify and separate infected or potentially infected persons should accompany infection control and preparedness measures within healthcare facilities — which are central to the effective treatment of cases and which are highly susceptible to nosocomial outbreaks in an epidemic situation. The experience of SARS was marked by numerous nosocomial outbreaks reported in affected countries (McDonald *et al.*, 2004). This has also translated to a culture and practice of clinical readiness in SARS-affected countries and regions such as Hong Kong, Taiwan and Singapore (Cheng *et al.*, 2020; Lum *et al.*, 2016; Wang *et al.*, 2020a).

6.5.5.1. *Measures and effectiveness*

Guidance on infection prevention and control for healthcare settings and in relation to COVID-19 have been developed by healthcare authorities and public health organizations such as CDC, Johns Hopkins Bloomberg School of Public Health's (JHSPH) Center for Health Security, and WHO (CDC, 2020d; Toner and Waldhorn, 2020; WHO, 2020b; Zhejiang University School of Medicine, 2020). These address measures across the different levels and layers of control such as healthcare worker training and compliance, surveillance mechanisms, hospital environment measures, and capacity planning preparations. The COVID-19 pandemic has also seen the development of such guidelines in the academic literature that are specific to practices involving higher transmission risk, such as dentistry, ophthalmology, radiology, anesthesia, operating room management and autopsy (Aquila *et al.*, 2020; Chandy *et al.*, 2020; Lai *et al.*, 2020; Meng *et al.*, 2019; Peng *et al.*, 2020; Zhao *et al.*, 2020).

Several COVID-19 studies have highlighted the importance of hospital-based infection control practices, such as use of personal protective equipment, hand hygiene, symptom screening and environmental disinfection and cleaning (Jones *et al.*, 2020; Liu *et al.*, 2020b; Rawlinson *et al.*, 2020; Wu *et al.*, 2020; Zhou *et al.*, 2020). Compliance to the measures was found to be associated with their risk perception, and organizational and environmental factors such as heavy workloads and lack of space or facilities are barriers to adherence (Houghton *et al.*, 2020; Parker and Goldman, 2006). Early hospital preparedness also plays a major role. A case study indicated how early surveillance adopted by public Hong Kong hospitals averted nosocomial transmission of SARS-CoV-2 (Cheng *et al.*, 2020). A patient who had visited a hospital in mainland China was included under the epidemiological criterion for surveillance on day 17 from announcement of a pneumonia cluster in China (31 December 2019), even though reported cases of SARS-CoV-2 were still confined to Wuhan until day 20. As a result of such early preparedness, no nosocomial transmission of SARS-CoV-2 had been reported in Hong Kong until March 2020 (Cheng *et al.*, 2020).

N95 respirators are generally recommended over surgical masks for more stringent protection of healthcare workers, and for airborne precautions in the case of novel respiratory virus. However, respirators have been associated with perceptions of being difficult to tolerate and they need appropriate fitting and usage. Attention should be paid to ensuring compliance with their correct usage (Balazy *et al.*, 2006; Makison Booth *et al.*, 2013; Chu *et al.*, 2020; Gostin, 2007; Ha, 2020; Iannone *et al.*, 2020; Jefferson *et al.*, 2009; Long *et al.*, 2020; Macintyre *et al.*, 2011, 2013). Worldwide shortages during a pandemic can compromise the traceability of their origins and quality check of supplies becomes important. For example, a protocol developed in a hospital in the Netherlands to test a minimum total inward leak (TIL) of 8% found that only 33% of tested respirators met the requirements (van Wezel *et al.*, 2020).

Global shortage of PPE during the COVID-19 pandemic in 2020 had also spurred research, guidelines and adoption of their risk-stratified use, and extended use or reuse of face masks (Cheng *et al.*, 2020; College of Radiologists, Singapore, 2020; Ha, 2020; Klompas *et al.*, 2020; Sun *et al.*, 2020; The National Institute for Occupational Safety and Health (NIOSH), 2018; Wong *et al.*, 2020). Disinfection techniques such as use of hydrogen peroxide plasma for respirators and simple steaming of medical masks, and methods to extend lifespan of masks were explored (Anderegg *et al.*, 2020; Carnino *et al.*, 2020; Cramer *et al.*, 2020; Ibáñez-Cervantes *et al.*, 2020; Widmer and Richner, 2020).

6.5.5.2. *Healthcare worker responsibilities and rights*

The critical role of healthcare workers and their exposure to psychological stress during a pandemic means providers and governments must be mindful of their workload and occupational safety (Morgantini *et al.*, 2020; WHO, 2020a). Measures such as redeployment of healthcare workers with elevated risks of severe infection from higher risk sites, use of telemedicine, and prioritization for testing, vaccination and treatment, can improve occupational health and alleviate concerns of heightened risks to themselves and family members (Jin *et al.*, 2020).

A pandemic can also call attention to the inherent conflict in the rights, roles and responsibilities of healthcare workers. The UK government's suggestion that retired NHS staff be activated to supplement COVID-19 patient care in March 2020 was met with resistance. A review article commented that while doctors' freedom of choice is protected in international law, arguments can be made that refusal represents the abdication of duty (Dunne *et al.*, 2020; Weaver, 2020).

6.6. General Measures

Most of the measures taken in this section are preventive and seek to slow disease spread rather than contain the epidemic. This is because the disease has usually already "seeded" itself in the community at this point, infectious persons are unknown to the government, and measures to segregate these individuals from non-infected groups are no longer possible.

6.6.1. *Community hygiene*

Hygiene measures — such as hand-washing, surface disinfection, use of PPE, and respiratory hygiene — are broadly accepted and widely used in outbreaks of influenza and respiratory diseases, with convincing supporting circumstantial evidence (Barker *et al.*, 2001; Biryukov *et al.*, 2020; CDC, 2005; Nelson *et al.*, 2021; NUS Saw Swee Hock School of Public Health, 2020a; Ong *et al.*, 2020; Rawlinson *et al.*, 2020; WHO, 2018b). Surface disinfection with 62–71% ethanol, 0.5% hydrogen peroxide or 0.1% sodium hypochlorite has been found to be effective on Coronaviruses (Kampf *et al.*, 2020). Alcoholic hand rubs and similar agents such as triclosan and chlorhexidine are effective against enveloped viruses which include Coronaviruses (Barker *et al.*, 2001; CEBM, 2020a; Gostin, 2007).

6.6.1.1. *Community masking*

While pre-COVID reviews indicated a lack of adequately designed studies to conclusively establish the protective effect of community masking, several COVID-19 studies noted that societal norms and government policies emphasizing mask-wearing are associated with low COVID-19 mortality (Chu *et al.*, 2020; Leffler *et al.*, 2020; Mitze *et al.*, 2020). Some Asian countries (Thailand, Japan, South Korea, Taiwan, Hong Kong, Vietnam, Malaysia, Cambodia, Philippines, Mongolia and Laos), where extensive mask usage was adopted, were associated with fairly lower mortality rates (Leffler *et al.*, 2020). Effectiveness is likely linked to early, consistent and correct usage, and being undertaken as part of a package of personal hygiene protective measures (Bin-Reza *et al.*, 2012; Brienen *et al.*, 2010; CDC, 2020b; Jefferson *et al.*, 2009; Sim *et al.*, 2014).

In view of the global shortage of surgical masks during the early stages of the epidemic, alternatives such as cloth masks were explored despite potential inadequacies (e.g. ill-fitting, non-disposable). Studies show that cloth masks provide lower degrees of protection compared to surgical masks or respirators, but can be used as a last resort or where a user is non-symptomatic (Chughtai *et al.*, 2020; Davies *et al.*, 2013; Shakya *et al.*, 2017; Kim, 2020b; van der Sande *et al*, 2008). WHO provides guidelines for the manufacturing of non-medical (fabric) masks (WHO, 2020d). Some governments and guidelines on masking adopt or recommend a risk-based approach for mask use by the general public, stratified by considerations of the type of setting and population groups (Hsieh *et al.*, 2020; WHO, 2020d).

6.6.1.2. *Population behavior and compliance*

Several studies noted strong adherence (over 70%) or increased uptake of community hygiene practices in the COVID-19 pandemic. Most of these studies were in countries which have successfully contained an initial outbreak situation, such as China, South Korea, and Vietnam. The studies also noted the role of public communications in influencing population behavior in some of these countries (Gharpure *et al.*, 2020; He *et al.*, 2021; Huang *et al.*, 2020b; Jang *et al.*, 2020; Muto *et al.*, 2020; Nguyen *et al.*, 2020). Some of the studies also noted that women were more likely to practice such behaviors than men, and that perceived risk towards COVID-19 infectivity (which is likely to motivate compliance with self-protective behaviors such as personal hygiene) was positively associated with females, the elderly, higher income groups, and people living with children (Hsieh *et al.*, 2020; Huynh, 2020).

Some studies noted a significant extent of incorrect mask usage (as high as 45% of users). Mask-wearing can create a false sense of security and result in more risk-taking behaviors such as less social distancing. Conversely, it can also help increase awareness of other NPIs and hygiene measures (de Araujo *et al.*, 2020; Doung-Ngern *et al.*, 2020; Gupta *et al.*, 2020; Klompas *et al.*, 2020; Yan *et al.*, 2020).

Such knowledge can help drive targeted delivery of public communications on community hygiene instructions to populations (Doung-Ngern *et al.*, 2020).

6.6.1.3. *Other hygiene measures*

The COVID-19 pandemic has seen the widespread adoption of environmental cleansing and disinfection measures by governments worldwide. An interesting observation is the quarantining and disinfection of bank notes by some governments such as South Korea and China, because they change hands frequently and can facilitate virus transmission (Bloomberg, 2020; Pietsch, 2020; Reuters, 2020). Such national disinfection efforts have spurred research on and adoption of adjunct technologies (such as UV-C light and antimicrobial surfaces) as easily deployable and affordable ways to inactivate viruses in aerosols or on actively used surfaces (García de Abajo *et al.*, 2020; Mantlo *et al.*, 2021).

Because of possible fecal transmission, it is also advisable to follow strict hand hygiene and regular disinfection of toilets, and for patients not to share toilets with their families even after being discharged (Amirian, 2020; Tian *et al.*, 2020b; Zhou *et al.*, 2020).

6.6.2. *Physical distancing*

Decreased social mixing has been a consistent response in past epidemics, and includes restrictions on mass gatherings and voluntary or imposed social separation (WHO, 2005). During the COVID-19 pandemic, multiple countries had gone into lockdown situations, and these have effectively curbed spread of the epidemic across the world and within the countries. Social distancing comprises a large component of lockdowns, effected through measures such as stay-at-home orders, closure of non-essential businesses (e.g. some shops, restaurants and sports facilities) and schools.

Studies have sought to evaluate which forms of physical distancing worked best through understanding the influencing transmission dynamics, contact volumes, mobility, and outbreak risks in different settings. Such evidence can inform policy on targeted distancing measures at specific "higher-risk" settings or population groups in the community, as a universal approach involves substantial economic and societal costs (CEBM, 2020a).

6.6.2.1. *Effectiveness and considerations*

Several studies tracking contacts made after the recent implementation of physical distancing measures in COVID-19 lockdowns noted clear association between decrease in cases and increasing social distancing. The studies also found that contacts per person generally reduced by about 70% or more to less than four (Charpentier *et al.*, 2020; Milne and Xie, 2020; NUS Saw Swee Hock School of Public Health, 2020a). The timing and duration of distancing measures play an important role (CEBM, 2020a), and physical distancing of one meter or more is associated with significantly lower risk of infection, with added benefits likely with even larger physical distances (Chu *et al.*, 2020).

For countries advocating social distancing practices without a mass "blanket" stay-at-home order, encouraging change in population behavior related to greeting habits and proximity to one another can be challenging. Some countries and organizations have employed visible markers to help consciously remind people to stand apart from each other in queues or meeting settings (*The Guardian*, 2020).

6.6.3. *School closures*

Several studies (Brauner *et al.*, 2021; Kucharski *et al.*, 2020; Leclerc *et al.*, 2020; Li *et al.*, 2020; NUS Saw Swee Hock School of Public Health, 2020a; Pullano *et al.*, 2020; Sypsa *et al.*, 2021; van Leeuwen *et al.*, 2021; Zhang *et al.*, 2020) have highlighted the comparatively larger volume of contacts recorded in schools and the significant reduction in transmission from school closures during COVID-19 lockdowns, with one study (Brauner *et al.*, 2021) estimating a reduction of 58% in the effective reproduction number (Rt). This aligns with the higher volume of contacts or higher proportion of contact reductions during lockdowns observed in school-age groups (around 5–20 years) noted in other studies (Prem *et al.*, 2017). Although some studies have suggested that the contribution of school contacts to epidemic impact was not apparently determinable (Guo *et al.*, 2021; Leclerc *et al.*, 2020), others have attributed this purported result to the longer transmission paths and the age group's mild symptomatology or lack of symptoms.

However, school closures remove the support structure of the school system and affects parents' work productivity, on top of the impact on children's education. The implications of extending school closures over months or longer can be considerable (Gostin, 2007; Moberly, 2020). Studies have also pointed to the impact on healthcare workers' productivity when their children have to stay home, which translates to compromised hospital capacity that may not be more than offset by reduced COVID-19 cases from the school closures (Bayham and Fenichel, 2020; Chin *et al.*, 2020b; Viner *et al.*, 2020).

Prolonged school closure and home confinement may also have negative effects on children's physical and mental health, due to reasons such as longer screen time, being physically less active, irregular sleep patterns, and reduced social interactions (Wang *et al.*, 2020b). Other secondary adverse effects include increased dropouts, child labor, violence against children, teen pregnancies, and widened inequality with children from lower income families not having access to home-based learning resources such as computers and the internet (Armitage and Nellums, 2020a). Considering children's significantly low risk for severe disease with COVID-19, it can be argued that the impact of school closure is almost entirely negative for this population group. It has also been pointed out that benefits of school closures may be marginal or less than projections from modeling studies, as contacts between children and adults continue as part of informal childcare with heightened transmission risk to older people (Viner *et al.*, 2020).

Decisions on school closures should be balanced against considerations of the high costs involved and accompany mitigating measures such as childcare subsidies for healthcare workers, leaving schools open for the children of healthcare and other essential workers, and provision of online education courses encouraging healthy home-based lifestyle. Policymakers can also look to examples of school social distancing interventions in countries that have reopened schools, kept schools open, or adopted partial closures (Viner *et al.*, 2020).

6.6.4. *Workplace closures*

Workplace closures present particularly difficult ethical issues, as workplaces are vital to the livelihoods of employers and employees, and their closure can cause severe financial hardship. Closure of workplaces sparked protests across various states in the US during the COVID-19 pandemic (BBC News, 2020; Bogel-Borroughs and Peters, 2020; Gostin and Berkman, 2007). Where workplace closures are necessary and legally enforced, it is preferable to subsidize lost profits and incomes (Rothstein *et al.*, 2003). For example, Singapore co-paid portions of local workers' wages during its "Circuit Breaker", a suite of significantly stricter islandwide measures and workplace closures to pre-empt escalating infections. These alleviated concerns on impact to livelihood and helped to promote compliance.

The economic impact and resources needed to compensate for lost income or profits for the closure duration can be enormous. Social separation, particularly for long durations, can also cause emotional detachment and disrupt social life (Cachero, 2020; China National Health Commission, 2020b). Other negative lifestyle changes include weight gain, increased appetite, decline in physical activity, and increased screen time and sedentary behaviors. A study examining the impact of COVID-19 isolation measures on lifestyle in Australia found that 24-hour total energy intake in 2020 was 9.5% higher than 2018/2019, and study participants walked less. Such lifestyle changes were actually sustained even after easing of restrictions (Gallo *et al.*, 2020).

Considering the economic and social costs of workplace closures, some countries (mostly in Europe) adopted tactical closures during the pandemic, such as closing only entities that most facilitate transmission and continuing operation of others via telecommuting (Germann *et al.*, 2006; Government of Netherlands, 2020; L&E Global, 2020; Post *et al.*, 2021). Some countries have also attempted less severe forms of school and workplace distancing. In Singapore, for example, before the more widespread availability of PCR testing, doctors were instructed to issue 5 days of stay-home sick leave to patients with respiratory symptoms, and 14-day leave of absence were issued to persons with higher risk of being infectious based on travel history and contact with prior cases.

6.7. "Higher Risk" Settings and Population Groups

Certain settings and population groups are associated with higher infection risk. Increased transmission risk is associated with higher volume of contacts, person-to-person interactions such as singing, speaking loudly, and conversations in close proximity (Leclerc *et al.*, 2020; Prakash, 2020; van Leeuwen *et al.*, 2021); poor sanitation (Tam *et al.*, 2018; United Nations, 1990); inadequate ventilation (Almilaji 2021; Azimi *et al.*, 2021; Morawska *et al.*, 2020); indoor and air-conditioned settings (Leclerc *et al.*, 2020; Lu *et al.*, 2020); and colder settings (Benedetti *et al.*, 2020; Biryukov *et al.*, 2020; CEBM, 2020a, 2020b). Young and middle-aged adults are also likely drivers of transmissibility with longer transmission path lengths, typically spreading the virus across multiple settings. It was also noted that female-to-female transmissions occurred more than male-to-male transmissions, with women shedding more virus over time than men (Harris, 2020; Kim and Jiang, 2020; Lau *et al.*, 2020; Muto *et al.*, 2020). For these reasons, populations contained in high-density accommodation (PCHDA), and places such as schools, choir practice sessions, weddings, gyms, bars, workplace settings involving lengthy meetings, and food processing plants, tend to involve clusters (Leclerc *et al.*, 2020).

Active, highly interactive, and likely asymptomatic or pre-symptomatic individuals who move across multiple disparate "high-risk" settings, are also more likely to become "super spreaders" — who as single cases infect especially large numbers and play a significant role in amplifying transmission. Occupations characterized by "super spreader" elements can therefore fall under "higher risk" population groups.

Some population groups are susceptible because of demographic factors or medical conditions, such as older adults or persons with multiple morbidities and chronic disease risk factors such as smoking, obesity, and poor nutrition.

The identification of risk areas supports targeting of containment efforts. Table 6.2 is an example of a framework that can be applied to support this identification process. Targeted social distancing, mass testing, and bio-surveillance of high-risk groups can improve the prevention of epidemic spread and conserve resources (Cleevely *et al.*, 2020; NUS Saw Swee Hock School of Public Health, 2020e; Public Health England, 2020; Reich *et al.*, 2020). However, social isolation among older adults can also be a serious public health concern because of their heightened risk of other health problems. Isolation can accompany home-based exercise programs and technology-assisted interventions (Armitage and Nellums, 2020b; CEBM, 2020a).

Efforts at identifying risk areas should be continuous, as definitions of higher risk settings and types of individuals can change as the epidemic evolves. In a continuing pandemic situation, targeted containment efforts at specific high-risk groups or settings should also be enforced vigilantly and reviewed regularly with a sensitivity to evolving changes, so that authorities do not get blindsided by unexpected developments. In July 2021, a large cluster in Singapore was traced to karaoke lounges which had not been allowed to reopen since the "Circuit Breaker" more than a year prior. The lounges — which were allowed to pivot to food and beverage only outlets to sustain their livelihoods — had operated illegally with the provision of hostess services or dice games that had evaded detection by enforcement officers (Aravindan and Chen, 2021; Khalik, 2021b).

6.7.1. *Populations contained in high-density accommodation*

The pandemic has seen PCHDAs such worker dormitories, correctional facilities, cruise ships, and military settings — facilitating rapid COVID-19 transmission as a result of mutually reinforcing factors like

Table 6.2. Risk considerations in identifying higher risk settings/individuals.

Settings/Situations/Individuals	Close/Multiple contacts	Ventilation/Enclosed Spaces	Sanitation	Loud/Exertive Communications/High Quality Interactions	Duration of Proximity	People with co-Morbidities	Poor Health-Seeking Behavior	"Hidden"	Cold, Dry Conditions	Young/Active People	Air-con Conditions/Airflow	Others
Populations contained in high-density accommodations	✓	✓	✓	✓	✓	✓	✓	✓				
Unlicensed brothels/rented rooms	✓	✓	✓	✓	✓	✓	✓	✓				
Drug-using networks	✓	✓	✓	✓	✓	✓	✓	✓				
Gangs/triads	✓	✓	✓	✓	✓	✓	✓	✓				
Dating apps	✓	✓			✓			✓				
Disability/eldercare day centers	✓	✓		✓	✓	✓	✓	✓				
Food processing/meat packing facilities	✓	✓		✓	✓				✓			
Distribution centers/warehouses	✓	✓		✓	✓							
Snow city/ice rink	✓	✓		✓	✓				✓	✓		
Swingers club	✓	✓		✓	✓		✓			✓		
Massage parlors	✓	✓			✓							

(Continued)

Table 6.2.　(*Continued*)

Settings/ Situations/ Individuals	Close/ Multiple contacts	Ventilation/ Enclosed Spaces	Sanitation	Loud/Exertive Communications/ High Quality Interactions	Duration of Proximity	People with co-Morbidities	Poor Health-Seeking Behavior	"Hidden"	Cold, Dry Conditions	Young/ Active People	Air-con Conditions/ Airflow	Others
Abattoirs	✓		✓	✓	✓							Mixing with animals
Poorly ventilated and confined shopping areas	✓	✓		✓						✓		
Gyms	✓	✓		✓	✓					✓	✓	
Choir practices	✓			✓	✓							
International schools	✓			✓	✓					✓		Less central control, and risk of imported cases
Call centers	✓	✓		✓	✓						✓	
Offices with open concept sitting and frequent/ more than hour-long meetings	✓	✓		✓	✓						✓	
Delivery workers	✓									✓		Movement across multiple locations/ communities
Cleaners	✓											
Taxi drivers	✓	✓			✓							
Private tutors	✓				✓							
Work-out instructors	✓			✓	✓					✓		

unavoidable close contact, shared facilities, and poor ventilation (Baettig *et al.*, 2021; Liu and Chang, 2020; Morawska *et al.*, 2020; Sloane, 2020). Studies on PCHDAs have recorded infection rates up to 25 times higher than the external community for COVID-19 (Henry, 2020). PCHDAs can become potential epicenters of outbreaks with implications for subsequent spread to the larger community, overwhelming of treatment facilities, crippling of national productivity, and resulting tensions between PCHDAs and society. In the event of an outbreak in a PCHDA, containment is extremely challenging as a result of exponential spread of infection, surge demand for resources, and space constraints — there needs to be buffer space to separate affected individuals (Guthrie *et al.*, 2012; Iglesias Osores, 2020; Jeger *et al.*, 2011; Kakimoto *et al.*, 2020; Lai *et al.*, 2021; Marcus *et al.*, 2020; Matthew *et al.*, 2020; Njuguna *et al.*, 2020).

For these reasons, public health preparedness of PCHDA settings should be part of national epidemic response plans, with the key guiding principles of all-inclusive stakeholder participation, close public health expert guidance or leadership, and the prevention of virus entry as a first principle. If the virus is already in circulation, there should be preparation for resource-intensive containment and for a heavy burden of disease (Akiyama *et al.*, 2020; Guthrie *et al.*, 2012; Iglesias Osores, 2020). As a case in point, preventive measures instituted early in Singapore's foreign worker dormitories may have averted the large clusters that emerged in April 2020 (Chen *et al.*, 2020).

Preventive and containment efforts in PCHDA settings involve surge demand resource planning, improved and organized access to healthcare services, structural interventions for the facilities, and the well-tested methods of contact tracing, isolation, quarantine, and physical distancing, with technical and administrative improvisation in view of the unique spatial constraints. PCHDA outbreaks are also characterized by a high prevalence of asymptomatic and pre-symptomatic cases being identifiable, and so testing with a broad-based and serialized approach is recommended (Arons *et al.*, 2020; Borras-Bermejo *et al.*, 2020; Dahl, 2020; Mizumoto *et al.*, 2020; Njuguna *et al.*, 2020; Sahu and Naqvi, 2020; Wallace *et al.*, 2020).

6.8. Risk Communication and Social Responsibility

Risk communication in use of containment measures is emphasized since misinformation can be rampant in epidemics, leading to substantial public anxiety, reliance on word-of-mouth for knowledge, and purchase of ineffective and expensive products (Rosling and Rosling, 2003; Tambyah and Tay, 2013; WHO, 2018a). General measures such as community hygiene also commonly accompany greater variability in adherence, and public education campaigns can help improve population compliance (Blendon *et al.*, 2006). Guiding principles in the literature have emphasized that public education campaigns should be clear, reassuring, and grounded in scientific evidence (Gostin, 2007; *The Economist*, 2020).

In the early days of the COVID-19 pandemic, many governments prioritized the management of communications. In Taiwan and Singapore, for example, frequent press briefings and public announcements were made by political leaders on outbreak developments and issues such as mask usage and handwashing. Concurrently, efforts are being made to tackle the propagation of misinformation in social media, e.g. WHO's Infodemic initiative (Channel News Asia, 2020a; Hsieh *et al.*, 2020; WHO-China Joint Mission, 2020; WHO, 2020e).

A strong sense of societal social responsibility can also help drive a whole-of-society approach and strengthen the national response (Ölcer *et al.*, 2020; Oosterhoff and Palmer, 2020). In China, the community largely accepted what has been described as "the most ambitious, agile and aggressive disease containment effort in history" from February to May 2020, and fully participated in the management of self-isolation and enhancement of public compliance. Civil society organizations were mobilized, and community volunteers were organized to support response activities and help solve practical difficulties for isolated residents. These contributed to the speed of implementation and efficacy of NPIs in reversing the escalating cases in Hubei and other provinces (WHO–China Joint Mission, 2020). Similarly, the Vietnamese Prime Minister's call to the public in August 2020 to download its national contact-tracing app was met with eager public acceptance and a sharp spike in downloads (An Luong, 2020). Well-coordinated public communications and a shared sense of inclusion can also be mutually reinforcing (Graffigna *et al.*, 2020; Nguyen *et al.*, 2020; Ölcer *et al.*, 2020).

6.9. Use of Technology

The laborious nature of containment measures, and the need for their swift execution, has led to the development and adoption of technologies to support public health processes. These include the integration of databases, collection of real-time location data, use of geofencing technology and AI to facilitate detection and contact tracing, compliance monitoring of community measures, and surveillance of at-risk regions. Examples include integration of Taiwan's National Health Insurance database with its migration and customs databases to facilitate case identification through generation of patient's travel and cluster-related information during clinical visits (Hsieh *et al.*, 2020; Wang *et al.*, 2020a), and China's deployment of AI facial scanning drones to detect non-compliance with mask wearing (Li, 2020).

Protection of privacy and the public's trust is a major step towards widespread uptake of such technologies. An outbreak in gay nightlife establishments in South Korea in May 2020 highlighted the sensitivity surrounding this issue in a country that has been effective using a centralized contact tracing database (Google, 2020; Kim, 2020a). Technologies should also go beyond merely augmenting manual processes. For example, contract tracing systems can transform the traditional interview-based and electronically mediated document-based process to an information systems-based approach. For communities and regions operating from a low digital baseline, an inclusive approach and alternative options should be considered for these populations.

The COVID-19 response has also seen the acceleration of pre-COVID-19 trends towards telemedicine to improve public and geographical access to treatment, triaging of COVID-19 cases, chronic disease management, general preventive screening and specialty services (CNA English News, 2020; Lim, 2020b; Pascoal *et al.*, 2020; Republic of the Philippines, Department of Health, Office of Secretary, 2020; WHO, 2020f). Credentialing issues, reimbursement principles, and pricing references need to be resolved and established to enable smooth continuation of the further digitalization of healthcare.

6.10. Multiple Intervention Strategies

The containment measures addressed in this chapter are not applied separately but must be used together as part of larger multi-intervention strategies. National responses are the deployment of the broad range of NPIs in varying forms of combination and levels of severity. The efficacy of any one measure depends in part on the extent and manner of implementation of other measures. The use of the measures should be flexible and agile to adjust to an evolving pandemic situation. Should the first level of containment fail or leak, measures supporting the next level ought to be strengthened to contain the situation. Maximizing the effectiveness of any one measure may entail costs that are too high to bear, while a combination of less stringent measures may serve the equal purpose more cost-effectively.

At the initial phase of the pandemic, governments of various countries adjusted travel restrictions when the source epidemic extended to autochthonous infections outside of Wuhan city and then mainland China (Russell *et al.*, 2021). When these failed to prevent importation and transmission within borders, several countries went into lockdown with full border closures and extensive general measures (Loewenthal *et al.*, 2020). South Korea — which was able to quickly establish and effect robust testing and contact tracing operations — could contain its epidemic spread with comparatively less stringent physical distancing orders and with its borders kept open with travel restrictions and post-arrival quarantine. On the other hand, Vietnam had comparatively more limited testing capacity but effected control through stricter nationwide movement restriction orders and mandated mask wearing at crowded places (AVIAN, 2020; Dezan Shira & Associates Staff in Vietnam, 2020; Nguyen, 2020; VOA News, 2020).

Various countries have also developed national response systems that coordinate across NPIs of varying forms and combinations of enforcement according to severity levels of epidemiological situation. These systems can help facilitate coordinated decision-making and implementation across measures and regions, and guided the phased lifting of measures from a lockdown situation for countries such as China, Switzerland, Czech Republic, Austria and New Zealand (NUS Saw Swee Hock School of Public Health, 2020c).

6.10.1. *Effectiveness studies*

Several studies have sought to quantify the impact of lockdowns and national responses across countries, and the deployment parameters that influence effectiveness. The studies indicate that combined application of measures yielded the strongest impact, while measures on their own may not reduce Rt sufficiently to less than one (Davies *et al.*, 2020;

Haug *et al.*, 2020; Kucharski *et al.*, 2020; Vokó and Pitter, 2020). Time to effectiveness (peaking and start of reduction of cases) averaged about 8–10 days after measures started for several of the countries studied (Alfano and Ercolano, 2020; Pan *et al.*, 2020; Zou *et al.*, 2020b). Earlier implementation timing was associated with lower mortality, lower Rt, and shorter time to effectiveness. The observation was that seemingly small delays in policy deployment can produce dramatically different health outcomes (Gerli *et al.*, 2020; Koh *et al.*, 2020; Loewenthal *et al.*, 2020; Turbé *et al.*, 2021; Wilasang *et al.*, 2020). A US study noted that regions where stay-at-home mandates were implemented late registered an extra 35 and 38 days before crossing the peak in number of cases and deaths, respectively (Medline *et al.*, 2020; Scullion and Scullion, 2020). Generally, there are also increased benefits, and reduction in infections as the lockdown duration and severity increases (Alfano and Ercolano, 2020; Cano *et al.*, 2020; Hsiang *et al.*, 2020; Hu *et al.*, 2020; Leffler *et al.*, 2020).

A few studies analyzed the comparative effectiveness of the NPIs on the COVID-19 outbreak. Generally, a strategy of detection and contact tracing with subsequent quarantine and isolation yields effective results with less detrimental economic impact than other measures such as blanket social distancing orders. Social distancing measures (including workplace and school closures and stay-home orders) are also effective and can reduce infection rates by up to 60–70 over percent, as well as reduce Rt to less than unity (Backer *et al.*, 2021; Sypsa *et al.*, 2021; Zhang *et al.*, 2020). Evidence on community hygiene measures is less definitive. Border control measures can delay and reduce the impact of local epidemics, and are effective at the earlier phase of an outbreak, but have limited impact over the rest of the course of an infection wave within national borders after community transmission has taken root (Aleta *et al.*, 2020). However, the continuation and management of border controls are important over the course of a prolonged pandemic in the prevention of subsequent waves of infection.

6.10.2. *Exiting from lockdowns*

Premature lifting of interventions may allow subsequent waves. The easing of lockdown measures should be accompanied by continuing community hygiene measures and the ramping up of robust surveillance, testing and contact tracing systems. Some countries (mostly European countries and US) that exited comparatively early from lockdowns *vis-à-vis* others in 2020, and effected less stringent post-lockdown measures, subsequently went on to experience large second waves of infection that necessitated re-entering lockdown towards the end of 2020.

Some countries and regions have also risk-stratified their exit such that vulnerable groups remain protected over a longer period while restrictions are lifted for other groups, avoiding the economic impact of a universal distancing approach. In New York, "Matilda's Law" requires that vulnerable populations stay home, with home visitations limited to immediate family members or close friends who require emergency help and pre-screening of visitors for flu-like symptoms (NY Forward, 2020; Yong, 2020).

Post-exit strategies of universal testing and immunity passports have been explored by policymakers and academics. On mass testing, limitations in test accuracy and the huge resources involved favor a more targeted testing approach of higher at-risk groups. There is hitherto also little scientific evidence on the optimal mass testing strategy (NUS Saw Swee Hock School of Public Health, 2020e). On immunity passports, the need for further validation of serological tests, uncertainty on how long immunity lasts, and ethical implications of discrimination and perverse incentives have slowed its implementation. Some countries such as Chile and Estonia which had earlier announced plans for the "passports" did not eventually proceed with the launch (Brown *et al.*, 2021; Lovelace, 2020).

Policy decisions on NPIs and the multi-intervention strategy undertaken are often driven by considerations of the transmission situation, scientific developments and evidence available, the economy, political concerns, and cultural norms. How well they are executed and their implementational dynamics ultimately depend on the epidemiological, healthcare, cultural and political factors unique to the context of each country.

6.10.3. *Arrival of vaccines*

The arrival of vaccines adds another dimension to the decision-making process. There should be a prioritization plan for vaccines with key principles for decisions on what population groups are most appropriate to vaccinate, in what proportions, and in what order. Beyond this, limitations and variability in the vaccines' efficacy, period of conferred immunity, and uptake, and the initially limited knowledge thereof, means that their arrival should not diminish the emphasis on ongoing containment measures (Miller, 2020; Subbarao, 2020; WHO, 2020g).

As scientific knowledge about the vaccines becomes more established, and national vaccination rates increase, countries can plan the easing of containment measures as higher levels of herd immunity are attained, and the risk of severe disease from COVID-19 and overwhelming hospital services becomes reduced. As per exiting from lockdowns, measures and sectors incurring lower socio-economic costs and yielding better cost-benefit ratios *vis-à-vis* transmission risks from their easing, should be prioritized for lifting and opening up. The pace of doing so, which measures or sectors to ease first, and the degree the easing is balanced against containment, ultimately depend on individual countries, regions and communities, in the contexts of epidemiological stage, healthcare capacity, socio-cultural and political environment, and what is deemed an acceptable extent of severe disease by them (de Courten and Calder, 2021; Khalik, 2021a; Mallapaty, 2021).

For some communities, some containment measures may remain indefinitely. As Singapore neared 70% in national vaccination rate in July 2021, her health minister had indicated that community masking would likely remain well into a COVID-19-endemic world (Sin, 2021). Singapore and UK, both having attained high vaccination rates, had been described to be taking dramatically different approaches to exit containment, in terms of speed and calibration (John and Nectar, 2021). Meanwhile, there are also countries with lower vaccination rates for various reasons such as resource limitations, and different approaches to vaccine risk-benefit evaluation and building population vaccine confidence (Pfortner, 2021), who will necessarily depend on containment measures over a longer time horizon.

6.11. The End of the Beginning

Since the beginning of the pandemic, the world looks increasingly diverse, with countries and regions in varying epidemiological stages of the outbreak, enabled with different response capacity, and attaining different vaccination uptake. The lifting of restrictions between countries will likely be risk-based, between countries with low and similar transmission rates, good surveillance, and transparent reporting. What is certain is the continued importance of NPIs as the pandemic continues to evolve.

The advent of the vaccines will be a major gamechanger in the world's continuing COVID-19 story. The prospective but yet somewhat uncertain ability to finally effectively and safely impart widespread immunity to COVID-19 to a major proportion of our populations (especially the vulnerable and the front-line healthcare workers) will mean that the narrative will change substantially from the end of the tumultuous year of 2020 to new global, national and community situations, for which much will have to stay the same in terms of social interactions and professional practices and much will evolve in potentially very different environments. That script is yet to be written and must await a further edition of this chapter.

Acknowledgments

This chapter draws heavily on the literature and insights in the NUS Saw Swee Hock School of Public Health COVID-19 Science Reports, written together with Ian YH Ang, Sharon HX Tan, Ruth Frances Lewis, Qian Yang, Rowena KS Yap, Bob XY Ng, and Hao Yi Tan.

References

Adekunle A, *et al.* Delaying the COVID-19 epidemic in Australia: Evaluating the effectiveness of international travel bans. *Aust N Z J Public Health* 2020; 44:257–259.

Ahmed W, *et al.* Detection of SARS-CoV-2 RNA in commercial passenger aircraft and cruise ship wastewater: A surveillance tool for assessing the presence of COVID-19 infected travelers. *J Travel Med* 2020; 27:taaa116.

Akiyama MJ, *et al.* Flattening the curve for incarcerated populations — COVID-19 in jails and prisons. *N Engl J Med* 2020; 382:2075–2077.

Aldedort J, *et al.* Non-pharmaceutical public health interventions for pandemic influenza: An evaluation of the evidence base. *BMC Public Health* 2007; 7:208.

Aleta A, *et al.* A data-driven assessment of early travel restrictions related to the spreading of the novel COVID-19 within mainland China. *Chaos Solitons Fractals* 2020; 139:110068.

Alfano V, Ercolano S. The efficacy of lockdown against COVID-19: A cross country panel analysis. *Appl Health Econ Health Policy* 2020; 18:509–517.

Alizon S, *et al.* Rapid spread of the SARS-CoV-2 Delta variant in some French regions, June 2021. *Euro Surveill* 2021; 26:2100573.

Almilaji O. Air recirculation role in the spread of COVID-19 onboard the Diamond Princess cruise ship during a quarantine period. *Aerosol Air Qual Res* 2021; 21:200495.

Amirian ES. Potential fecal transmission of SARS-CoV-2: Current evidence and implications for public health. *Int J Infect Dis* 2020; 95:363–370.

An Luong DN. Vietnam's Coronavirus app Bluezone treads grey line between safety, privacy. *South China Morning Post* 2020; 24 August.

Anderegg L, *et al.* A scalable method of applying heat and humidity for decontamination of N95 respirators during the COVID-19 crisis. *PLoS One* 2020; 15:e0234851.

Anderson C, *et al.* Pooling nasopharyngeal swab specimens to increase testing capacity for SARS-CoV-2. *Med J (Ft Sam Houst Tex)* 2021; (PB 8-21-01/02/03):8–11.

Anderson RM, *et al.* How will country-based mitigation measures influence the course of the COVID-19 epidemic? *Lancet* 2020; 395:931–934.

Ang P. Jurong Fishery Port COVID-19 cluster likely spread from Indonesian or other fishing boats; fish in S'pore still safe to eat: Kenneth Mak. *The Straits Times* 2021; 21 July.

Annas GJ. Your liberty or your life. Talking Point on public health versus civil liberties. *EMBO Rep* 2007; 8:1093–1098.

Aquila I, *et al.* Severe acute respiratory syndrome Coronavirus 2 pandemic. *Arch Pathol Lab Med* 2020; 144:1048–1056.

Aravindan A, Chen L. Singapore races to find guests, hostesses in karaoke lounge virus cluster. *Reuters* 2021; 15 July.

Armitage R, Nellums LB. Considering inequalities in the school closure response to COVID-19. *Lancet Glob Health* 2020a; 8:e644.

Armitage R, Nellums LB. COVID-19 and the consequences of isolating the elderly. *Lancet Public Health* 2020b; 5:e256.

Arons MM, *et al.* Presymptomatic SARS-CoV-2 infections and transmission in a skilled nursing facility. *N Engl J Med* 2020; 382:2081–2090.

Aschwanden D, *et al.* Psychological and behavioural responses to Coronavirus disease 2019: The role of personality. *Eur J Pers* 2020; 10.1002/per.2281.

AVIAN, 2020. Partially Open South Korea. https://www.tripsguard.com/ destination/south-korea/ (accessed 4 December 2020).

Azimi P, *et al.* Mechanistic transmission modeling of COVID-19 on the Diamond Princess cruise ship demonstrates the importance of aerosol transmission. *Proc Natl Acad Sci USA* 2021; 118:e2015482118.

Backer J, *et al.* Incubation period of 2019 novel Coronavirus (2019-nCoV) infections among travellers from Wuhan, China. *Euro Surveill* 2020; 25: 2000062.

Backer JA, *et al.* Impact of physical distancing measures against COVID-19 on contacts and mixing patterns: Repeated cross-sectional surveys, the

Netherlands, 2016-17, April 2020 and June 2020. *Euro Surveill* 2021; 26:2000994.

Baettig SJ, *et al*. Case series of Coronavirus (SARS-CoV-2) in a military recruit school: Clinical, sanitary and logistical implications. *BMJ Mil Health* 2021; 167:251–254.

Balazy A, *et al*. Do N95 respirators provide 95% protection level against airborne viruses, and how adequate are surgical masks? *Am J Infect Control* 2006; 34:51–57.

Barker J, *et al*. Spread and prevention of some common viral infections in community facilities and domestic homes. *J Appl Microbiol* 2001; 91:7–21.

Bayham J, Fenichel EP. Impact of school closures for COVID-19 on the US health-care workforce and net mortality: A modelling study. *Lancet Public Health* 2020; 5:e271–e278.

BBC News. Coronavirus lockdown protest: What's behind the US demonstrations? *BBC News* 2020; 21 April.

Benedetti F, *et al*. Inverse correlation between average monthly high temperatures and COVID-19-related death rates in different geographical areas. *J Transl Med* 2020; 18:251.

Billah MA, *et al*., Reproductive number of Coronavirus: A systematic review and meta-analysis based on global level evidence. *PLoS One* 2020; 15:e0242128.

Bin-Reza F, *et al*. The use of masks and respirators to prevent transmission of influenza: A systematic review of the scientific evidence. *Influenza Other Respir Viruses* 2012; 6:257–267.

Biryukov J, *et al*. Increasing temperature and relative humidity accelerates inactivation of SARS-CoV-2 on surfaces. *mSphere* 2020; 5:e00441–20.

Blendon RJ, *et al*. Attitudes toward the use of quarantine in a public health emergency in four countries. *Health Aff (Millwood)* 2006; 25:w15–w25.

Bloomberg. China sanitises, quarantines millions of bank notes in COVID-19 fight. *New Straits Times* 2020 16 Feb.

Bogel-Borroughs N, Peters J. "You Have to Disobey": Protesters gather to defy stay-at-home orders. *The New York Times* 2020; 20 April.

Borras-Bermejo B, *et al*. Asymptomatic SARS-CoV-2 infection in nursing homes, Barcelona, Spain, April 2020. *Emerg Infect Dis* 2020; 26: 2281–2283.

Bourouiba L. Turbulent gas clouds and respiratory pathogen emissions: Potential implications for reducing transmission of COVID-19. *JAMA* 2020; 323:1837–1838.

Boyd M, *et al*. Protecting an island nation from extreme pandemic threats: Proof-of-concept around border closure as an intervention. *PLoS One* 2017; 12:e0178732.

Brauner JM, *et al*. Inferring the effectiveness of government interventions against COVID-19. *Science* 2021; 371:eabd9338.

Brienen NC, *et al.* The effect of mask use on the spread of influenza during a pandemic. *Risk Anal* 2010; 30:1210–1218.

Brooks SK, *et al.* The psychological impact of quarantine and how to reduce it: Rapid review of the evidence. *Lancet* 2020; 395:912–920.

Brown RCH, *et al.* The scientific and ethical feasibility of immunity passports. *Lancet Infect Dis* 2021; 21:e58–e63.

Business Insider. South Korea is testing 200,000 members of a doomsday church that is the source of more than 60% of its Coronavirus cases. *Business Insider* 2020; 25 February.

Cachero P. Isolated and sequestered in their homes, Chinese citizens report anxiety and depression while on lockdown amid the coronavirs outbreak. *Business Insider US* 2020; 24 February.

Cano OB, *et al.* COVID-19 modelling: The effects of social distancing. *Interdiscip Perspect Infect Dis* 2020; 2020:2041743.

Carnino JM, *et al.* Pretreated household materials carry similar filtration protection against pathogens when compared with surgical masks. *Am J Infect Control* 2020; 48:883–889.

Carter ED. When outbreaks go global: Migration and public health in a time of Zika. *Migration Policy Institute* 2016; 7 July.

Caruso BA, Freeman MC. Shared sanitation and the spread of COVID-19: Risks and next steps. *Lancet Planet Health* 2020; 4:e173.

CDC (Centers for Disease Control and Prevention, USA), 2005. Public Health Guidance for Community-Level Preparedness and Response to Severe Acute Respiratory Syndrome (SARS). https://www.cdc.gov/sars/guidance/index.html (accessed 3 March 2020).

CDC (Centers for Disease Control and Prevention, USA), 2020. History of Quarantine. https://www.cdc.gov/quarantine/historyquarantine.html#:~:text=Ships%20arriving%20in%20Venice%20from,giorni%20which%20mean%2040%20days (accessed 14 January 2021).

CDC (Centers for Disease Control and Prevention, USA), 2020a. When to Quarantine. https://www.cdc.gov/coronavirus/2019-ncov/if-you-are-sick/quarantine.html#:~:text=CDC%20continues%20to%20endorse%20quarantine,and%20update%20recommendations%20as%20needed (accessed 4 December 2020).

CDC (Centers for Disease Control and Prevention, USA), 2020b. Interim Guidance Issued for the Use of Facemasks and Respirators in Public Settings During an Influenza Pandemic. https://www.cdc.gov/media/pressrel/2007/r070503.htm (accessed 12 February 2020).

CDC (Centers for Disease Control and Prevention, USA), 2020c. Interim Guidance: Healthcare Professionals 2019-nCoV: Evaluating and Reporting Persons Under Investigation (PUI). https://www.cdc.gov/coronavirus/2019-nCoV/hcp/clinical-criteria.html (accessed 2 March 2020).

CDC (Centers for Disease Control and Prevention, USA), 2020d. Interim Infection Prevention and Control Recommendations for Patients with Confirmed Coronavirus Disease 2019 (COVID-19) or Persons Under Investigation for COVID-19 in Healthcare Settings. https://www.cdc.gov/coronavirus/2019-ncov/infection-control/control-recommendations.html (accessed 2 March 2020).

CEBM (Centre for Evidence-Based Medicine), 2020a. Oxford COVID-19 Evidence Service. https://www.cebm.net/oxford-covid-19/ (accessed 23 March 2020).

CEBM (Centre for Evidence-Based Medicine), 2020b. Do Weather Conditions Influence the Transmission of the Coronavirus (SARS-CoV-2)? https://www.cebm.net/covid-19/do-weather-conditions-influence-the-transmission-of-the-coronavirus-sars-cov-2/ (accessed 7 June 2020).

Cencetti G, *et al*. 2021. Digital proximity tracing on empirical contact networks for pandemic control. *Nat Commun* 2021; 12:1655.

Chandy PE, *et al*. Interventional radiology and COVID-19: Evidence-based measures to limit transmission. *Diagn Interv Radiol* 2020; 26:236–240.

Channel News Asia. Health Minister orders POFMA correction directions to States Times Review, Facebook over COVID-19 post. *CNA* 2020a; 14 February.

Channel News Asia. Singapore confirms 2 COVID-19 cases linked to new Science Park cluster; 3 more discharged. *CNA* 2020b; 28 February.

Charpentier A, *et al*. COVID-19 pandemic control: Balancing detection policy and lockdown intervention under ICU sustainability. *Math Model Nat Phenom* 2020; 15:57.

Chen JI, *et al*. COVID-19 and Singapore: From early response to circuit breaker. *Ann Acad Med Singapore* 2020; 49:561–572.

Cheng VCC, *et al*. Escalating infection control response to the rapidly evolving epidemiology of the coronavirus disease 2019 (COVID-19) due to SARS-CoV-2 in Hong Kong. *Infect Control Hosp Epidemiol* 2020; 41:493–498.

Chin A, *et al*. Stability of SARS-CoV-2 in different environmental conditions. *Lancet Microbe* 2020a; 1:e10.

Chin ET, *et al*. Projected geographic disparities in healthcare worker absenteeism from COVID-19 school closures and the economic feasibility of child care subsidies: A simulation study. *BMC Med* 2020b; 18:218.

China National Health Commission, 2020a. Chinese Clinical Guidance for COVID-19 Pneumonia Diagnosis and Treatment (7th edition). http://kjfy.meetingchina.org/msite/news/show/cn/3337.html (accessed 14 January 2021).

China National Health Commission, 2020b. Guidelines for Local Authorities to Promote Psychological Crisis Intervention Related to COVID-19. www.nhc.gov.cn/jkj/s3577/202001/6adc08b966594253b2b791be5c3b9467.shtml (accessed 29 February 2020).

Chinazzi M, *et al*. The effect of travel restrictions on the spread of the 2019 novel Coronavirus (COVID-19) outbreak. *Science* 2020; 368:395–400.

Chu DK, *et al*. Physical distancing, face masks, and eye protection to prevent person-to-person transmission of SARS-CoV-2 and COVID-19: A systematic review and meta-analysis. *Lancet* 2020; 395:1973–1987.

Chughtai AA, *et al*. Effectiveness of cloth masks for protection against severe acute respiratory syndrome Coronavirus 2. *Emerg Infect Dis* 2020; 26:e200948.

Cleevely M, *et al*., 2020. A Workable Strategy for COVID-19 Testing: Stratified Periodic Testing rather than Universal Random Testing — Summary. https:// https://www.inet.ox.ac.uk/publications/a-workable-strategy-for-covid-19-testing-stratified-periodic-testing-rather-than-universal-random-testing/ (accessed 15 April 2020).

CNA English News. CORONAVIRUS/Over 3,000 institutions providing tele-medicine for quarantined: NHIA. *Focus Taiwan CNA English News* 2020; 3 July.

Cochrane, 2020. Coronavirus (COVID-19) Resources: Can Travel-related Control Measures Contain the Spread of the COVID-19 Pandemic? https:// www.cochrane.org/CD013717/PUBHLTH_can-travel-related-control-measures-contain-spread-covid-19-pandemic (accessed 14 January 2021).

College of Radiologists, Singapore, 2020. Resource site for Radiology & Imaging. https://www.ams.edu.sg/colleges/radiologists/covid-19-resource-site-for-radiology-imaging (accessed 10 March 2020).

Cook AR, *et al*. Differential household attack rates mirror the ability to control Coronavirus disease 2019 (COVID-19). *Clin Infect Dis* 2021; 72: e1166–e1167.

Costantino V, *et al*. The effectiveness of full and partial travel bans against COVID-19 spread in Australia for travellers from China during and after the epidemic peak in China. *J Travel Med* 2020; 27:taaa081.

Cramer A, *et al*. Assessment of the qualitative fit test and quantitative single-pass filtration efficiency of disposable n95 masks following gamma irradiation. *JAMA Netw Open* 2020; 3:e209961.

Crotty F, *et al*. Nursing homes: The titanic of cruise ships — Will residential aged care facilities survive the COVID-19 pandemic? *Intern Med J* 2020; 50:1033–1036.

Currie DJ, *et al*. Stemming the flow: How much can the Australian smartphone app help to control COVID-19? *Public Health Res Pract* 2020; 30:3022009.

Dahl E. Coronavirus (COVID-19) outbreak on the cruise ship Diamond Princess. *Int Marit Health* 2020; 71:5–8.

Davies A, *et al*. Testing the efficacy of homemade masks: Would they protect in an influenza pandemic? *Disaster Med Public Health Prep* 2013; 7: 413–418.

Davies NG, *et al*. Effects of non-pharmaceutical interventions on COVID-19 cases, deaths, and demand for hospital services in the UK: A modelling study. *Lancet Public Health* 2020; 5:e375–e385.

Davis EL, *et al*., 2020. An imperfect tool: Contact tracing could provide valuable reductions in COVID-19 transmission if good adherence can be achieved and maintained. https://www.ndm.ox.ac.uk/publications/1113028 (accessed 12 June 2020).

Day T, *et al*. When is quarantine a useful control strategy for emerging infectious diseases? *Am J Epidemiol* 2006; 163:479–485.

de Araujo ESA, *et al*. Teach, and teach and teach: Does the average citizen use masks correctly during daily activities? Results from an observational study with more than 12,000 participants. *medRxiv* 2020; 2020.06.25.20139907.

de Courten M, Calder RV. We probably can't eliminate COVID in Australia forever. As we vaccinate, we should move to a more sustainable strategy. *The Conversation* 2021; 7 July.

De Salazar PM, *et al*., 2020. Using Predicted Imports of 2019-nCoV Cases to Determine Locations that may not be Identifying all Imported Cases. https://dash.harvard.edu/handle/1/42639518 (accessed 4 December 2020).

Dezan Shira & Associates Staff in Vietnam, 2020. Vietnam Business Operations and the Coronavirus: Updates. https://www.vietnam-briefing.com/news/vietnam-business-operations-and-the-coronavirus-updates.html/ (accessed 4 December 2020).

Dickens BL, *et al*. Strategies at points of entry to reduce importation risk of COVID-19 cases and reopen travel. *J Travel Med* 2020a; 27:taaa141.

Dickens BL, *et al*. Institutional, not home-based, isolation could contain the COVID-19 outbreak. *Lancet* 2020b; 395:1541–1542.

Doung-Ngern P, *et al*. Case-control study of use of personal protective measures and risk for SARS-CoV 2 infection, Thailand. *Emerg Infect Dis* 2020; 26:2607–2616.

Dunne CP, *et al*. 2020. COVID-19: Is it Reasonable to Ask Retired Doctors to Return to "Duty". https://blogs.bmj.com/bmj/2020/03/05/covid-19-is-it-reasonable-to-ask-retired-doctors-to-return-to-duty/ (accessed 5 March 2020).

Eberhardt JN, *et al*. Multi-Stage group testing improves efficiency of large-scale COVID-19 screening. *J Clin Virol* 2020; 128:104382.

Ekong I, *et al*. COVID-19 mobile positioning data contact tracing and patient privacy regulations: Exploratory search of global response strategies and the use of digital tools in Nigeria. *JMIR Mhealth Uhealth* 2020; 8:e19139.

Farrell M, *et al*. Influenza risk management: Lessons learned from an A(H1N1) pdm09 outbreak investigation in an operational military setting. *PLoS One* 2013; 8:e68639.

Ferretti L, *et al*. Quantifying SARS-CoV-2 transmission suggests epidemic control with digital contact tracing. *Science* 2020; 368:eabb6936.

Fiore VG, *et al*. Containment of COVID-19: Simulating the impact of different policies and testing capacities for contact tracing, testing, and isolation. *PLoS One* 2021; 16:e0247614.

Fong MW, *et al*. Nonpharmaceutical measures for pandemic influenza in non-healthcare settings — Social distancing measures. *Emerg Infect Dis* 2020; 26:976–984.

Fraser C, Riley S, Anderson RM, Ferguson NM. Factors that make an infectious disease outbreak controllable. *Proc Natl Acad Sci USA* 2004; 101: 6146–6151.

Frieden TR, Lee CT. Identifying and interrupting superspreading events — Implications for control of severe acute respiratory syndrome Coronavirus 2. *Emerg Infect Dis* 2020; 26:1059–1066.

Gallo LA, *et al*. The impact of isolation measures due to COVID-19 on energy intake and physical activity levels in Australian University students. *Nutrients* 2020; 12:1865.

Gandhi M, *et al*. Asymptomatic transmission, the Achilles' heel of current strategies to control COVID-19. *N Engl J Med* 2020; 382:2158–2160.

García de Abajo FJ, *et al*. Back to normal: An old physics route to reduce SARS-CoV-2 transmission in indoor spaces. *ACS Nano* 2020; 14: 7704–7713.

Gerli AG, *et al*. COVID-19 mortality rates in the European Union, Switzerland, and the UK: Effect of timeliness, lockdown rigidity, and population density. *Minerva Med* 2020; 111:308–314.

Germann TC, *et al*. Mitigation strategies for pandemic influenza in the United States. *Proc Natl Acad Sci USA* 2006; 103:5935–5940.

Gharpure R, *et al*. Knowledge and practices regarding safe household cleaning and disinfection for COVID-19 prevention — United States, May 2020. *MMWR Morb Mortal Wkly Rep* 2020; 69:705–709.

Giri B, *et al*. Review of analytical performance of COVID-19 detection methods. *Anal Bioanal Chem* 2021; 413:35–48.

Google. Apple and Google partner on COVID-19 contact tracing technology. Google The Keyword 2020; 10 April.

Gostin LO. *Public Health Law: Power, Duty, Restraint* (2nd edn.). Milbank Memorial Fund and University of California Press, New York and Berkeley, 2007.

Gostin LO, Berkman BE. *Preparing for Pandemic Influenza: Legal and Ethical Challenges*. National Academies Press (US), Washington (DC), 2007.

Gostin LO, Hodge JG. US emergency legal responses to novel Coronavirus: Balancing public health and civil liberties. *JAMA* 2020; 323:1131–1132.

Government of Netherlands, 2020. Partial Lockdown to Continue. https://www.government.nl/latest/news/2020/11/17/partial-lockdown-to-continue (accessed 4 December 2020).

Graffigna G, *et al.* Measuring Italian citizens' engagement in the first wave of the COVID-19 pandemic containment measures: A cross-sectional study. *PLoS One* 2020; 15:e0238613.

Guan WJ, *et al.* Clinical characteristics of Coronavirus disease 2019 in China. *N Engl J Med* 2020; 382:1708–1720.

Guo M, 2020. Coronavirus Detected on Doorknob in S. China's Guangzhou. https://news.cgtn.com/news/2020-02-03/Coronavirus-detected-on-doorknob-in-S-China-s-Guangzhou-NMua1LcOWY/index.html (accessed 3 February 2020).

Guo S, *et al.* Mitigation interventions in the United States: An exploratory investigation of determinants and impacts. *Res Soc Work Pract* 2021; 31:26–41.

Gupta M, *et al.* The use of facemasks by the general population to prevent transmission of COVID 19 infection: A systematic review. *medRxiv* 2020; 2020.05.01.20087064.

Guthrie JA, *et al.* Influenza control can be achieved in a custodial setting: Pandemic (H1N1) 2009 and 2011 in an Australian prison. *Public Health* 2012; 126:1032–1037.

Ha JF. The COVID-19 pandemic, personal protective equipment and respirator: A narrative review. *Int J Clin Pract* 2020; 74:e13578.

Hafstad V. Antibody Testing Begins in Iceland. *Iceland Monitor* 2020; 12 May.

Hagen A, 2021. How Dangerous is the Delta Variant (B.1.617.2)? https://asm.org/Articles/2021/July/How-Dangerous-is-the-Delta-Variant-B-1-617-2 (accessed 30 July 2021).

Harris JE. Data from the COVID-19 epidemic in Florida suggest that younger cohorts have been transmitting their infections to less socially mobile older adults. *Rev Econ Househ* 2020; Aug 22:1–19.

Hastings DL, *et al.* Mycoplasma pneumoniae outbreak in a long-term care facility — Nebraska, 2014. *MMWR — Morb Mortal Wkly Rep* 2015; 64:296–299.

Haug N, *et al.* Ranking the effectiveness of worldwide COVID-19 government interventions. *Nat Hum Behav* 2020; 4:1303–1312.

He S, *et al.* Analysis of risk perceptions and related factors concerning COVID-19 epidemic in Chongqing, China. *J Community Health* 2021; 46:278–285.

He X, *et al.* Temporal dynamics in viral shedding and transmissibility of COVID-19. *Nat Med* 2020; 26:672–675.

Heijmans PJ, Bloomberg. Singapore's Coronavirus response has contained the outbreak — But its strategy is hard to replicate. *Fortune* 2020, 28 February.

Henry BF. Social distancing and incarceration: Policy and management strategies to reduce COVID-19 transmission and promote health equity through decarceration. *Health Educ Behav* 2020; 47:536–539.

Heyman D, 2005. Model Operational Guidelines for Disease Exposure Control. Center for Strategic & International Studies (CSIS). http://citeseerx.ist.psu.

edu/viewdoc/download?doi=10.1.1.357.2252&rep=rep1&type=pdf (accessed 3 March 2020).

Hinch R, *et al*, 2020. Effective Configurations of a Digital Contact Tracing App: A report to NHSX. https://cdn.theconversation.com/static_files/files/1009/Report_-_Effective_App_Configurations.pdf?1587531217 (accessed 12 June 2020).

Hoang MV. Fighting against COVID-19 in Vietnam: The value of rapid antibody testing should not be confused. *Health Promot Perspect* 2020; 10:168.

Hollingsworth TD, *et al*. Will travel restrictions control the international spread of pandemic influenza? *Nat Med* 2006; 12:497–499.

Houghton C, *et al*. Barriers and facilitators to healthcare workers' adherence with infection prevention and control (IPC) guidelines for respiratory infectious diseases: A rapid qualitative evidence synthesis. *Cochrane Database Syst Rev* 2020; 4:CD013582.

Hsiang S, *et al*. The effect of large-scale anti-contagion policies on the COVID-19 pandemic. *Nature* 2020; 584:262–267.

Hsieh CC, *et al*. The outcome and implications of public precautionary measures in Taiwan — Declining respiratory disease cases in the COVID-19 pandemic. *Int J Environ Res Public Health* 2020; 17:4877.

Hsieh YH, *et al*. Impact of quarantine on the 2003 SARS outbreak: A retrospective modeling study. *J Theor Biol* 2007; 244:729–736.

Hu Z, *et al*. Evaluating the effect of public health intervention on the global-wide spread trajectory of COVID-19. *medRxiv* 2020; 2020.03.11.20033639.

Huang L, *et al*. Rapid asymptomatic transmission of COVID-19 during the incubation period demonstrating strong infectivity in a cluster of youngsters aged 16–23 years outside Wuhan and characteristics of young patients with COVID-19: A prospective contact-tracing study. *J Infect* 2020a; 80:e1–e13.

Huang Y, *et al*. Measures undertaken in China to avoid COVID-19 infection: Internet-based, cross-sectional survey study. *J Med Internet Res* 2020b; 22:e18718.

Huynh TLD. The COVID-19 risk perception: A survey on socioeconomics and media attention. *Econ Bull* 2020; 40:758–764.

Iannone P, *et al*. The need of health policy perspective to protect Healthcare Workers during COVID-19 pandemic. A GRADE rapid review on the N95 respirators effectiveness. *PLoS One* 2020; 15:e0234025.

Ibáñez-Cervantes G, *et al*. Disinfection of N95 masks artificially contaminated with SARS-CoV-2 and ESKAPE bacteria using hydrogen peroxide plasma: Impact on the reutilization of disposable devices. *Am J Infect Control* 2020; 48:1037–1041.

ICAO (International Civil Aviation Organization), 2020. Manual on Testing and Cross-border Risk Management Measures.

Iglesias Osores S. Transmission and prevention of SARS-CoV-2 (COVID-19) in prisons. *Rev Esp Sanid Penit* 2020; 22:87–90.

James A, *et al*. Successful contact tracing systems for COVID-19 rely on effective quarantine and isolation. *PLoS One* 2021; 16:e0252499.

Jang WM, *et al*. Social distancing and transmission-reducing practices during the 2019 Coronavirus disease and 2015 Middle East respiratory syndrome Coronavirus outbreaks in Korea. *J Korean Med Sci* 2020; 35:e220.

Jefferson T, *et al*. Physical interventions to interrupt or reduce the spread of respiratory viruses: Systematic review. *BMJ* 2009; 339:b3675.

Jeger V, *et al*. H1N1 outbreak in a Swiss military boot camp — Observations and suggestions. *Swiss Med Wkly* 2011; 141:w13307.

Jiang AB, *et al*. Significantly longer COVID-19 incubation times for the elderly, from a case study of 136 patients throughout China. *medRxiv* 2020; 2020.04.14.20065896.

Jin YH, *et al*. Perceived infection transmission routes, infection control practices, psychosocial changes, and management of COVID-19 infected healthcare workers in a tertiary acute care hospital in Wuhan: A cross-sectional survey. *Mil Med Res* 2020; 7:24.

John T, Nectar G. Singapore and the UK are both planning to "live with Covid". They are worlds apart on how to do that. *CNN* 2021; 17 July.

Jones NK, *et al*. Effective control of SARS-CoV-2 transmission between healthcare workers during a period of diminished community prevalence of COVID-19. *Elife* 2020; 9:e59391.

Kakimoto K, *et al*. Initial investigation of transmission of COVID-19 among crew members during quarantine of a cruise ship — Yokohama, Japan, February 2020. *MMWR Morb Mortal Wkly Rep* 2020; 69:312–313.

Kampf G, *et al*. Persistence of Coronaviruses on inanimate surfaces and their inactivation with biocidal agents. *J Hosp Infect* 2020; 104:246–251.

Katul GG, *et al*. Global convergence of COVID-19 basic reproduction number and estimation from early-time SIR dynamics. *PLoS One* 2020; 15:e0239800.

Keeling MJ, *et al*. Efficacy of contact tracing for the containment of the 2019 novel Coronavirus (COVID-19). *J Epidemiol Community Health* 2020; 74:861–866.

Kenyon C. Flattening-the-curve associated with reduced COVID-19 case fatality rates — An ecological analysis of 65 countries. *J Infect* 2020; 81:e98–e99.

Khalik S. Moving from COVID-19 pandemic to endemic: Singapore's strategy and how it can unfold. *The Straits Times* 2021a; 3 July.

Khalik S. Spike in COVID-19 cases raises disturbing questions, but also carries lessons for Singapore. *The Straits Times* 2021b; 19 July.

Kim MJ. Tracing South Korea's latest virus outbreak shoves LGBTQ community into unwelcome spotlight. *The Washington Post* 2020a; 11 May.

Kim MN. What type of face mask is appropriate for everyone-mask-wearing policy amidst COVID-19 pandemic? *J Korean Med Sci* 2020b; 35:e186.

Kim Y, Jiang X. Evolving transmission network dynamics of COVID-19 cluster infections in South Korea: A descriptive study. *medRxiv* 2020; 2020.05.07.20091769.

Klompas M *et al.* Universal masking in hospitals in the COVID-19 era. *N Engl J Med* 2020; 382:e63.

Koh WC *et al.* Estimating the impact of physical distancing measures in containing COVID-19: An empirical analysis. *Int J Infect Dis* 2020; 100:42–49.

Korea Centers for Disease Control and Prevention, 2020. Findings from Investigation and Analysis of Re-Positive Cases. https://www.cdc.go.kr/board/board.es?mid=a30402000000&bid=0030&act=view&list_no=367267&nPage=1 (accessed 3 June 2020).

Korevaar HM *et al.* Quantifying the impact of US state non-pharmaceutical interventions on COVID-19 transmission. *medRxiv* 2020; 2020.06.30.20142877.

Kucharski AJ *et al.* Effectiveness of isolation, testing, contact tracing, and physical distancing on reducing transmission of SARS-CoV-2 in different settings: A mathematical modelling study. *Lancet Infect Dis* 2020; 20:1151–1160.

L&E Global, 2020. Germany: Latest Developments in German Employment Law with Regard to COVID-19, Minimum Wage and Mobile Work. https://knowledge.leglobal.org/germany-latest-developments-in-german-employment-law-with-regard-to-covid-19-minimum-wage-and-mobile-work/ (accessed 4 December 2020).

Lai CC *et al.* The Bayesian susceptible-exposed-infected-recovered model for the outbreak of COVID-19 on the Diamond Princess cruise ship. *Stoch Environ Res Risk Assess* 2021 Jan 26; 35:1–15.

Lai THT *et al.* Stepping up infection control measures in ophthalmology during the novel Coronavirus outbreak: An experience from Hong Kong. *Graefes Arch Clin Exp Ophthalmol* 2020; 258:1049–1055.

Lau MSY *et al.* Characterizing superspreading events and age-specific infectiousness of SARS-CoV-2 transmission in Georgia, USA. *Proc Natl Acad Sci USA* 2020; 117:22430–22435.

Leclerc QJ *et al.* What settings have been linked to SARS-CoV-2 transmission clusters? *Wellcome Open Res* 2020; 5:83.

Leffler CT *et al.* Association of country-wide Coronavirus mortality with demographics, testing, lockdowns, and public wearing of masks. *Am J Trop Med Hyg* 2020; 103:2400–2411.

Li J. China's facial-recognition giant says it can crack masked faces during the Coronavirus. *QUARTZ* 2020; 18 February.

Li B *et al.* Viral infection and transmission in a large well-traced outbreak caused by the Delta SARS-CoV-2 variant. *medRxiv* 2021; 2021.07.07.21260122.

Li ML *et al*. Forecasting COVID-19 and analyzing the effect of government interventions. *medRxiv* 2020; 2020.06.23.252+42356-53*345620138693.

Liebig J *et al*. The current state of COVID-19 in Australia: Importation and spread. *medRxiv* 2020; 2020.03.25.20043877.

Lim J. Singapore's Experience — COVID-19. https://sph.nus.edu.sg/2020/03/singapores-experience-tackling-covid-19/; 2020a. (accessed 24 March 2020).

Lim J. Coronavirus: More doctors attending to patients through video call. *The Straits Times* 2020b; 4 May.

Linton NM *et al*. Incubation period and other epidemiological characteristics of 2019 novel Coronavirus infections with right truncation: A statistical analysis of publicly available case data. *J Clin Med* 2020; 9:538.

Liu X, Chang YC. An emergency responding mechanism for cruise epidemic prevention — Taking COVID-19 as an example. *Mar Policy* 2020; 119: 104093.

Liu Y, Rocklöv J. The reproductive number of the Delta variant of SARS-CoV-2 is far higher compared to the ancestral SARS-CoV-2 virus. *J Travel Med* 2021; 28:taab124.

Liu F *et al*. Using the contact network model and Metropolis-Hastings sampling to reconstruct the COVID-19 spread on the "Diamond Princess". *Sci Bull (Beijing)* 2020a; 65:1297–1305.

Liu M *et al*. Use of personal protective equipment against Coronavirus disease 2019 by healthcare professionals in Wuhan, China: Cross sectional study. *BMJ* 2020b; 369:m2195.

Liu Y *et al*. Aerodynamic analysis of SARS-CoV-2 in two Wuhan hospitals. *Nature* 2020c; 582:557–560.

Loewenthal G *et al*. COVID-19 pandemic-related lockdown: Response time is more important than its strictness. *EMBO Mol Med* 2020; 12:e13171.

Long Y *et al*. Effectiveness of N95 respirators versus surgical masks against influenza: A systematic review and meta-analysis. *J Evid Based Med* 2020; 13:93–101.

Lovelace B, 2020. WHO doesn't recommend Coronavirus passports because immunity remains questionable. *CNBC* 2020; 16 September.

Lu J *et al*. COVID-19 outbreak associated with air conditioning in restaurant, Guangzhou, China, 2020. *Emerg Infect Dis* 2020; 26:1628–1631.

Lum LH *et al*. Pandemic preparedness: Nationally-led simulation to test hospital systems. *Ann Acad Med Singapore* 2016; 45:332–337.

MacIntyre CR *et al*. A cluster randomized clinical trial comparing fit-tested and non-fit-tested N95 respirators to medical masks to prevent respiratory virus infection in health care workers. *Influenza Other Respir Viruses* 2011; 5:170–179.

MacIntyre CR *et al*. A randomized clinical trial of three options for N95 respirators and medical masks in health workers. *Am J Respir Crit Care Med* 2013; 187:960–966.

Makison Booth C *et al*. Effectiveness of surgical masks against influenza bio-aerosols. *J Hosp Infect* 2013; 84:22–26.

Mallapaty S. How many COVID deaths are acceptable in a post-pandemic world? *Nature* 2021; 593:326–327.

Mangosing F. PH gov't, private sector in rush to build field hospitals for COVID-19 cases. *INQUIRER.NET* 2020; 13 April.

Mantlo EK *et al*. Luminore coppertouch surface coating effectively inactivates SARS-CoV-2, Ebola Virus, and Marburg virus *in vitro*. *Antimicrob Agents Chemother* 2021; 65:e0139020.

Marchand-Senécal X *et al*. Diagnosis and management of first case of COVID-19 in Canada: Lessons applied from SARS-CoV-1. *Clin Infect Dis* 2020; 71:2207–2210.

Marcus JE *et al*. COVID-19 monitoring and response among U.S. Air Force Basic military trainees — Texas, March–April 2020. *MMWR Morb Mortal Wkly Rep* 2020; 69:685–688.

Markovits D. Quarantines and distributive justice. *J Law Med Ethics* 2005; 33:323–344.

Marshall DL *et al*. Sentinel Coronavirus environmental monitoring can contribute to detecting asymptomatic SARS-CoV-2 virus spreaders and can verify effectiveness of workplace COVID-19 controls. *Microb Risk Anal* 2020; 16:100137.

McDonald LC *et al*. SARS in healthcare facilities, Toronto and Taiwan. *Emerg Infect Dis* 2004; 10:777–781.

Medline A *et al*. Evaluating the impact of stay-at-home orders on the time to reach the peak burden of COVID-19 cases and deaths: Does timing matter? *BMC Public Health* 2020; 20:1750.

Meng L *et al*. Coronavirus disease 2019 (COVID-19): Emerging and future challenges for dental and oral medicine. *J Dent Res* 2020; 99:481–487.

Miller AM. WHO: Herd immunity is a long way off stopping COVID-19. *World Economic Forum* 2020; 21 August.

Milne GJ, Xie S. The effectiveness of social distancing in mitigating COVID-19 spread: A modelling analysis. *medRxiv* 2020; 2020.03.20.20040055.

MOH (Ministry of Health), Singapore, 2020a. Revised Discharge Criteria for COVID-19 Patients (accessed 28 May 2020).

MOH (Ministry of Health), Singapore, 2020b. MOH Circular 54A/2020: Revision of Suspect Case Definition for Coronavirus Disease 2019 (COVID-19) (accessed 23 February 2020).

MOH (Ministry of Health), Singapore, 2020c. MOH Circular: Availability of COVID-19 serology testing for determination of previous COVID-19 infection in the outpatient setting.

Ministry of Manpower, Singapore, 2020. Measures to Contain the COVID-19 Outbreak in Migrant Worker Dormitories. https://www.mom.gov.sg/newsroom/press-releases/2020/1214-measures-to-contain-the-covid-19-outbreak-in-migrant-worker-dormitories (accessed 20 January 2021).

Mitze T *et al*. Face masks considerably reduce COVID-19 cases in Germany. *Proc Natl Acad Sci USA* 2020; 117:32293–32301.

Miyamae Y *et al*. Duration of viral shedding in asymptomatic or mild cases of novel Coronavirus disease 2019 (COVID-19) from a cruise ship: A single-hospital experience in Tokyo, Japan. *Int J Infect Dis* 2020; 97:293–295.

Mizumoto K *et al*. Estimating the asymptomatic proportion of Coronavirus disease 2019 (COVID-19) cases on board the Diamond Princess cruise ship, Yokohama, Japan, 2020. *Euro Surveill* 2020; 25:2000180.

Moberly T. COVID-19: school closures and bans on mass gatherings will need to be considered, says England's CMO. *BMJ* 2020; 368:m806.

Moghadas SM *et al*. The implications of silent transmission for the control of COVID-19 outbreaks. *Proc Natl Acad Sci USA* 2020; 117:17513–17515.

Morawska L *et al*. How can airborne transmission of COVID-19 indoors be minimised? *Environ Int* 2020; 142:105832.

Morgantini LA *et al*. Factors contributing to healthcare professional burnout during the COVID-19 pandemic: A rapid turnaround global survey. *PLoS One* 2020; 15:e0238217.

Moriarty LF *et al*. Public health responses to COVID-19 outbreaks on cruise ships — Worldwide, February-March 2020. *MMWR Morb Mortal Wkly Rep* 2020; 69:347–352.

Mubayi A *et al*. A cost-based comparison of quarantine strategies for new emerging diseases. *Math Biosci Eng* 2010; 7:687–717.

Muto K *et al*. Japanese citizens' behavioral changes and preparedness against COVID-19: An online survey during the early phase of the pandemic. *PLoS One* 2020; 15:e0234292.

NCID, Academy of Medicine Singapore, Chapter of Infectious Disease Physicians, 2020. Position Statement from the National Centre for Infectious Diseases and the Chapter of Infectious Disease Physicians, Academy of Medicine, Singapore. https://www.ams.edu.sg/view-pdf.aspx?file=media%5c5558_fi_168.pdf&ofile=Period+of+Infectivity+Position+Statement (accessed 2 June 2020).

Nelson A *et al*. Environmental detection of severe acute respiratory syndrome Coronavirus 2 (SARS-CoV-2) from medical equipment in long-term care facilities undergoing COVID-19 outbreaks. *Am J Infect Control* 2021; 49:265–268.

Ng Y *et al*. Evaluation of the effectiveness of surveillance and containment measures for the first 100 patients with COVID-19 in Singapore — 2 January–29 February, 2020. *MMWR Morb Mortal Wkly Rep* 2020; 69:307–311.

Nguyen M. Vietnam's war against COVID-19. *The Diplomat* 2020; 19 October.

Nguyen NPT *et al*. Preventive behavior of Vietnamese people in response to the COVID-19 pandemic. *PLoS One* 2020; 15:e0238830.

Niehus R *et al.* Quantifying bias of COVID-19 prevalence and severity estimates in Wuhan, China that depend on reported cases in international travelers. *medRxiv* 2020; 2020.02.13.20022707.

NIOSH (The National Institute for Occupational Safety and Health), 2018. Recommended Guidance for Extended Use and Limited Reuse of N95 Filtering Facepiece Respirators in Healthcare Settings. https://www.cdc.gov/niosh/topics/hcwcontrols/recommendedguidanceextuse.html (accessed 10 March 2020).

Nishiura H *et al.* Quarantine for pandemic influenza control at the borders of small island nations. *BMC Infect Dis* 2009; 9:27.

Njuguna H *et al.* Serial laboratory testing for SARS-CoV-2 infection among incarcerated and detained persons in a correctional and detention facility — Louisiana, April-May 2020. *MMWR — Morb Mortal Wkly Rep* 2020; 69:836–840.

Nortajuddin A. Cruise Industry Sinking in a Pandemic? *The Asean Post* 2020; 5 November.

NUS Saw Swee Hock School of Public Health, 2020a. COVID-19 Science Report: Containment Measures. https://doi.org/10.25540/pr8t-dzrn (accessed 2 August 2020).

NUS Saw Swee Hock School of Public Health, 2020b. COVID-19 Science Report: Clinical Characteristics. https://doi.org/10.25540/32s7-wc9p (accessed 7 June 2020).

NUS Saw Swee Hock School of Public Health, 2020c. COVID-19 Science Report: Country Journeys. https://doi.org/10.25540/086b-6k94 (accessed 4 December 2020).

NUS Saw Swee Hock School of Public Health, 2020d. COVID-19 Science Report: Diagnostics. https://doi.org/10.25540/e3y2-aqye (accessed 27 July 2020).

NUS Saw Swee Hock School of Public Health, 2020e. COVID-19 Science Report: Exit Strategies. https://doi.org/10.25540/g7z2-sy92 (accessed 5 June 2020).

NY Forward. *A Guide to Reopening New York and Building Back Better.* NY Forward, New York, 2020.

Ölcer S *et al.* Lay perspectives on social distancing and other official recommendations and regulations in the time of COVID-19: A qualitative study of social media posts. *BMC Public Health* 2020; 20:963.

Ong SWX *et al.* Air, surface environmental, and personal protective equipment contamination by severe acute respiratory syndrome Coronavirus 2 (SARS-CoV-2) from a symptomatic patient. *JAMA* 2020; 323:1610–1612.

Ooi PL *et al.* Use of quarantine in the control of SARS in Singapore. *Am J Infect Control* 2005; 33:252–257.

Oosterhoff B, Palmer CA. Attitudes and psychological factors associated with news monitoring, social distancing, disinfecting, and hoarding behaviors among US adolescents during the Coronavirus disease 2019 pandemic. *JAMA Pediatr* 2020; 174:1184–1190.

Pan A *et al.* Association of public health interventions with the epidemiology of the COVID-19 outbreak in Wuhan, China. *JAMA* 2020; 323:1915–1923.

Park M *et al.* A systematic review of COVID-19 epidemiology based on current evidence. *J Clin Med* 2020; 9:967.

Parker MJ, Goldman RD. Paediatric emergency department staff perceptions of infection control measures against severe acute respiratory syndrome. *Emerg Med J* 2006; 23:349–353.

Pascoal FB *et al.*, 2020. The Rise of Telemedicine in Indonesia. https://www.dentons.com/en/insights/articles/2020/july/20/the-rise-of-telemedicine-in-indonesia (accessed 31 January 2021).

Peak CM *et al.* Individual quarantine versus active monitoring of contacts for the mitigation of COVID-19: A modelling study. *Lancet Infect Dis* 2020; 20:1025–1033.

Peeling RW *et al.* Serology testing in the COVID-19 pandemic response. *Lancet Infect Dis* 2020; 20:e245–e249.

Peng X *et al.* Transmission routes of 2019-nCoV and controls in dental practice. *Int J Oral Sci* 2020; 12:9.

Pfortner S. Why Germany is embroiled in a row over vaccinating children against Covid. *Germany's News in English* 2021; 2 August.

Pietsch B. Cash could be spreading the Coronavirus, warns the World Health Organisaton. *The Telegraph* 2020; 5 March.

Port JR *et al.* Increased aerosol transmission for B.1.1.7 (alpha variant) over lineage A variant of SARS-CoV-2. *bioRxiv* 2021; 2021.07.26.453518.

Post RAJ *et al.* How did governmental interventions affect the spread of COVID-19 in European countries? *BMC Public Health* 2021; 21:411.

Prakash M. Eat, Pray, Work: A meta-analysis of COVID19 transmission risk in common activities of work and leisure. *medRxiv* 2020; 2020.05.22.20110726.

Prem K *et al.* Projecting social contact matrices in 152 countries using contact surveys and demographic data. *PLoS Comput Biol* 2017; 13:e1005697.

Public Health England, 2016. Infection Control Precaution to Minimize Transmission of Acute Respiratory Tract Infections in Healthcare Settings. https://assets.publishing.service.gov.uk/government/uploads/system/uploads/attachment_data/file (accessed 12 February 2020).

Public Health England, 2020. Guidance on Social Distancing for Everyone in the UK. https://www.gov.uk/government/publications/covid-19-guidance-on-social-distancing-and-for-vulnerable-people/guidance-on-social-distancing-for-everyone-in-the-uk-and-protecting-older-people-and-vulnerable-adults (accessed 23 March 2020).

Pulia MS *et al.* Multi-tiered screening and diagnosis strategy for COVID-19: A model for sustainable testing capacity in response to pandemic. *Ann Med* 2020; 52:207–214.

Pullano G *et al.* Evaluating the effect of demographic factors, socioeconomic factors, and risk aversion on mobility during the COVID-19 epidemic in France under lockdown: A population-based study. *Lancet Digit Health* 2020; 2:e638–e649.

Qian G *et al.* COVID-19 transmission within a family cluster by presymptomatic carriers in China. *Clin Infect Dis* 2020; 71:861–862.

Rahman B *et al.* The basic reproduction number of SARS-CoV-2 in Wuhan is about to die out, how about the rest of the World? *Rev Med Virol* 2020; 30:e2111.

Rawlinson S *et al.* COVID-19 pandemic — Let's not forget surfaces. *J Hosp Infect* 2020; 105:790–791.

Reardon S. How the Delta variant achieves its ultrafast spread. *Nature* 2021; July 21.

Reich O *et al.* Modeling COVID-19 on a network: Super-spreaders, testing and containment. *medRxiv* 2020; 2020.04.30.20081828.

Republic of the Philippines, Department of Health, Office of the Secretary, 2020. Department of Health — National Privacy Commission (DOHNPC) Joint Memorandum Circular No. 2020-0001. https://www.privacy.gov.ph/wp-content/uploads/2020/10/DOH-mc2020-0016.pdf (accessed 31 January 2021).

Reuters. South Korea burns, quarantines bank notes as COVID-19 rages. *New Straits Times* 2020; 6 March.

Rocklöv J *et al.* COVID-19 outbreak on the Diamond Princess cruise ship: Estimating the epidemic potential and effectiveness of public health counter-measures. *J Travel Med* 2020; 27:taaa030.

Rosling L, Rosling M. Pneumonia causes panic in Guangdong province. *BMJ* 2003; 326:416.

Rothstein M *et al.*, 2003. Quarantine and Isolation: Lessons Learned from SARS. A Report to the Centers for Disease Control and Prevention. https://biotech.law.lsu.edu/blaw/cdc/SARS_REPORT.pdf (accessed 3 March 2020).

Royal Caribbean International, 2020. Healthy Cruising Panel: Cruising Safely with Royal Caribbean. https://www.royalcaribbean.com/sgp/en/healthy-cruising-panel (accessed 26 September 2020).

Rubin D *et al.* Association of social distancing, population density, and tempera-ture with the instantaneous reproduction number of SARS-CoV-2 in counties across the United States. *JAMA Netw Open* 2020; 3:e2016099.

Russell TW *et al.* Effect of internationally imported cases on internal spread of COVID-19: A mathematical modelling study. *Lancet Public Health* 2021; 6:e12–e20.

Ryu S *et al*. Nonpharmaceutical measures for pandemic influenza in nonhealth-care settings-international travel-related measures. *Emerg Infect Dis* 2020; 26:961-966.

Sahu A, Naqvi WM. Floating countries and corona pandemic: Impact of COVID-19 on stranded cruise ships. *Int J Res Pharm Sci* 2020; 1(11):219–223.

Sawano T *et al*. Limiting spread of COVID-19 from cruise ships: Lessons to be learnt from Japan. *QJM* 2020; 113:309–310.

Scullion F, Scullion G. Testing the effects of the timing of application of preventative procedures against COVID-19: An insight for future measures such as local emergency brakes. *medRxiv* 2020; 2020.06.02.20120352.

Sekizuka T *et al*. Haplotype networks of SARS-CoV-2 infections in the Diamond Princess cruise ship outbreak. *Proc Natl Acad Sci USA* 2020; 117: 20198–20201.

Shakya KM *et al*. Evaluating the efficacy of cloth facemasks in reducing particulate matter exposure. *J Expo Sci Environ Epidemiol* 2017; 27:352–357.

Sim D, Kok X. "Far from out of the woods": How a COVID-19 variant put Singapore back in defensive mode. *South China Morning Post* 2021; 23 May.

Sim SW *et al*. The use of facemasks to prevent respiratory infection: A literature review in the context of the Health Belief Model. *Singapore Med J* 2014; 55:160–167.

Sin Y. Masks to remain key even in COVID-19 new normal: Ong Ye Kung. *The Straits Times* 2021; 1 July.

Sloane PD. Cruise ships, nursing homes, and prisons as COVID-19 epicenters: A "Wicked Problem" with breakthrough solutions? *J Am Med Dir Assoc* 2020; 21:958–961.

Subbarao K. COVID-19 vaccines: Time to talk about the uncertainties. *Nature* 2020; 586:475.

Summan A, Nandi A. Timing of non-pharmaceutical interventions to mitigate COVID-19 transmission and their effects on mobility: A cross-country analysis. *Eur J Health Econ* 2021; 7:1–13.

Sun Y *et al*. Scenarios to manage the demand for N95 respirators for healthcare workers during the COVID-19 pandemic. *Risk Manag Health Policy* 2020; 13:2489–2496.

Sypsa V *et al*. Effects of social distancing measures during the first epidemic wave of severe acute respiratory syndrome infection, Greece. *Emerg Infect Dis* 2021; 27:452–462.

Tam CC *et al*. Epidemiology and transmission of respiratory infections in Thai army recruits: A prospective cohort study. *Am J Trop Med Hyg* 2018; 99:1089–1095.

Tambyah PA, Tay J. The Middle East respiratory syndrome Coronavirus (MERS-CoV) and Singapore. *Ann Acad Med Singapore* 2013; 42:376–378.

Tan A. 550 COVID-19 cases infected with Delta variant detected in Singapore so far. *The Straits Times* 2021; 9 June.

The Economist. The virus is coming. *The Economist* 2020; 27 February.

The Guardian, 2020. Coronavirus live: Coronavirus Outbreak. https://www. theguardian.com/world/live/2020/mar/18/coronavirus-live-news-updates-outbreak-us-states-uk-australia-europe-eu-self-isolation-lockdown-latest-update?page=with:block-5e720aa58f088d7575595a15 (accessed 19 March 2020).

The Novel Coronavirus Pneumonia Emergency Response Epidemiology Team. The epidemiological characteristics of an outbreak of 2019 novel Coronavirus diseases (COVID-19) — China, 2020. *China CDC Wkly* 2020; 2:113–122.

The Royal Caribbean and Norwegian Cruise Line, 2020. Recommendations from the Healthy Sail Panel. https://nclhltdcorp.gcs-web.com/static-files/5492d5db-6745-4b21-b952-49d3639f6e79 (accessed 26 September 2020).

The Straits Times, 2020. Coronavirus: Support offered to Malaysian workers staying in Singapore after lockdown, says Iswaran. *The Straits Times* 2020; 18 March.

Tian H *et al.* An investigation of transmission control measures during the first 50 days of the COVID-19 epidemic in China. *Science* 2020a; 368:638–642.

Tian Y *et al.* Review article: Gastrointestinal features in COVID-19 and the possibility of faecal transmission. *Aliment Pharmacol Ther* 2020b; 51:843–851.

Tindale LC *et al.* Evidence for transmission of COVID-19 prior to symptom onset. *Elife* 2020; 9:e57149.

Today. "In-principle understanding" that M'sian work permit holders can enter S'pore during lockdown: Lawrence Wong. *Today* 2020; 20 March.

Toner E, Waldhorn R, 2020. What US Hospitals Should Do Now to Prepare for a COVID-19 Pandemic. www.centerforhealthsecurity.org/cbn/2020/cbnre-port-02272020.html (accessed 2 March 2020).

Turbé H *et al.* Adaptive time-dependent priors and Bayesian inference to evaluate SARS-CoV-2 public health measures validated on 31 Countries. *Front Public Health* 2021; 8:583401.

UNICEF, 2020. COVID-19 Preparedness and Emergency Response. https://www.unicef.org/media/66371/file/WASH-COVID-19-infection-prevention-and-control-in-households-and-communities-2020.pdf (accessed 4 February 2021).

United Nations, 1990. Basic principles for the treatment of prisoners, Adopted and Proclaimed by General Assembly resolution 45/111. https://www.ohchr.org/en/professionalinterest/pages/basicprinciplestreatmentofprisoners.aspx (accessed 6 April 2020).

UNWTO, 2020. Impact of COVID-19 on Global Tourism made Clear as UNWTO Counts the Cost of Standstill. https://www.unwto.org/news/impact-of-covid-19-on-global-tourism-made-clear-as-unwto-counts-the-cost-of-standstill (accessed 4 December 2020).

US Department of Health and Human Services, 2017. HHS Pandemic Influenza Plan. https://www.cdc.gov/flu/pandemic-resources/pdf/pan-flu-report-2017v2.pdf (accessed 2 March 2020).

van der Sande M *et al*. Professional and home-made face masks reduce exposure to respiratory infections among the general population. *PLoS One* 2008; 3:e2618.

van Doremalen N *et al*. Aerosol and surface stability of SARS-CoV-2 as compared with SARS-CoV-1. *N Engl J Med* 2020; 382:1564–1567.

van Leeuwen E *et al*. Augmenting contact matrices with time-use data for fine-grained intervention modelling of disease dynamics: A modelling analysis. *Stat Methods Med Res* 2021; Sep 1:9622802211037078.

van Wezel RAC *et al*. In hospital verification of non CE-marked respiratory protective devices to ensure safety of healthcare staff during the COVID-19 outbreak. *J Hosp Infect* 2020; 105:447–53.

Vera DM *et al*. Assessing the impact of public health interventions on the transmission of pandemic H1N1 influenza a virus aboard a Peruvian navy ship. *Influenza Other Respir Viruses* 2014; 8:353–359.

Viner RM *et al*. School closure and management practices during Coronavirus outbreaks including COVID-19: A rapid systematic review. *Lancet Child Adolesc Health* 2020; 4:397–404.

VOA News. Vietnam Orders National Isolation After Initial Containment of Coronavirus. VOA News 2020; 31 March.

Vokó Z, Pitter JG. The effect of social distance measures on COVID-19 epidemics in Europe: An interrupted time series analysis. *Geroscience* 2020; 42: 1075–1082.

Wallace M *et al*. Public Health Response to COVID-19 cases in correctional and detention facilities — Louisiana, March-April 2020. *MMWR Morb Mortal Wkly Rep* 2020; 69:594–598.

Wang CJ *et al*. Response to COVID-19 in Taiwan: Big data analytics, new technology, and proactive testing. *JAMA* 2020a; 323:1341–1342.

Wang G *et al*. Mitigate the effects of home confinement on children during the COVID-19 outbreak. *Lancet* 2020b; 395:945–947.

Wang K *et al*. Real-time estimation of the reproduction number of the novel Coronavirus disease (COVID-19) in China in 2020 based on incidence data. *Ann Transl Med* 2020c; 8:689.

Weaver M. Majority of retired NHS staff don't want to return to tackle COVID-19 crisis. *The Guardian* 2020; 4 March.

Webster RK *et al*. How to improve adherence with quarantine: Rapid review of the evidence. *Public Health* 2020; 182:163–169.

Wei WE *et al*. Presymptomatic transmission of SARS-CoV-2 — Singapore, January 23–March 16, 2020. *MMWR — Morb Mortal Wkly Rep* 2020; 69:411–415.

Wells CR *et al*. Impact of international travel and border control measures on the global spread of the novel 2019 Coronavirus outbreak. *Proc Natl Acad Sci USA* 2020; 117:7504–7509.

WHO (World Health Organization), 2005. Avian influenza: Assessing the pandemic threat.

WHO (World Health Organization), 2018a. Managing Epidemics: Key Facts about Major Deadly Diseases. https://www.who.int/emergencies/diseases/managing-epidemics-interactive.pdf?ua=1 (accessed 2 March 2020).

WHO (World Health Organization), 2018b. Influenza (Avian and other zoonotic). https://www.who.int/news-room/fact-sheets/detail/influenza-(avian-and-other-zoonotic (accessed 20 February 2020).

WHO (World Health Organization), 2020a. Coronavirus Disease (COVID-19) Outbreak: Rights, Roles and Responsibilities of Health Workers, Including Key Considerations for Occupational Safety and Health. https://www.who.int/docs/default-source/coronaviruse/who-rights-roles-respon-hw-covid-19.pdf?sfvrsn=bcabd401_0 (accessed 2 March 2020).

WHO (World Health Organization), 2020b. Infection Prevention and Control During Health Care when Novel Coronavirus (nCoV) Infection is Suspected.

WHO (World Health Organization), 2020c. Considerations for Quarantine of Individuals in the Context of Containment for Coronavirus Disease (COVID-19): Interim Guidance.https://www.who.int/publications/i/item/considerations-for-quarantine-of-individuals-in-the-context-of-containment-for-coronavirus-disease-(covid-19) (accessed 9 March 2020).

WHO (World Health Organization), 2020d. Mask use in the Context of COVID-19. https://apps.who.int/iris/bitstream/handle/10665/337199/WHO-2019-nCov-IPC_Masks-2020.5-eng.pdf?sequence=1&isAllowed=y (accessed 4 December 2020).

WHO (World Health Organization), 2020e. Managing the COVID-19 infodemic: Promoting Healthy Behaviours and Mitigating the Harm from Misinformation and Disinformation. https://www.who.int/news/item/23-09-2020-managing-the-covid-19-infodemic-promoting-healthy-behaviours-and-mitigating-the-harm-from-misinformation-and-disinformation (accessed 4 December 2020).

WHO (World Health Organization), 2020f. Innovative Ways to Care for NCD Patients in Thailand in COVID-19 time. https://www.who.int/thailand/news/feature-stories/detail/innovative-ways-to-care-for-ncd-patients-in-thailand-in-covid-19-time (accessed 31 January 2021).

WHO (World Health Organization), 2020g. How are Vaccines Developed? https://www.who.int/news-room/feature-stories/detail/how-are-vaccines-developed (accessed 2 February 2021).

WHO-China Joint Mission, 2020. Report of the WHO-China Joint Mission on Coronavirus Disease 2019 (COVID-19).

Widmer AF, Richner G. Proposal for a EN 149 acceptable reprocessing method for FFP2 respirators in times of severe shortage. *Antimicrob Resist Infect Control* 2020; 9:88.

Wilasang C *et al.* Reduction in effective reproduction number of COVID-19 is higher in countries employing active case detection with prompt isolation. *J Travel Med* 2020; 27:taaa095.

Wölfel R *et al.* Virological assessment of hospitalized patients with COVID-19. *Nature* 2020; 581:465–469.

Wong J *et al.* Preparing for a COVID-19 pandemic: A review of operating room outbreak response measures in a large tertiary hospital in Singapore. *Can J Anaesth* 2020; 67:732–745.

Wu S *et al.* Environmental contamination by SARS-CoV-2 in a designated hospital for Coronavirus disease 2019. *Am J Infect Control* 2020; 48:910–914.

Xia W *et al.* Transmission of corona virus disease 2019 during the incubation period may lead to a quarantine loophole. *medRxiv* 2020; 2020.03.06.20031955.

Xiao J *et al.* Nonpharmaceutical measures for pandemic influenza in nonhealthcare settings — Personal protective and environmental measures. *Emerg Infect Dis* 2020; 26:967–975.

Yan Y *et al.* Do face masks create a false sense of security? A COVID-19 dilemma. *medRxiv* 2020; 2020.05.23.20111302.

Yang L *et al.* Estimation of incubation period and serial interval of COVID-19: analysis of 178 cases and 131 transmission chains in Hubei province, China. *Epidemiol Infect* 2020; 148:e117.

Yang Q *et al.* Saliva TwoStep for rapid detection of asymptomatic SARS-CoV-2 carriers. *Elife* 2021; 10:e65113.

Yong C. Coronavirus: Seniors, vulnerable groups to get own priority shopping hours at NTUC FairPrice, Cold Storage and Giant supermarkets. *The Straits Times* 2020; 24 March.

Yuan HY *et al.* Effectiveness of quarantine measure on transmission dynamics of COVID-19 in Hong Kong. *medRxiv* 2020; 2020.04.09.20059006.

Zhang J *et al.* Changes in contact patterns shape the dynamics of the COVID-19 outbreak in China. *Science* 2020; 368:1481–1486.

Zhao S *et al.* Anesthetic management of patients with COVID 19 infections during emergency procedures. *J Cardiothorac Vasc Anesth* 2020; 34:1125–1131.

Zhejiang University School of Medicine. *Handbook of COVID-19 Prevention.* Zhejiang University, China, 2020.

Zhou J *et al.* Infection of bat and human intestinal organoids by SARS-CoV-2. *Nat Med* 2020; 26:1077–1083.

Zhou J *et al.* Investigating severe acute respiratory syndrome Coronavirus 2 (SARS-CoV-2) surface and air contamination in an acute healthcare setting during the peak of the Coronavirus Disease 2019 (COVID-19) pandemic in London. *Clin Infect Dis* 2021; 73:e1870–e1877.

Zhu CQ *et al.* A COVID-19 case report from asymptomatic contact: Implication for contact isolation and incubation management. *Infect Dis Poverty* 2020; 9:70.

Zlojutro A *et al.* A decision-support framework to optimize border control for global outbreak mitigation. *Sci Rep* 2019; 9:2216.

Zou L *et al.* SARS-CoV-2 viral load in upper respiratory specimens of infected patients. *N Engl J Med* 2020a; 382:1177–1179.

Zou Y *et al.* Outbreak analysis with a logistic growth model shows COVID-19 suppression dynamics in China. *PLoS One* 2020b; 15:e0235247.

https://doi.org/10.1142/9789811254338_0007

Chapter 7

COVID-19 Vaccines: Overview, Efficacy, Safety and Challenges

Poh Lian Lim

National Centre for Infectious Diseases, Tan Tock Seng Hospital, Singapore 308442, Singapore

poh_lian_lim@ttsh.com.sg

Abstract

The rapid and extraordinary development and deployment of Coronavirus disease 2019 (COVID-19) vaccines worldwide represent an unprecedented achievement in the history of vaccine development. This chapter provides an overview of COVID-19 vaccine strategies, platforms, clinical trials, and regulatory frameworks. Vaccine safety, efficacy, herd immunity, and severe acute respiratory syndrome Coronavirus 2 (SARS-CoV-2) variants are also discussed. Real world challenges confronted include the ethics of vaccine allocation, vaccine nationalism, vaccine hesitancy, and vaccine passports.

Keywords: COVID-19 vaccines; vaccine platforms; clinical trials; regulatory frameworks; vaccine safety; vaccine efficacy; herd immunity; SARS-CoV-2 variants; vaccine allocation; vaccine nationalism; vaccine hesitancy; vaccine passports

7.1. Background

The respiratory virus outbreak which evolved into the Coronavirus disease 2019 (COVID-19) pandemic emerged in the news in January 2020. Transmitted primarily through droplets, with some contribution via aerosols and fomites, severe acute respiratory syndrome Coronavirus 2 (SARS-CoV-2) spread rapidly through travel. Although the origins of the virus remain somewhat controversial, and the subject of two World Health Organization (WHO) missions to date, epidemiologic evidence indicates that the 2020 pandemic was initially seeded around the world by travelers from its epicenter in Wuhan, China (WHO, 2021a).

The pandemic has caused unprecedented disruption worldwide, with severe economic, social and personal impact to billions of people. Developing successful vaccines against COVID-19 was therefore an urgent priority for the global scientific, medical and public health communities. However, there was no guarantee of success. For the top three infectious diseases with global impact — HIV/AIDS, tuberculosis and malaria — there are still no truly effective vaccines available, even after decades of research and massive investment of resources. It took over 40 years after pathogen identification to develop a deployable Ebola vaccine. Until now, there are no commercially available vaccines against SARS and Middle East respiratory syndrome (MERS), diseases caused by the two human viruses phylogenetically closest to SARS-CoV-2, despite the emergence of these outbreak pathogens in 2003 and 2012, respectively.

The development of vaccines against COVID-19 — able to be deployed for population-wide vaccinations within 12 months of pathogen discovery — is therefore an extraordinary achievement, and completely unprecedented in the history of vaccine development.

7.2. COVID-19 Immunology and Vaccine Strategies

Virus entry into the body is through the respiratory tract mucosa, utilizing the angiotensin-converting enzyme-2 (ACE2) receptor on bronchial and alveolar epithelial cells. The virus interacts with the ACE2 receptor through its spike (S) protein receptor-binding domain (RBD). Neutralizing antibodies which can protect against experimental infection appear to primarily target the S protein. Individuals infected with SARS-CoV-2 also produce antibody responses to other proteins such as nucleocapsid (N) protein, but anti-N antibodies may not provide protective immunity — so most targeted strategies have focused on the S protein for vaccine development efforts.

The S protein consists of two domains, S1 and S2. The S1 domain contains the RBD, so antibodies to S1 block the virus from binding to the ACE2 receptor, whereas the S2 domain controls membrane fusion; and antibodies to S2 inhibit conformational changes to block membrane fusion (Jeyanathan *et al.*, 2020).

In addition to B-cell-mediated humoral immunity with measurable antibody levels, studies have also shown T-cell immunity in individuals who have recovered from symptomatic and asymptomatic infection (Sekine *et al.*, 2020). T-cell responses have also been elicited by various vaccine candidates, in addition to neutralizing antibody responses. Mucosal immunity in convalescent patients may also play an important role for protective immunity.

Evidence for the duration of protective immunity after natural infection continues to emerge, with current data showing at least 8 months of immunological memory after COVID-19, with distinctly different kinetics to the components represented by circulating antibodies, memory B-cells, memory CD4 cells, and memory CD8 cells (Dan *et al.*, 2021).

7.3. COVID-19 Vaccine Platforms, Clinical Trials, and Regulatory Frameworks

Vaccine development efforts can be grouped broadly into six major vaccine technology platforms:

(a) Inactivated vaccines;
(b) Protein subunit vaccines;
(c) Non-replicating viral vectored vaccines;
(d) Nucleic acid vaccines (mRNA or DNA);
(e) Live attenuated vaccines;
(f) Viral-like particles (VLPs).

The COVID-19 vaccine landscape — consisting of over 76 candidates in clinical evaluation and 182 candidates in pre-clinical development — was summarized by the World Health Organization as of 2 March 2021 (WHO, 2021b). Of the different vaccine platforms, live attenuated vaccines and VLPs have not featured prominently among

COVID-19 vaccine candidates so far. To date, successful vaccines have been developed from the mRNA, viral vectored and inactivated vaccine categories, with RNA vaccines providing the highest vaccine efficacy rates for prevention of symptomatic laboratory-confirmed infections.

The vaccine development process typically consists of pre-clinical studies in cells (*in vitro*) and in animals (*in vivo*) before vaccines can undergo research in human volunteers. Vaccine clinical trials consist of Phase 1–3 studies, the data from which are then submitted for review by health regulators in different countries, in order to obtain regulatory approval, or Emergency Use Authorization (EUA). Typically, the data are also submitted for publication in the medical literature after rigorous peer review.

Below is the overview of the clinical trial process for vaccine development:

(a) Pre-clinical trials: Studies in cells (*in vitro*) or in animals (*in vivo*);
(b) Phase 1: Humans; dose-ranging for safety, small numbers (dozens);
(c) Phase 2: Humans; efficacy and safety at varying doses and intervals, larger (hundreds);
(d) Phase 3: Humans; placebo-controlled, efficacy and safety, very large (thousands);
(e) Phase 4: Post-marketing pharmacovigilance; effectiveness and safety (millions).

In USA, EUA is intended to allow the use of an unregistered product (one that has not yet received full regulatory approval) on the basis of compelling public health needs. It is analogous to the "Expanded Access or Compassionate Use" route for individual patients facing serious or life-threatening diseases to have access to an investigational product or device. This regulatory mechanism may not exist in many countries. For Singapore, a "Pandemic Special Access Route" (PSAR) had to be put in place for the Health Sciences Authority (HSA) to facilitate rigorous but expedited review of data, a rolling data submission process, and authorization of COVID-19 vaccines for use at the direction of the Ministry of Health or MOH (HSA, 2021). The WHO is not a health regulator *per se*, but it has an analogous process of "Emergency Use Listing" (EUL) which is being used for COVID-19 vaccines and serves as a reference point for countries. Regulatory authorities have committed to careful review of

Table 7.1. Summary of COVID-19 vaccines used in mass vaccinations.

Vaccine Platform	Company (Country)	Clinical Trials Status	Regulator Authorization Status
mRNA	Pfizer-BioNTech (USA/Germany)	Phase 1, 2, 3, 4 Phase 3 Published	UK, USA, Singapore WHO EUL
mRNA	Moderna (USA)	Phase 1, 2, 3, 4 Phase 3 Published	USA, UK, Singapore
Adenovirus vectored ChAdOx1	AstraZeneca (UK)	Phase 1, 2, 3, 4 Phase 3 Published	UK WHO EUL
Adenovirus vectored Ad26	Janssen (USA)	Phase 1, 2, 3	USA
Adenovirus vectored Ad26/Ad5	Gamaleya (Russia)	Phase 1, 2, 3 Phase 3 Published	Russia
Adenovirus vectored Ad5	CanSino (China)	Phase 1, 2, 3	China
Inactivated	Sinovac (China)	Phase 1, 2, 3, 4	China
Inactivated	Sinopharm (China)	Phase 1, 2, 3 Phase 3 Published	China
Inactivated	Bharat (India)	Phase 1, 2, 3	India

safety signals and enhanced post-marketing pharmacovigilance, to balance public concerns around EUAs.

As of March 2021, there are at least nine vaccines from three vaccine platforms currently being used in mass vaccinations, having completed Phase 3 clinical trials. These are summarized in Table 7.1, along with their authorization status by selected health regulatory authorities.

Although the speed of vaccine development has caused public anxiety and added to vaccine hesitancy, this astounding achievement was enabled by many factors that came together. Firstly, the pandemic presented a clear and present global threat, which affected health, business, daily life and travel on an unprecedented scale — thus, it mobilized governments and industry to pour resources into developing countermeasures including diagnostics, therapeutics and vaccines. Pharmaceutical companies that would normally wait for successful results from a Phase 1 or Phase 2 trial before planning a Phase 3 trial, plunged into planning all three clinical trial phases in rapid sequence. Countries and companies competed to produce the first effective COVID-19 vaccines. Secondly,

COVID-19 galvanized health authorities with the political will to reduce regulatory hurdles that make normal product licensing a slow and cumbersome process. For example, HSA has expedited rolling submissions of clinical trial data, rather than requiring complete dossiers before review. Thirdly, ongoing high rates of COVID-19 transmission allowed vaccine efficacy data to accrue quickly, and conclusively demonstrate high rates of protection.

7.4. COVID-19 Vaccine Efficacy

In designing clinical trials, the most important decisions are the primary and secondary endpoints for the study. Sample size calculations depend on the endpoint selected. The costs and resources needed for the study, even ease of recruitment depend on how feasible or onerous it is to obtain data for the endpoints selected. The relevance and applicability of the study also depend on whether the endpoints chosen are meaningful and useful in answering clinical needs and public health questions.

The fatality rate for COVID-19 hovers at about 2.2% globally, with more than 4.2 million deaths out of over 200 million cases, as of 6 August 2021 (WHO, 2021c). The clinical spectrum of disease ranges from severe respiratory failure requiring intensive care unit (ICU) admission and ventilator support, to pneumonia, mild upper respiratory infections, and completely asymptomatic persons who can still transmit infection.

Hence, the primary and secondary endpoints selected for Phase 3 studies for vaccine candidates developed by US pharmaceutical companies were decided in consultation with their regulatory authority, the US Food and Drug Administration (FDA). Primary endpoints for vaccine efficacy were reductions in symptomatic, laboratory-confirmed COVID-19 disease, with reductions in severe disease and death as secondary endpoints by specific timepoints after getting vaccinated.

The studies would have been much harder to conduct using asymptomatic infection as an endpoint, and would have required repeatedly testing asymptomatic persons in the midst of a raging pandemic with lockdowns. However, data on vaccine efficacy in reducing asymptomatic infection are needed to inform policy decisions about how vaccination status should be factored into public health interventions such as safe distancing, quarantine and travel restrictions. Hence, those data are now being collected in smaller subsets of ongoing Phase 3 studies.

The fact that there was ongoing transmission of COVID-19 allowed for rapid accrual of infections in the placebo group, as the comparator for COVID-19 vaccines. If vaccines are like an umbrella to protect you from the rain, then you will see how good the protection is only if it is raining hard, and the umbrella keeps you dry. Hence, the vaccine studies had to be conducted in countries where many COVID-19 infections were happening.

Large Phase 3 trials are essential for authorization and licensure because Phase 1 and Phase 2 primarily report on immunogenicity, using measures of humoral and cell-mediated immunity as correlates of protective immunity. Phase 3 studies are the "proof of the pudding" — does vaccination protect you from actual disease? — candidates that performed well in Phase 2 studies may well stumble and fizzle out at Phase 3. Phase 3 results also help validate immunological correlates of protection by seeing if they are consistent with observed vaccine efficacy. If immunogenicity can be used as validated surrogate markers of vaccine efficacy, this will potentially minimize the need for large, resource-intensive trials for later iterations of the same vaccine product.

On 9 November 2020, **Pfizer-BioNTech** announced that its candidate vaccine, BNT162b2, had met the first interim analysis threshold with an evaluable case count of 94 cases of COVID-19, and that the vaccine arm demonstrated over 90% protection by 7 days after the second dose (Pfizer, 2021a). Very shortly thereafter, on 18 November 2020, Pfizer-BioNTech announced that BNT162b2 had met its Phase 3 clinical trial primary endpoint outcomes with 170 cases, 162 of which were in the placebo arm, and 8 in the vaccine arm, yielding a vaccine efficacy rate of 95% against symptomatic, laboratory-confirmed COVID-19 by 28 days after the first dose (Pfizer, 2021b).

Moderna released the pre-specified first interim analysis of its Phase 3 COVE study of mRNA-1273 on 16 November 2020, showing 90 cases in their placebo group, compared to 5 in their vaccinated group, with a similar vaccine efficacy rate of 94.5% (Moderna, 2021a). Its Phase 3 clinical trial results were announced on 30 November 2020, with 185 cases in the placebo group, compared to 11 in the vaccinated group, giving a vaccine efficacy of 94.1%. Of the 30 severe cases, all occurred in the placebo group, and none in the vaccinated group (Moderna, 2021b).

AstraZeneca announced the interim analysis findings for its ChAdOx1 vaccine on 23 November 2020, with an overall efficacy of

70%. One dosing regimen in 2,741 participants (who had inadvertently received a half-dose followed by the full dose 1 month later) showed 90% efficacy, while the remaining 8,895 participants who had received 2 full doses 1 month apart showed 62% efficacy at 14 days after the second dose (AstraZeneca, 2021). Subsequent analysis has shown that a longer interval ($\geq$12 weeks) between standard doses yielded a higher vaccine efficacy of 81%, compared to 55% vaccine efficacy if the second dose was given at a shorter interval of less than 6 weeks (Voysey *et al.*, 2021). However, there was a relative paucity of data for older adults.

Janssen's Phase 3 ENSEMBLE trial interim analysis was announced on 29 January 2021 (NIH, 2021). Utilizing an adenovirus type 26 recombinant vectored vaccine, it was 66% effective in preventing moderate and severe COVID-19 at 28 days after a single dose, with evidence of effectiveness varying by location: 72% in the US, 66% in Latin America, and 57% in South Africa. The analysis examined 468 cases of symptomatic COVID-19 from 44,325 adult volunteers.

Gamaleya published the Phase 3 analysis for its Sputnik V vaccine on 2 February 2021, which utilized a heterologous prime-boost approach with recombinant adenovirus type 26 (rAd26) vectored vaccine, followed by a second dose 21 days later, using recombinant adenovirus type 5 (rAd5). Unlike the other studies, its Phase 3 trial utilized a 3:1 randomization. The study showed 91.6% vaccine efficacy for its primary outcome of PCR-confirmed COVID-19 from day 21 after the first dose, with 16 cases out of the 14,964 in the vaccine group, and 62 cases out of the 4,902 in the placebo group (Logunov *et al.*, 2021).

Sinovac conducted Phase 3 clinical trials in Brazil, Turkey, Indonesia, Chile, utilizing an inactivated vaccine with two doses given 14 days apart. It announced partial Phase 3 results on 5 February 2021 from Brazil and Turkey, with 50% efficacy for all cases from 14 days after completing the second dose, but details were incomplete and data from all sites were not combined (Sinovac, 2021).

Bharat announced on 3 March 2021 the first interim analysis of 43 cases for its Covaxin Phase 3 study with 25,800 participants, with 36 cases from the placebo group, and 7 cases from the vaccinated group, giving an efficacy of 80.6%. Using a 2-dose adjuvanted inactivated virus vaccine given 2 weeks apart, its primary outcome was PCR-confirmed symptomatic COVID-19 at least 14 days after receiving the second dose (Bharat Biotech, 2021).

Vaccine efficacy has been consistent across gender, age-groups and ethnicities for the mRNA vaccines by Pfizer and Moderna (Baden *et al.*, 2021; Polack *et al.*, 2020). Less data is available at this time for some of the other vaccines for different age-groups, especially older adults.

7.5. Variants of Concern and Vaccine Efficacy

Unfortunately, the SARS-CoV-2 virus has continued to mutate. This was a biological and mathematical inevitability, as human infections surge past 200 million and the virus circulated and passaged through person after person. Even as the first doses of the Pfizer-BioNTech vaccine started to be administered in the United Kingdom in early December, variants of concern (VOCs) had begun to emerge.

On 14 December 2020, the UK announced that a new and more readily transmissible VOC, B.1.1.7 or Alpha, had emerged and quickly become the dominant circulating strain (Public Health England, 2021). By January 2021, B.1.1.7 had been detected in over 30 countries, as well as 12 states in USA (Galloway *et al.*, 2021). More VOCs are being reported, the clinical and public health significance of which are still being evaluated. First identified in Brazil, the P1 or Gamma variant (B.1.1.28.1) also carries the N501Y mutation which may increase transmission, and the E484K mutation which may allow immune evasion of antibodies from prior COVID-19 infection. Another VOC, B.1.351 or Beta, first identified in South Africa, also carries similar mutations, including N501Y and E484K (Yuan *et al.*, 2021). First documented in India, the B.1.617.2 or Delta variant was designated a VOC in May 2021 — a highly transmissible variant that became dominant in many parts of the world (Callaway, 2021). Initially reported from South Africa, the B.1.1.529 or Omicron variant was designated a VOC in November 2021 — it has more mutations and greater transmissibility than the Delta variant (Callaway and Ledford, 2021).

It is likely that reinfections may occur more readily with VOCs that carry the E484K and other mutations — indeed, current vaccines (based on the original virus strain) have reduced efficacy rates against variants such as Beta, Gamma, Delta, and Omicron. Countries may have different variants circulating at varying levels, and a VOC can rapidly become the dominant circulating virus strain within 3 months — which occurred in many countries. Furthermore, countries vary in surveillance capabilities to detect emerging VOCs. This will make it much more challenging to assess vaccine efficacy results from Phase 3 trials. Data on vaccine efficacy will become an increasingly complex interaction between vaccine platforms, doses, intervals, as well as circulating variants. Further information is available from the US CDC surveillance of VOC (CDC, 2021).

7.6. COVID-19 Vaccine Safety

Vaccine safety is paramount when undertaking population-wide immunization, because without public trust, vaccination campaigns will fail. Even if a vaccine is extremely effective, serious safety concerns may terminate its usefulness.

The vaccine platforms with which we have had the most experience are the inactivated vaccines, live attenuated vaccines, and protein subunit vaccines. Adenovirus vectored vaccines have been used less often, and until COVID-19, mRNA vaccines had not been used for vaccines against infectious diseases.

When evaluating new vaccines, safety issues to consider include:

(a) **Serious adverse events (SAE)** which may include death, hospitalization, anaphylaxis. Common side-effects such as fever may also be classified as severe if they meet the pre-specified criteria for Grade 3 or Grade 4 in intensity, but severe adverse effects may not necessarily be classified as SAE.
(b) **Adverse events of special interest (AESI)** which are of medical or scientific concern, and linked to specific vaccines or vaccine components. These include a wide range of possible events such as thrombocytopenia, Guillain-Barre syndrome, autoimmune disease, and vaccine-induced enhanced disease. AESI may range from mild to severe, and from immediate to delayed onset.
(c) **Common side-effects** seen with other vaccines as well, such as fever, injection site redness, pain or swelling, headache, myalgia, and fatigue. These can affect vaccine tolerability and may make vaccine recipients less willing to complete the second dose or return for boosters later.

At the outset, stringent regulatory authorities such as the US FDA set out the requirement for a 2-month waiting period after completing the second dose of vaccination, to allow detection of autoimmune and other AESI, most of which would be expected to emerge within 4 to 6 weeks after the vaccine. For vaccines with a 28-day interval between both doses (such as the Moderna mRNA-1273 vaccine), this effectively resulted in a 3-month observation period after receiving the first dose of vaccine before Phase 3 results could be submitted to the regulatory authorities.

The other aspect of safety that is occasionally under-appreciated is the importance of large numbers in detecting rare SAE. To have a reasonable chance of detecting an event that occurs at frequency X, a sample size of at least 3X is needed. If an SAE occurs at a rate of 1 per 10,000 vaccine doses, then a trial randomized 1:1 between vaccine and placebo groups would need to recruit at least 60,000 participants, and evaluate at least 30,000 recipients in the vaccine group in order to have a reasonable chance of detecting an SAE at that frequency. The sample size for most COVID-19 vaccine Phase 3 trials have been 30,000–40,000 participants for vaccine efficacy and safety endpoints, which provides the statistical power to detect SAE occurring at 1 per 5,000 to 1 per 7,000, assuming an equal randomization between vaccine and placebo. However, regulatory authorities recognize that post-marketing pharmacovigilance, after population-wide vaccinations have started, will be required to detect extremely rare SAE at a rate of 1 per 100,000, or even 1 per million.

This has proved true for anaphylaxis reactions to COVID-19 vaccines. Anaphylaxis to influenza vaccination occurs at ~1.3 per million doses. For the Pfizer-BioNTech COVID-19 vaccine, anaphylaxis rates are currently 4.7 per million (~1 per 200,000); while for the Moderna vaccine, anaphylaxis rates are 2.5 per million (~1 per 400,000).

The common side-effects of vaccines — injection site pain/redness/swelling, fever, headache, myalgia, fatigue — generally resolve within 2 to 3 days. Lymphadenopathy in the axilla or neck area have been reported at ~1 per 1,000 to 1 per 100, but resolve spontaneously within 7 to 10 days. Bell's palsy has been reported in both vaccine and placebo recipients, but does not appear to exceed normal baseline rates and fluctuations in data. Similarly, no major safety signals or excess deaths related to vaccine have been detected on rigorous analysis, although deaths have been reported in both placebo and vaccine recipients in vaccine clinical trials, as well as in the population-wide vaccination campaigns.

Vaccine safety has been generally consistent across gender, age-groups and ethnicities, but it should be noted that Asians comprised only 4% of the participants for the Pfizer and Moderna Phase 3 trials. Singapore has reported an anaphylaxis rate of 2.7 per 100,000 doses of Pfizer vaccine (Ministry of Health Singapore, 2021). Anaphylaxis and allergic reactions to the mRNA vaccines appeared to be more common among female and younger individuals, although that remains to be confirmed.

Given that there are less Phase 3 data for various subgroups including medical comorbidities and immune-suppressed individuals, there is less certainty for vaccine efficacy and safety for these groups. Similarly, because recruitment excluded children below 5, the vaccines currently cannot be recommended for this segment of the population until more clinical trial data become available. Safety data will continue to be collected for Phase 3 trial participants for the mRNA vaccines over a period of 2 years. This has become more complex because withholding a highly effective vaccine from the placebo group has become ethically untenable — thus, it may become more challenging to compare vaccine with placebo arms for long-term safety.

7.7. Real World Rollouts

The UK became the first country in the world to authorize the Pfizer-BioNTech vaccine on 2 December 2020. The US FDA authorized the Pfizer-BioNTech vaccine on 11 December 2020, the Moderna vaccine on 18 December 2020, and the Janssen vaccine on 27 February 2021. Singapore became the first country in Asia to authorize the Pfizer-BioNTech vaccine on 14 December 2020, and the Moderna vaccine on 3 February 2021, under the HSA's PSAR framework. The WHO granted EUL status to the Pfizer-BioNTech vaccine on 31 December 2020, and to the AstraZeneca vaccine on 15 February 2021.

The first shipment of the Pfizer-BioNTech vaccines arrived in Singapore on 21 December 2020, and the first doses were administered to 40 healthcare workers at the National Centre for Infectious Diseases (NCID) on 30 December 2020. The first delivery of Moderna vaccines arrived in Singapore on 17 February 2021, 2 weeks after PSAR authorization. Sinovac's first delivery of vaccines arrived in Singapore on 23 February 2021, and were authorized for administration in Singapore under the special access route in June 2021.

Vaccine rollouts in the real world are a function of getting practical details to work together, including cold chain management, supply chain management (shelf-life of vaccines at freezer and refrigerator temperatures, consumables such as needles, syringes), the safe use of multi-dose vials, the logistics of mass vaccinations including safe distancing for the post-vaccination observation period, information management of vaccination data, and surveillance systems for adverse events following immunizations.

For the Pfizer vaccine, requiring ultra-cold freezers at $-70°C$ has been a major challenge, with the short half-life of 5 days at fridge temperatures. Moderna requires only ordinary freezer temperatures of $-20°C$. The AstraZeneca, Janssen and Sinovac vaccines have the advantage of being able to be stored at refrigerator temperatures of 2 to $8°C$.

Table 7.2 summarizes the two main vaccines currently authorized for use in Singapore.

Table 7.2.   Two currently authorized COVID-19 vaccines in Singapore.

Detail	Pfizer-BioNTech	Moderna
Vaccine type	mRNA	mRNA
Vaccine efficacy	95%	94%
Anaphylaxis rate	1 per 200,000	1 per 400,000
Freezer temperatures	$-70°C$	$-20°C$
Shelf-life in fridge (2–8°C)	5 days	30 days
Shelf-life out of fridge (<25°C)	6 hours	12 hours
Vaccine dosage	0.3 mL 30 mcg	0.5 mL 100 mcg
Dilution needed	Yes	No
Gentle mixing	Do not shake vaccine vial	Do not shake vaccine vial
Number of doses per vial (Recipients to schedule)	5 to 6 per vial	10 per vial
Eligibility Contraindications	Persons >5 years old Anaphylaxis, severe reactions	Persons >18 years old Anaphylaxis, severe reactions
Dose #2 Allowable range	Day 21 Day 17–28	Day 28 Day 24–36

7.8. Challenges Ahead

Although proof of concept has now been achieved, many questions remain:

(a) How long does vaccine protection last, and how many boosters will be needed?
(b) How well does each vaccine protect against the various emerging VOCs?
(c) What are the optimal and accepted dosing intervals for validity and protection?
(d) What is the protective efficacy of each vaccine against asymptomatic, symptomatic, severe and fatal COVID-19?
(e) What is the efficacy and safety of each vaccine for specific groups: pregnant women, children, different co-morbidities, immunosuppression, older adults?
(f) What is the efficacy for various heterologous prime-boost vaccine combinations?

Although COVID-19 vaccines have been delivered to populations at scale within a year from pathogen discovery, many daunting challenges remain. The following issues are briefly sketched out as many developments continue to unfold.

7.8.1. *Variants and herd immunity*

The advent of safe and highly effective COVID-19 vaccines has brought real hope — if enough of the human population can achieve herd immunity through vaccination rather than infection, it may be possible to bring this devastating pandemic under control. There are precedents with other respiratory infections; even measles with a basic reproductive number (R0) of 15 was eliminated in many regions through vaccination. For certain SARS-CoV-2 strains with R0 estimated at 3, herd immunity would be achieved if 67% of the population became immune (1–1/R0). With vaccines that have 95% efficacy, it means at least 70% of the population would have to get vaccinated to achieve the herd immunity threshold of 67%.

However, if new variants emerge with N501Y and other mutations that confer higher transmissibility, then a higher proportion of the population would have to be vaccinated in order to achieve herd immunity.

For example, a 33% increase in transmissibility, raising R0 to 4, would therefore raise the herd immunity threshold to 75% — and so on.

On the other hand, there is emerging data that certain mutations (e.g. E484K) confer to variants the ability to evade vaccine immunity, resulting in varying reductions in vaccine efficacy for different vaccine products. If vaccine efficacy is significantly reduced, as emerging data would indicate with several vaccine-variant pairs such as Sinovac-P1 and AstraZeneca-B.1.351, then herd immunity may not achievable, even with very high vaccine coverage rates.

7.8.2. *Ethics of vaccine allocation*

Allocation of the scarce resource of COVID-19 vaccines within countries and between countries has been a major challenge from the standpoint of ethics, equity, and public health impact. Anticipating this, the WHO Strategic Advisory Group of Experts (SAGE) issued a framework to guide member states in prioritizing the allocation of COVID-19 vaccines (WHO, 2021d). Based on ethical principles of equal worth of persons, optimizing protection for those at highest risk of getting infected, and those most vulnerable to severe morbidity and mortality, SAGE recommended that the highest priority for vaccination should be given to health-care workers, older adults, and persons with medical co-morbidities.

7.8.3. *Vaccine nationalism*

Allocating vaccines between countries has also become a difficult issue. Export controls on vaccines have been proposed by countries or regions producing vaccines such as India or the European Union (EU) in response to shortages in vaccine supplies for their own populations facing COVID-19 surges.

Many developed countries have made arrangements to purchase vaccine supplies directly from companies producing vaccines, leaving poorer or less pro-active countries with inadequate access to vaccines. The COVAX facility was formed to address this problem of access to COVID-19 vaccines. COVAX is a collaborative platform between Gavi, the Vaccine Alliance, the Coalition for Epidemic Preparedness Innovations (CEPI) and the WHO, which serves to risk-pool the procurement of vaccines and distribute them in an equitable manner (Gavi, 2021).

An Independent Allocation of Vaccines Group (IAVG) has been formed to oversee and advise on this process (WHO, 2021e).

7.8.4. *Vaccine hesitancy*

Vaccine hesitancy — defined as the reluctance or refusal to get vaccinated despite the availability of vaccine services — was listed among the top ten threats to global health by the WHO in 2019. At this stage of global COVID-19 vaccination efforts, vaccine hesitancy plays a less prominent role while vaccine demand far exceeds vaccine supply. Many questions are already being asked about vaccine safety and efficacy, durability of protection, and long-term side-effects. Many of those questions will be answered as data are collected and studies are completed. However, vaccine hesitancy will remain a formidable challenge to COVID-19 vaccination roll-outs, and factors fueling vaccine hesitancy will vary between different regions and population groups. Engagement with the general public and specific communities must take many forms, ranging from media campaigns and social media forums to faith-based organizations and door-to-door visits. Infodemic management will require resources to monitor and respond to rumors, and to counter misinformation.

7.8.5. *Vaccine passports*

As countries struggle to reopen borders and revive economies, "vaccine passport" systems are under active consideration and implementation by regional groupings such as the EU and ASEAN, as well as aviation authorities. Major implementation challenges include: how to authenticate these vaccine passports, which vaccines and dosing intervals will be considered valid, how to authenticate prior infection for recovered individuals who may require only one vaccine dose or none, and who adjudicates these questions. The WHO has also raised questions around the ethics of using these vaccine passports in border controls when there is still such unequal access to COVID-19 vaccines.

7.9. Summary

COVID-19 has become the pandemic of our century. The successful development of vaccines within a year is the result of productive competition and collaboration among scientists, clinicians, companies, and governments. Leadership by international agencies such as the WHO and non-governmental organizations provide a necessary counter-weight of ethical and public health considerations. Both perspectives are complementary and both drives are needed, as we move forward to provide humanity with the means to push back this pandemic.

References

AstraZeneca Press Release, 2021. https://www.astrazeneca.com/media-centre/press-releases/2020/azd1222hlr.html (accessed 5 April 2021).

Baden LR *et al*. Efficacy and Safety of the mRNA-1273 SARS-CoV-2 Vaccine. *N Engl J Med* 2021; 384:403–416.

Bharat Biotech Press Release, 2021. http://www.sinovac.com/?optionid=754&auto_id=922 (accessed 5 April 2021).

Callaway E. Delta Coronavirus variant: Scientists brace for impact. *Nature* 2021; 595:17–18.

Callaway E, Ledford H. How bad is Omicron? What scientists know so far. *Nature* 2021; 600:197–199.

CDC (Centers for Disease Control and Prevention, USA), 2021. https://www.cdc.gov/coronavirus/2019-ncov/variants/about-variants.html (accessed 8 December 2021).

Dan JM *et al*. Immunological memory to SARS-CoV-2 assessed for up to 8 months after infection. *Science* 2021; 371:eabf4063.

Galloway SE *et al*. Emergence of SARS-CoV-2 B.1.1.7 lineage — United States, December 29, 2020 — January 12, 2021. *MMWR Morb Mortal Wkly Rep* 2021; 70:95–99.

Gavi, the Vaccine Alliance, 2021. https://www.gavi.org/covax-facility?gclid=CjwKCAjwx6WDBhBQEiwA_dP8rUXb15r9AWocQqWIHpkEwmSt97x7AioDS6btQG8HNpoH75eJ1JufhhoCH3sQAvD_BwE (accessed 5 April 2021).

HSA (Health Sciences Authority) of Singapore, 2021. https://www.who.int/publications/m/item/draft-landscape-of-covid-19-candidate-vaccines (accessed 5 April 2021).

Jeyanathan M *et al*. Immunological considerations for COVID-19 strategies. *Nat Rev Immunol* 2020; 20:615–632.

Logunov DY *et al*. Safety and efficacy of an rAd26 and rAd5 vector-based heterologous prime-boost COVID-19 vaccine: An interim analysis of a randomised controlled phase 3 trial in Russia. *Lancet* 2021; 397:671–681.

Ministry of Health Singapore, 2021. https://www.cdc.gov/coronavirus/2019-ncov/cases-updates/variant-surveillance/variant-info.html (accessed 5 April 2021).

Moderna Press Release, 2021a. https://investors.modernatx.com/news-releases/news-release-details/modernas-covid-19-vaccine-candidate-meets-its-primary-efficacy (accessed 5 April 2021).

Moderna Press Release, 2021b. https://investors.modernatx.com/news-releases/news-release-details/moderna-announces-primary-efficacy-analysis-phase-3-cove-study (accessed 5 April 2021).

NIH (National Institutes of Health), 2021. https://www.nih.gov/news-events/news-releases/janssen-investigational-covid-19-vaccine-interim-analysis-phase-3-clinical-data-released (accessed 5 April 2021).

Pfizer Press Release, 2021a. https://www.pfizer.com/news/press-release/press-release-detail/pfizer-and-biontech-announce-vaccine-candidate-against (accessed 5 April 2021).

Pfizer Press Release, 2021b. https://www.pfizer.com/news/press-release/press-release-detail/pfizer-and-biontech-conclude-phase-3-study-covid-19-vaccine (accessed 5 April 2021).

Polack FP *et al*. Safety and efficacy of the BNT162b2 mRNA COVID-19 vaccine. *N Engl J Med* 2020; 383:2603–2615.

Public Health England, 2021. https://www.gov.uk/government/news/phe-investigating-a-novel-variant-of-covid-19 (accessed 5 April 2021).

Sekine T *et al*. Robust T cell immunity in convalescent individuals with asymptomatic or mild COVID-19. *Cell* 2020; 183:158–168.e14.

Sinovac Press Release, 2021. http://www.sinovac.com/?optionid=754&auto_id=922 (accessed 5 April 2021).

Voysey M *et al*. Single-dose administration and the influence of the timing of the booster dose on immunogenicity and efficacy of ChAdOx1 nCoV-19 (AZD1222) vaccine: A pooled analysis of four randomised trials. *Lancet* 2021; 397:881–891.

WHO (World Health Organization), 2021a. Novel Coronavirus (2019-nCoV) Situation Report-1, 21 January 2020. https://www.who.int/docs/default-source/coronaviruse/situation-reports/20200121-sitrep-1-2019-ncov.pdf (accessed 5 April 2021).

WHO (World Health Organization), 2021b. The COVID-19 Candidate Vaccine Landscape and Tracker. https://www.who.int/publications/m/item/draft-landscape-of-covid-19-candidate-vaccines (accessed 2 March 2021).

WHO (World Health Organization), 2021c. WHO Coronavirus (COVID-19) Dashboard. https://covid19.who.int (accessed 6 August 2021).

WHO (World Health Organization), 2021d. https://www.who.int/publications/m/item/who-sage-roadmap-for-prioritizing-uses-of-covid-19-vaccines-in-the-context-of-limited-supply (accessed 5 April 2021).

WHO (World Health Organization), 2021e. https://www.who.int/groups/iavg (accessed 5 April 2021).

Yuan M *et al*. Structural and functional ramifications of antigenic drift in recent SARS-CoV-2 variants. *Science* 2021; 373:818–823.

Chapter 8

Pathophysiology of SARS-CoV-2 Infection and COVID-19

Teluguakula Narasaraju,[*,§] **Marko Radic,**[†,¶] **and Anil Kaul**[‡,‖]

[*]*Adichunchanagiri Institute of Medical Sciences, Center for Research and Innovation, Adichunchanagiri University, BG Nagara, Karnataka, India*

[†]*Department of Microbiology, Immunology and Biochemistry, College of Medicine, University of Tennessee Health Science Center, Memphis, Tennessee, USA*

[‡]*School of Health Care Administration, Oklahoma State University, Tulsa, Oklahoma, USA*

[§]*narasa@acu.ac.in*
[¶]*mradic@uthsc.edu*
[‖]*anil.kaul@okstate.edu*

Abstract

A detailed understanding of the pathophysiologic mechanisms of severe acute respiratory syndrome Coronavirus-2 (SARS-CoV-2) infection and Coronavirus disease 2019 (COVID-19) is vital for improving patient management — to facilitate prompt recognition of progression to severe disease and effective therapeutic strategies. This chapter summarizes the underlying pathophysiology in the lungs and other organs of COVID-19 patients. The roles of the cytokine storm culminating in exaggerated inflammatory responses and formation of neutrophil extracellular traps

(NETs) are discussed. Pathological features of the various stages from the onset of COVID-19 are outlined — progressing from early mild infection to severe clinical illness to the critically ill phase.

Keywords: COVID-19 pathophysiology; lungs; gross pathology; histopathology; cytokine storm; cytokines; chemokines; hyperinflammatory responses; immune cells; neutrophilia; neutrophil extracellular traps; acute respiratory distress syndrome; early mild SARS-CoV-2 infection; severe clinical illness; critically ill phase; COVID-19 pathology in liver, heart, blood vessels

8.1. Lung Pathology in SARS-CoV-2 Infection

The majority of patients with Coronavirus disease 2019 (COVID-19) recover with mild to moderate symptoms. However, about 10–15% of patients develop progressive pneumonia with severe to critical pulmonary lesions, and a significant number of these patients succumb to infection with pathologic manifestations of acute respiratory distress syndrome (ARDS) (Li and Ma, 2020; Pan *et al.*, 2020). The current management of COVID-19 relies mainly on clinical characteristics and lung computed tomography (CT) imaging that provide the basis for determining severity of illness and requirement for ventilator support (Wang *et al.*, 2020; Wu *et al.*, 2020). Although lung CT analysis can reveal consolidation and bilateral ground-glass opacities, the progressive pathologic changes occurring at different stages of COVID-19 have yet to be fully understood.

Numerous lung biopsy and autopsy studies have described the pathophysiology in severe acute respiratory syndrome Coronavirus-2 (SARS-COV-2) infection (Barton *et al.*, 2020; Suess and Hausmann, 2020; Tian *et al.*, 2020; Zhang *et al.*, 2020). The gross pathologic analyses commonly show highly edematous lungs with focal or diffuse congestion. Variable degrees of hemorrhagic and necrotic lesions are observed, with bronchi filled with fluid, without prominent mucus plugging, and with patent vasculature (Zhang *et al.*, 2020). The parenchymal tissues appear pale pink to dark red in color with ill-defined hemorrhagic lesions (Barton *et al.*, 2020). Several autopsy studies show that upper airways (including trachea and large bronchi) are normally widely patent without mucus plugs, while focal white patches are observed with mucosal ulceration, along with histologic evidence of mixed inflammatory cell infiltration including neutrophils and fibrin. The microscopic lung pathology analyses prominently exhibit wide-spread diffuse alveolar damage with hemorrhagic effusions, inflammatory exudation, epithelial denudation, coagulopathy, and widespread formation of hyaline membrane and intra-alveolar fibrin deposition (Barton *et al.*, 2020; Suess and Hausmann, 2020; Tian *et al.*, 2020). In addition, extensive numbers of degenerative neutrophils filling the bronchioles and alveoli are observed (Barnes *et al.*, 2020). Different anatomic areas of the lower respiratory tract including airways, alveoli, and vascular bed frequently display necrotic areas with the presence of inflammation and hyaline membranes with or without alveolar type 2 cell proliferation. In another post-mortem analysis, needle core biopsies demonstrated unusual lung tissue remodeling with alveolar type 2 epithelial cell regeneration and widespread fibrotic lesions, suggesting that critical ill patients may develop long-term abnormalities after recovery from SARS-CoV-2 infection (Barnes *et al.*, 2020). Massive neutrophil influx has been associated with increased pulmonary pathology in severely ill COVID-19 patients (Divani *et al.*, 2020; Feng *et al.*, 2020; Fox *et al.*, 2020).

Early epithelial cytotoxicity induced by SARS-CoV-2 triggers excessive release of cytokines and chemokines. In normal response to viral infection, the type I interferon (IFN) response is key in orchestrating antiviral defense. The type I IFN subtypes including IL-1α and IL-1β are induced upon recognition of viral nucleotides by pattern recognition receptors such as toll-like receptors (TLRs), or retinoic acid-inducible gene I (RIG-I). IL-1α and IL-1β exert antiviral effects via tyrosine kinase 2/JAK signaling-mediated expression of signal transducer and activator of transcription 1 and 2 (STAT1 and STAT2) that induce IFN-stimulated genes (ISGs). Further, ISGs orchestrate antiviral components such as protein kinase R, Mx proteins, and 2′,5′-oligoadenylate synthetase that degrade viral RNA (Suess and Hausmann, 2020). Interestingly, SARS-CoV-2 infection suppresses type I IFN response — critically ill patients lack efficient type I IFN response (Acharya *et al.*, 2020), but instead show augmented type II IFN response and production of IFN-γ, which stimulates pro-inflammatory cytokine induction that exacerbates pulmonary injury (Tay *et al.*, 2020). SARS-CoV-2 has been documented to be a poor inducer of type I IFN both *in vitro* as well as in animal models of infection compared with other respiratory RNA virus infections (Blanco-Melo *et al.*, 2020; Chu *et al.*, 2020). Accordingly, low ISG levels are found in severely ill COVID-19 patients with impaired type I IFN response. Interestingly, SARS-CoV-2 proteins such as ORF3b inhibit the type I IFN response, thereby preventing the host-induced antiviral response (Sa Ribero *et al.*, 2020). Furthermore, SARS-CoV-2 proteins including NSP13 and NSP15 interact with TANK-binding kinase 1 (TBK1) and the TBK1 activator ring finger protein 41 (RNF41 or NRDP1), respectively (Gordon *et al.*, 2020). NSP15 is a highly conserved endoribonuclease among Coronaviruses (Deng *et al.*, 2018; Frieman *et al.*, 2009; Ivanov *et al.*, 2004), that antagonizes the induction of IFN-I by cleaving the 5'-polyuridines of the negative-sense viral RNA. SARS-CoV-2 infection causes strong induction of the type II IFN-γ response, which is associated with exacerbated lung pathology. In addition, virus-inflicted early epithelial necrosis induces the release of excessive amounts of plasma IFN-γ, interleukin-2 (IL-2), IL-7, IL-10, granulocyte colony-stimulating factor (G-CSF), and monocyte chemoattractant protein (MCP), causing the rapid progression of ARDS and septic shock in patients, and eventually leading to multiple organ failure (Huang *et al.*, 2020).

Overwhelming immune cell influx is reported in pathologic manifestations during the progressive complication of ARDS in severely ill COVID-19 patients. Histopathologic analyses of lung autopsies of patients who died from COVID-19 display massive peri-bronchial cuffing of inflammatory cells, including neutrophils and lymphocytes (Zuo *et al.*, 2020). Activated and degenerated neutrophils are noted to fill interstitial spaces, along with neutrophil plugs in the small pulmonary capillaries and blood vessels within the damaged areas of the lungs. Exaggerated T-cell immune responses are also linked to acute lung injury in COVID-19. Severe COVID-19 patients exhibit excessive influx of T-cells including CD4 and CD8 cells, which accumulate in the interstitial spaces, with exudative diffuse alveolar damage and bronchopneumonia (Xu *et al.*, 2020). Strong staining of neutrophil elastase (NE) is observed in the injured COVID-19 lungs, whereas NE staining is absent in lungs from patients who died from other causes.

Evidence is accumulating that uncontrolled activation of neutrophils and their released NETs play central roles in disrupting the alveolar-capillary barrier that culminates in impaired gaseous exchange and severe hypoxemia, which is a prominent clinical manifestation in critically ill patients (Arcanjo *et al.*, 2020; Radermecker *et al.*, 2020; Zuo *et al.*, 2020). Furthermore, NETs released in response to SARS-CoV-2 infection can induce epithelial damage and apoptosis *in vitro*, indicating that activated neutrophils and accumulated NETs disrupt the alveolar epithelial barrier during the course of infection. In support of this, high and persistent neutrophilia is observed among patients who succumbed to severe COVID-19, compared to those survived with mild to moderate illness (Arcanjo *et al.*, 2020; Barnes *et al.*, 2020; Zuo *et al.*, 2020). Hence, elevated neutrophil-lymphocyte ratio can serve as an early prognostic marker in COVID-19. Accordingly, in severe COVID-19, greater neutrophilia may drive heightened pulmonary influx of neutrophils and stimulate excessive release of NETs, which can exacerbate alveolar-capillary damage and lead to pathologic manifestations of ARDS. Containing large amounts of extracellular histones, the released chromatin of NETs can disrupt the epithelial lining and stimulate platelet aggregation, leading to pulmonary vascular thrombosis. Over time, the accumulated cellular debris may aggravate inflammation and magnify the cytokine storm (Pedersen and Ho, 2020). Interestingly, NETs are mainly associated with the inflammatory interstitial lesions and the airways, while NETs-prone primed neutrophils are found in the pulmonary microcirculation (Wu *et al.*, 2020). Studies support the hypothesis that NETs may contribute to lung pathology in severe COVID-19, and therefore represent putative therapeutic targets (Teluguakula Narasaraju, 2021; Narasaraju *et al.*, 2011, 2020).

However, most of these pathology reports from COVID-19 patients were derived from samples collected post-mortem, and data are lacking on how these pathologic lesions evolve during progression of the disease. Based on the pathology reports, clinical features, and laboratory findings, pathologic lesions of COVID-19 can reasonably be categorized into three stages from the onset of the illness, i.e. mild, severe and critical, as outlined in Figure 8.1.

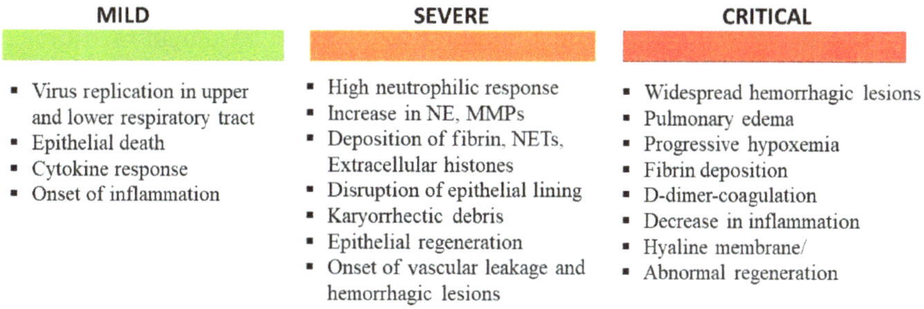

MILD	SEVERE	CRITICAL
• Virus replication in upper and lower respiratory tract • Epithelial death • Cytokine response • Onset of inflammation	• High neutrophilic response • Increase in NE, MMPs • Deposition of fibrin, NETs, Extracellular histones • Disruption of epithelial lining • Karyorrhectic debris • Epithelial regeneration • Onset of vascular leakage and hemorrhagic lesions	• Widespread hemorrhagic lesions • Pulmonary edema • Progressive hypoxemia • Fibrin deposition • D-dimer-coagulation • Decrease in inflammation • Hyaline membrane/ • Abnormal regeneration

Figure 8.1.   Model of changes in pathologic signatures at different stages of progression of COVID-19.

8.1.1. *Stage 1: Early mild infection*

During the early stage, the virus spreads from the upper respiratory tract into deeper lungs, and represents the active phase of virus replication. SARS-CoV-2 binds to angiotensin-converting enzyme 2 (ACE2) receptors on respiratory epithelial cells and immune cells such as macrophages. This stage of virus infection causes cytopathic effects, and induces robust cytokine and chemokine responses, which eventually trigger overwhelming inflammation. Although the cellular tropism of SARS-CoV-2 is yet to be fully elucidated, the virus can infect bronchiolar ciliated epithelium, goblet cells, alveolar type I and type II pneumocytes, macrophages, and dendritic cells (Acharya *et al.*, 2020). Infected patients at this stage may serve as a potential source of transmission of the virus.

8.1.2. *Stage 2: Severe clinical illness*

As the virus migrates into the deeper lungs and aggravates cytopathic effects, it also causes extensive influx of immune cells. This second phase can be defined as the inflammatory exudative stage during which massive numbers of neutrophils, macrophages and histiocytes are recruited into the infected lungs. These lesions have been reported in both lung biopsies and autopsies from COVID-19 patients (Barton *et al.*, 2020; Suess and Hausmann, 2020). The activated neutrophils likely instigate acute alveolar-capillary damage by generating toxic granule proteins (such as NE and matrix metalloproteinases including MMP-9 and MMP-2) and components of NETs (such as extracellular histones or ECH). Indeed, higher proportions of neutrophils and macrophages are found in bronchoalveolar lavage fluid samples from severely ill COVID-19 patients. The released neutrophil proteases can also disrupt extracellular matrix protein in the basement membrane, causing epithelial sloughing. Exposure of basement membrane and underlying pulmonary tissue can be a potential target by ECH, which interact and activate platelets to form aggregates. Widespread thrombotic complications are associated with severe pulmonary embolism and vascular pathology in COVID-19 patients (Suess and Hausmann, 2020; Zhang *et al.*, 2020). A combination of aggravated inflammatory and cytokine responses together with NETs components and thrombotic factors drive severe pulmonary pathology in SARS-COV-2 infection. Epithelial cells damaged during influenza pneumonia are regenerated by growth factors such as hepatocyte growth factor, produced simultaneously by myeloid lineage cells (Narasaraju *et al.*, 2010). Therefore, it is likely that epithelial hyperplasia and fibroblast proliferation begin during this stage, and become more obvious at the critical stages of infection. During this phase, the lung CT scan would likely appear as focal ground-glass opacities, and may be regarded as the "early stage" of ARDS pathophysiology.

8.1.3. *Stage 3: Critically ill phase*

COVID-19 patients who develop critical illness likely display progressive manifestations of ARDS. The lung autopsies or post-mortem biopsies from these patients reveal widespread hemorrhagic effusions, evident by alveoli filled with red blood cells and cellular debris. Extensive diffuse alveolar damage with pulmonary edema, fibrotic proliferation, hyaline membrane formation are reflected by impaired gaseous exchange — these patients may succumb to infection with respiratory failure despite ventilation therapy (Blanco-Melo *et al.*, 2020). Furthermore, heightened levels of D-dimers indicate pro-thrombotic status in the pulmonary vasculature. It is likely that these severe pathologic lesions arise from cumulative effects of prior inflammation, epithelial necrosis, protease-mediated extracellular matrix degradation, and vascular injury. The increased endothelial necrosis, platelet activation and aggregation may eventually progress into disseminated pulmonary vascular thrombosis in patients with severe COVID-19. In conclusion, developing therapeutic strategies that target crucial pathologic events at the severe phase, especially targeting epithelial loss and blocking protease-mediated alveolar-capillary damage will likely prevent or ameliorate the progressive pathologic complications of ARDS, thus effectively mitigating morbidity and mortality in severely ill COVID-19 patients.

8.2. Pathophysiology in Other Organs

SARS-CoV-2 infection can also impact other organs including the heart, liver, gastrointestinal tract, and kidneys (Barnes *et al.*, 2020; Feng *et al.*, 2020; Fox *et al.*, 2020). Extensive liver damage is reported in severely ill COVID-19 patients as evidenced by elevated levels of plasma bilirubin, and liver enzymes including alanine transaminase and aspartate aminotransferase (Prasad and Prasad, 2020). Autopsy liver specimens exhibit moderate macro- and micro-vesicular steatosis as well as some necrotic hepatocytes around the central veins without portal or lobular inflammation. Biopsy specimens taken from the heart reveal patchy non-specific pericardial infiltration with aggregates of inflammatory cells, including lymphocytes and plasma cells. In the heart, inflammatory infiltrates are found in either the endocardium, myocardium, and/or epicardial fat, occasionally associated with fibrosis, suggesting an early onset of manifestations. Inflammatory changes in the myocardium are characterized by accumulations of histiocytes, CD3+ T-cells, and neutrophils, together with platelet-fibrin thrombosis in small intra-myocardial blood vessels and endocardial mural blood vessels (Solomon *et al.*, 2020). Taken together, severe heart pathology increases the risk for cardiac failure (Freaney *et al.*, 2020).

References

Acharya D *et al.* Dysregulation of type I interferon responses in COVID-19. *Nat Rev Immunol* 2020; 20:397–398.

Arcanjo A *et al.* The emerging role of neutrophil extracellular traps in severe acute respiratory syndrome Coronavirus 2 (COVID-19). *Sci Rep* 2020; 10:19630.

Barnes BJ *et al.* Targeting potential drivers of COVID-19: Neutrophil extracellular traps. *J Exp Med* 2020; 217:e20200652.

Barton LM *et al.* COVID-19 autopsies, Oklahoma, USA. *Am J Clin Pathol* 2020; 153:725–733.

Blanco-Melo D *et al.* Imbalanced host response to SARS-CoV-2 drives development of COVID-19. *Cell* 2020; 181:1036–1045.

Chu H *et al.* Comparative replication and immune activation profiles of SARS-CoV-2 and SARS-CoV in human lungs: An ex vivo study with implications for the pathogenesis of COVID-19. *Clin Infect Dis* 2020; 71:1400–1409.

Deng X, Baker SC. An "Old" protein with a new story: Coronavirus endoribonuclease is important for evading host antiviral defenses. *Virology* 2018; 517:157–163.

Divani AA *et al.* Coronavirus disease 2019 and stroke:Clinical manifestations and pathophysiological insights. *J Stroke Cerebrovasc Dis* 2020; 29:104941.

Feng G *et al.* COVID-19 and liver dysfunction: current insights and emergent therapeutic strategies. *J Clin Transl Hepatol* 2020; 8:18–24.

Freaney PM *et al.* COVID-19 and heart failure with preserved ejection fraction. *JAMA* 2020; 324:1499–1500.

Frieman M *et al.* Severe acute respiratory syndrome Coronavirus papain-like protease ubiquitin-like domain and catalytic domain regulate antagonism of IRF3 and NF-kappaB signaling. *J Virol* 2009; 83:6689–6705.

Fox SE *et al*. Pulmonary and cardiac pathology in African American patients with COVID-19: An autopsy series from New Orleans. *Lancet Respir Med* 2020; 8:681–686.

Gordon DE *et al*. A SARS-CoV-2 protein interaction map reveals targets for drug repurposing. *Nature* 2020; 583:459–468.

Huang C *et al*. Clinical features of patients infected with 2019 novel Coronavirus in Wuhan, China. *Lancet* 2020; 395:497–506.

Ivanov KA *et al*. Major genetic marker of nidoviruses encodes a replicative endoribonuclease. *Proc Natl Acad Sci USA* 2004; 101:12694–12699.

Li X, Ma X. Acute respiratory failure in COVID-19: is it "typical" ARDS? *Crit Care* 2020; 24:198.

Narasaraju T *et al*. MCP-1 antibody treatment enhances damage and impedes repair of the alveolar epithelium in influenza pneumonitis. *Am J Respir Cell Mol Biol* 2010; 42:732–743.

Narasaraju T *et al*. Excessive neutrophils and neutrophil extracellular traps contribute to acute lung injury of influenza pneumonitis. *Am J Pathol* 2011; 179:199–210.

Narasaraju T *et al*. Neutrophilia and NETopathy as key pathologic drivers of progressive lung impairment in patients with COVID-19. *Front Pharmacol* 2020; 11:870.

Pan C *et al*. Lung recruitability in COVID-19-associated acute respiratory distress syndrome: A single-center observational study. *Am J Resp Crit Care Med* 2020; 201:1294–1297.

Pedersen SF, Ho YC. SARS-CoV-2: A storm is raging. *J Clin Invest* 2020; 130:2202–2205.

Prasad A, Prasad M. Single virus targeting multiple organs: What we know and where we are heading? *Front Med* 2020; 7:370.

Radermecker C *et al*. Neutrophil extracellular traps infiltrate the lung airway, interstitial, and vascular compartments in severe COVID-19. *J Exp Med* 2020; 217:e20201012.

Sa Ribero M *et al*. Interplay between SARS-CoV-2 and the type I interferon response. *PLoS Pathog* 2020; 16:e1008737.

Solomon MD *et al*. The COVID-19 pandemic and the incidence of acute myocardial infarction. *N Engl J Med* 2020; 383:691–693.

Suess C, Hausmann R. Gross and histopathological pulmonary findings in a COVID-19 associated death during self-isolation. *Int J Legal Med* 2020; 134:1285–1290.

Tay MZ *et al*. The trinity of COVID-19: Immunity, inflammation and intervention. *Nat Rev Immunol* 2020; 20:363–374.

Teluguakula N. Neutrophils set extracellular traps to injure lungs in coronavirus disease 2019. *J Infect Dis* 2021; 223:1503–1505.

Tian S *et al*. Pathological study of the 2019 novel Coronavirus disease (COVID-19) through postmortem core biopsies. *Mod Pathol* 2020; 33:1007–1014.

Wang Y *et al*. Temporal changes of CT findings in 90 patients with COVID-19 pneumonia: A longitudinal study. *Radiology* 2020; 296:E55–E64.

Wu C *et al*. Risk factors associated with acute respiratory distress syndrome and death in patients with Coronavirus disease 2019 pneumonia in Wuhan, China. *JAMA Intern Med* 2020; 180:934–943.

Xu Z *et al*. Pathological findings of COVID-19 associated with acute respiratory distress syndrome. *Lancet Respir Med* 2020; 8:420–422.

Zhang H *et al*. Histopathologic changes and SARS-CoV-2 immunostaining in the lung of a patient with COVID-19. *Ann Intern Med* 2020; 172:629–632.

Zuo Y *et al*. Neutrophil extracellular traps in COVID-19. *JCI Insight* 2020; 5:e138999.

Chapter 9

Antagonism and Evasion of Cellular Innate Immunity by SARS-CoV-2

Shachee Swaraj[*,‡], **Tanisha Malpani**[†,§],
and Shashank Tripathi[*,‖]

*Centre for Infectious Disease Research,
Department of Microbiology & Cell Biology,
Indian Institute of Science,
Bengaluru, India*

†*Division of Biological Sciences, Indian Institute of Science,
Bengaluru, India*

‡*shachees@iisc.ac.in*
§*tanisham@iisc.ac.in*
‖*shashankt@iisc.ac.in*

Abstract

The replication cycle of severe acute respiratory syndrome Coronavirus 2 (SARS-CoV-2) shares many features with other human Coronaviruses such as SARS-CoV and Middle East respiratory syndrome Coronavirus (MERS-CoV). Recent studies have elucidated the viral strategies of antagonizing the host immune response, including a multitude of mechanisms by which SARS-CoV-2 can dampen the interferon-mediated innate immunity. Furthermore, an imbalance and delay in interferon production, and exaggerated secretion of pro-inflammatory cytokines contribute to the severe immunopathology of Coronavirus disease 2019 (COVID-19). This chapter summarizes our current understanding of the intimate relationship between SARS-CoV-2 and the host innate and adaptive immune responses. The strategies that the virus utilizes to exploit cellular resources and to evade the innate immune system are described. The chapter provides a detailed discussion of interferon-mediated innate immunity, interferon evasion and antagonism by SARS-CoV-2 and human Coronaviruses.

Keywords: SARS-CoV-2; COVID-19; innate immunity; interferon induction; interferon signaling; viral evasion; viral antagonism; cytokine storm; virus–host interactions

9.1. Introduction

Viruses are obligate intracellular parasites that enter the host cell and hijack the cellular machinery for their own replication. In retaliation, the host cell elicits a formidable antiviral response, mediated by interferons (IFNs) which are often sufficient to prevent establishment of viral infection. The host cellular innate immunity is the first line of defense against viral infections, and is therefore a target of various viral proteins for modulation, resulting in a continuous molecular "arms race" between virus and host. This chapter will discuss the process of IFN production and signaling, followed by lessons learnt from previous Coronaviruses, and end with a detailed discussion on the current knowledge of severe acute respiratory syndrome Coronavirus-2 (SARS-CoV-2) proteins and their interactions with the cellular innate immune machinery.

9.2. Host Cell and Virus: A Toxic Relationship

The host cell is innately equipped with an arsenal of tools to target the virus at almost all the stages of its infection cycle. It does so in a two-step operation. Firstly, the viral pathogen is recognized, and secondly, a signaling cascade is triggered to block infection and eliminate the pathogen. In 1989, Charles Janeway conceived the idea of receptors that may recognize patterns in microbes or pathogens. The host cell recognizes the virus using these receptors known as pattern recognition receptors (PRRs). Generally, three families of PRRs play the most important roles in recognizing viral pathogen-associated molecular patterns (PAMPs), namely toll-like receptors (TLRs), retinoic acid inducible gene-I (RIG-I)-like receptors (RLRs) or MDA5, and NOD-like receptors (NLRs) (Seth *et al.*, 2006). These receptors recognize viral molecular patterns, such as viral nucleic acids (DNA, ssRNA, or dsRNA) or proteins, which are common in a range of different viruses (Seth *et al.*, 2006; Weber, 2021). Most RNA viruses, like SARS-CoV-2, are recognized by cytosolic RNA sensors, RIG-I, and melanoma differentiation-associated gene 5 (MDA5). An intracellular receptor, RIG-I is an ATP-dependent DExD/H box-containing RNA helicase. It is very likely that SARS-CoV-2 is also recognized by this RLR. Upon recognizing viral RNA via the C-terminal, the caspase activation and recruitment domain (CARD) on the N-terminal recruits and activates the mitochondrial antiviral signaling protein (MAVS, also known as CARDIF, VISA, IPS-1) present on the mitochondrial membrane. Activated MAVS interacts with tumor necrosis factor receptor-associated factor 3 (TRAF3) leading to the activation of kinases such as IKK and TBK1. These kinases phosphorylate the inhibitor of NF-κB (I-κB) and interferon regulatory factors (IRF3/7). The activated transcription factors NF-κB or IRF3/7 translocate to the nucleus from cytoplasm, leading ultimately to expression of type I interferons (IFNs) and pro-inflammatory cytokines (Braciale and Hahn, 2013; Weber, 2021). Endosomal TLRs (namely TLR3, 7, 8, 9) play roles in SARS-CoV-2 antiviral innate immunity. Viral dsRNA is recognized by TLR3, and ssRNA by TLR7 and TLR8. After recognition, downstream signaling proteins are activated, including adaptor proteins (MyD88 or TRIF), protein kinases, and RING domain ubiquitin ligase TRAF6. TRAF6 activates several protein kinases leading to the activation of transcription factors NF-κB, IRF3 or IRF7. These activated transcription factors translocate into the nucleus to induce the expression of type I IFNs. The nucleotide-binding oligomerization domain-like receptors (NLRs) are cytoplasmic PRRs that oligomerize with an adaptor, ASC (apoptosis-associated speck-like protein containing a caspase recruitment domain) to form inflammasome complexes. These complexes are needed to establish the antiviral state against SARS-CoV-2 (Braciale and Hahn, 2013).

The IFNs produced further mediate immune reactions — an efficient IFN response is very crucial to provide protection against any viral infection. Discovered by Alick Isaacs and Jean Lindenmann, IFNs are secreted out of the virus-infected cell, and act in a paracrine and autocrine fashion. They essentially act as "message-bearers" for the surrounding cells, alerting them on the impending danger (Weber, 2021). Although type I IFNs act via IFNAR1/2, and type III IFNs act via IFNLR1 and IL10RB, both IFN types trigger similar downstream signaling. The membrane-anchored receptors recruit Janus kinases (JAK) to activate STAT1/2 that translocate into the nucleus along with IRF9 in the form of the ISGF3 complex. This complex binds to IFN-stimulated response elements (ISREs) to induce the transcription of many genes responsive to IFN stimulation, designated as IFN-stimulated genes (ISGs). These ISGs are the key players in mounting an antiviral innate immune response against the virus (Seth *et al.*, 2006). Some ISGs function to upregulate the signaling proteins — they enhance the signaling and further activate ISGs, serving as positive regulators of pathogen-sensing and IFN sensitization. Examples of sensors that serve to fortify IFN response include OAS/RNaseL, ALR, PKR, cGAS, IRFs, STAT1/2 proteins. On the other hand, some ISGs (e.g. SOCS, USP18) may act as negative regulators of IFN signaling and cause IFN desensitization, thereby maintaining homeostasis. Yet other ISGs exert direct antiviral effects either by interfering with the viral replication machinery or by inhibiting virus entry, viral component assembly and virion release — examples include Mx, viperin, tetherin, IFITMs, CH25H (Seth *et al.*, 2006; Weber, 2021). Together, these hundreds of antiviral effectors establish a state of viral resistance that interferes with the normal virus infection cycle. IFNs as well as ISGs also activate the second arm of immune system by prompting the adaptive immune response. Therefore, timely and sufficient production of IFNs in and around the site of infection is very critical for resolving the disease. In order to successfully infect the host, viruses need to exploit novel as well as conservative strategies to combat the host immune response. They express proteins to help escape host detection as well as to counter the various host effector proteins to be able to finally establish the disease.

9.3. Human Coronaviruses

Before 2000, Coronaviruses were considered for many years to be pathogens that merely cause mild common cold in the human population. However, the emergence of SARS-CoV in 2003 thrust human Coronaviruses (HCoV) into the spotlight, and became acknowledged as a genuine threat. Therefore, most of the HCoV research since 2003 was concentrated on SARS-CoV. With the MERS-CoV outbreak several years later, and the SARS-CoV-2 pandemic starting in 2019, it is highly likely that the world has not yet seen the last of Coronaviruses. Of the seven HCoVs, four of them (HCoV-229E, HCoV-NL63, HCoV-OC43 and HCoV-HKU1) contribute to about one-third of common cold infections in humans across the world (van der Hoek, 2007) — they are considerably less pathogenic compared to SARS-CoV, MERS-CoV, and SARS-CoV-2.

As described, IFN induction occurs due to the recognition of viral RNA by the RLRs, TLRs, and other PRRs. HCoVs avoid this recognition by forming double membrane vesicles (DMVs) in which only replication, transcription, and other processes occur. The DMVs shield the PAMPs of the virus from any cytosolic host sensors (Kindler and Thiel, 2014). For SARS-CoV and MERS-CoV, the creation of DMVs involves the recruitment of the transmembrane proteins NSP3, NSP 4 and NSP 6 to the endoplasmic reticulum or ER (Knoops *et al.*, 2008). However, MERS-CoV is able to form DMVs in the absence of NSP6 as well (Oudshoorn *et al.*, 2017). Viral RNAs are also prevented from detection by the N protein of HCoVs — it sequesters the viral RNA, protecting it from interactions with PRRs (Lu *et al.*, 2011). The viral RNAs also use the disguise of a cap to stay hidden — this cap is a methylated guanine molecule linked to the 5′ end that is present in host mRNA (Kindler and Thiel, 2014). Initially, NSP13 of HCoVs cleaves the triphosphate end, and a host GTase adds GTP to the same end — this is followed by methylation by NSP14 and NSP10/NSP16 complex to form a cap (Totura and Baric, 2012). NSP15 endoribonuclease also cleaves the viral RNA at certain points such that it escapes detection by the PRRs (Kindler and Thiel, 2014). MERS-CoV 4b protein has a phosphodiesterase domain that degrades the 2-5A bond of 2′,5′-oligoadenylate synthetase (OAS) which is known to induce innate immunity (Thornbrough *et al.*, 2016). Once identified by PRRs, HCoVs deploy additional proteins to block the signaling for IFNs. The activation of MAVS by RLRs is inhibited by the SARS-CoV 3b and 9b proteins as they localize to mitochondria and disrupt RLR/MAVS complex formation (Freundt *et al.*, 2009; Shi *et al.*, 2014). MAVS is also hindered by the SARS-CoV N protein which induces degradation of MAVS and TRAF6 via binding with E3 ligase TRIM25 (Hu *et al.*, 2017). MERS-CoV 4a protein binds with PACT to inhibit RLR-induced activation of MAVS — it also hinders NF-κB translocation to the nucleus by binding to dsRNA (Siu *et al.*, 2014).

HCoVs also target MAVS-related complexes formed by kinases and other factors that aid signal transfer from MAVS to IRF and NF-κB. MERS-CoV M protein interrupts the binding of TRAF3 with TBK1 by co-localizing with them, while SARS-CoV M protein inhibits the TRAF3/TANK/TBK1/IKKe complex formation by binding with these molecules (Lui *et al.*, 2016; Siu *et al.*, 2009). However, the M protein of HCoV-HKU1 does not show these properties, suggesting that this activity is not conserved among all HCoVs (Lim *et al.*, 2016). MERS-CoV 4b protein inhibits the TBK1/IKKe complex association, while ORF8b protein causes the disruption of IKKe activation through binding with HSP70 chaperone (Wong *et al.*, 2020, Yang *et al.*, 2015). These strategies inhibit IRF3 translocation to the nucleus, and its mediated activation of IFN translation. SARS-CoV and MERS-CoV NSP3 (PLpro) protein targets IRF3 by obstructing phosphorylation, dimerization, and nuclear translocation of IRF3 — the DUB domain of NSP3 is essential for this process (Frieman *et al.*, 2009). DUB also plays an important role in deubiquitinating or deISGylating antiviral factors which marks them for degradation or deactivates them (Shokri *et al.*, 2018). HCoV-NL63 NSP 3 also causes STING/MAVS-mediated IFN inhibition (Sun *et al.*, 2012). SARS-CoV proteins 8a and 8b also interact with and degrade IRF3 in an ubiquitin-proteosome-dependent manner (Wong *et al.*, 2017). MERS-CoV 4b protein harbors a nuclear localization signal (NLS) which binds with the α-karyopherin, KPNA4 — the latter is responsible for the translocation of NF-κB to the nucleus (Canton *et al.*, 2018). When activated, NF-κB and IRF3/7 induce translation of IFNs and ISGs — SARS-CoV and MERS-CoV possess proteins that abrogate this response. SARS-CoV NSP1 and ORF6 proteins inhibit phosphorylation and translocation of STAT1 respectively, which prevents the signal from reaching the nucleus (Frieman *et al.*, 2007; Wathelet *et al.*, 2007). To achieve this, ORF6 binds to important nuclear import factors like KPNA2 and KPNB1 — these factors are also required by NF-κB for translocation. SARS-CoV ORF3a also induces the PERK unfolded protein response (UPR) pathway. A key feature of PERK-mediated UPR is the lysosome-mediated degradation of IFNAR receptors (Minakshi *et al.*, 2009). One important strategy of SARS-CoV and MERS-CoV is mediated by NSP1 which selectively inhibits translation of cellular mRNAs and targets them for degradation. This translational shut-off is the final strategy deployed to prevent production of IFNs and ISGs (Huang *et al.*, 2011, Lokugamage *et al.*, 2015). Another means to suppress IFN signaling exploited by SARS-CoV is to use the host genes for its own benefit. By promoting upregulation of negative regulators of IFN pathway, such as SOCS1/3, the S protein inhibits IFN translation (Sa Ribero *et al.*, 2020). The above strategies of IFN antagonism reveal some of the mechanisms by which HCoVs mount a robust attack against the host immune system. Since SARS-CoV-2 is genetically similar to these HCoVs, our current understanding of HCoVs is of utmost importance.

9.4. SARS-CoV-2: A Novel Foe of Humankind

Over recent decades, there has been escalating concern over the increasing number of viruses that newly emerge, giving rise to previously unrecognized infections and epidemics among humans and wildlife. Under such a scenario, the most essential part of science is to identify aspects of the disease process and progression that can offer new approaches for treatment and prevention. SARS-CoV-2, the novel Coronavirus that emerged in December 2019, mainly infects the alveolar epithelial cells in the respiratory tract of humans. It causes a previously unrecognized infection designated as Corona Virus Disease 2019 (COVID-19) which is characterized by mild flu-like symptoms in most of the cases — however, some cases may progress to an acute respiratory distress syndrome (ARDS). SARS-CoV-2 has a single-stranded positive-sense RNA (+ssRNA) genome of 30 kilobases (kb) that encodes all the proteins from 15 open reading frames (ORFs) required by the virus to cause infection. The two-thirds (20 kb) of the genome from the 5′ end codes for non-structural proteins (NSP1–16) within two ORFs (ORF1a and ORF1b). The other one-third of the genome encodes four structural proteins comprising spike (S), envelope (E), membrane (M) and nucleocapsid (N) proteins, and nine different accessory proteins (ORF3a, 3b, 6, 7a, 7b, 8, 9b, 9c, 10). These proteins carry out all the viral processes for successful infection. Like other RNA viruses, SARS-CoV-2 is recognized by the intracellular RNA sensors. The innate immune response, mediated by the lung epithelial cells, alveolar macrophages, dendritic cells, and neutrophils spring into action upon detecting these viral particles (Bouayad, 2020; Sa Ribero *et al.*, 2020). Most of the SARS-CoV-2 proteins are dedicated to countering the host IFN response. These mechanisms are very well-studied and documented in SARS-CoV and MERS-CoV. The ensuing delicate interactions between host and virus decide the ultimate balance between the severity of infection and the probability of recovery to normal health.

9.5. Teeny Tiny Virus Troops: Render the Host Defense Defenseless

Here we address the mechanisms of IFN antagonism by SARS-CoV-2 to target various pathways of antiviral response during infection. Such mechanisms include strategies to avoid detection by PRRs, to inhibit induction of type I and III IFNs, to prevent IFN signaling to block production of ISGs, or to suppress the antiviral effector ISG functions. Many viruses utilize specific viral proteins as "armors" to evade the host immune response. SARS-CoV, MERS-CoV and SARS-CoV-2, which are capable of causing epidemics or pandemics, share many common proteins and may also share many mechanisms for host immune antagonism. However, SARS-CoV-2 has evolved to acquire certain novel ORFs and proteins with characteristics unique among HCoVs. Hence, it is plausible that this virus may have novel tactics for evading host IFN responses other than the known conserved strategies (Bouayad, 2020; Sa Ribero *et al.*, 2020). Several SARS-CoV-2 proteins are identified as potent IFN antagonists, including, NSP13 (RNA helicase), NSP14 (exonuclease), NSP15 (endoribonuclease) and accessory proteins ORF6 (Yuen *et al.*, 2020). NSP1, NSP3, NSP12, NSP14, ORF3, ORF6 and membrane (M) proteins are also found to inhibit the production of IFN-β (Lei *et al.*, 2020; Sa Ribero *et al.*, 2020; Xia *et al.*, 2020; Yuen *et al.*, 2020; Zheng *et al.*, 2020). Studies further elucidated the different mechanisms by which SARS-CoV-2 proteins counteract the host immune response. Other than directly "attacking" host cellular defense, viral proteins can also manipulate host cellular proteins either by proteolytic cleavage of immune effector proteins or via covalent modifications such as ubiquitination, deubiquitinylation, phosphorylation, dephosphorylation, or degradation. They can also shield their recognition by covalent modifications of their own proteins, e.g. glycosylation of viral structural proteins. The viral proteins hijack many cellular processes for the virus' own benefit, and affects almost all cellular pathways directly or indirectly to create a favorable environment for viral replication. Some viral proteins also utilize the host's genetic and epigenetic factors for expropriating salient cellular pathways (Khan and Islam, 2020). The molecular mechanisms of host immune evasion exploited by these SARS-CoV-2 proteins will be further elaborated.

9.6. SARS-CoV-2 Evasion of Host Detection

The inhibition of IFN by SARS-CoV-2 is more potent than its previous Coronavirus counterparts. In fact, a distinguishing feature of COVID-19 is the strong suppression of IFNs followed by a surge in pro-inflammatory cytokines from neutrophils and macrophages that incites a cytokine storm in the body. This contributes to the severity of the disease. Through evolutionary processes, another key characteristic of SARS-CoV-2 is that it has acquired a reduced percentage of CpG dinucleotides in its genome. The repeated CpG motif in viruses is recognized by zinc finger antiviral protein (ZAP), which then recruits various host components to degrade the genome as well as to initiate the innate immune signaling pathway. Over time, SARS-CoV-2 has developed a genome comprising the least amount of CpG compared to other known Coronaviruses. This confers an advantage to SARS-CoV-2 to remain undetected in the cell (Xia, 2020). Thus, to evade detection by PRRs and other pathogen receptors, SARS-CoV-2 not only employs many of the proteins previously studied in SARS-CoV and MERS-CoV, but it also has evolved its own innovative strategies.

9.7. Double Membrane Vesicles and Replication–Transcription Complexes

Although HCoVs recognize different receptors which facilitate their entry into the susceptible cell, all HCoVs, including SARS-CoV-2, induce the formation of DMVs which are formed with the help of ER membranes. Replication–Transcription complexes formed by different NSPs of the virus are present in the DMVs. Hence, these DMVs shield the dsRNA and ssRNA replicative and transcriptive intermediates of the virus from PRRs, PKR, and OAS. NSPs 3, 4 and 6, each have 2, 4 and 6 transmembrane domains, respectively. These domains localize to the ER and contribute to the formation of DMVs by helping in the generation of double membranes as well as the budding off into vesicles (Santerre *et al.*, 2020). Although not much is known about SARS-CoV-2 DMVs, by extrapolating from our knowledge of SARS-CoV proteins, one can hypothesize that NSP3 is necessary for membrane proliferation to fulfill the need for formation of multiple DMVs. On the other hand, NSP4 is needed for the pairing of the membranes derived from the ER since NSP4 and NSP3 are known to interact and pair up with each other. This action can be compared to joining the two elements of a zipper. NSP6 is equally important for the creation of DMVs as it causes the double-membraned ER-bodies to bud out as vesicles. The exact mechanism by which NSP6 induces sphere formation is not clear (Knoops *et al.*, 2008). However, autophagy-related factors (e.g. LC-3) and EDEMosome-related factors (e.g. OS-9) localize with NSP6 of the murine Coronavirus, mouse hepatitis virus or MHV (Reggiori *et al.*, 2010). Hence, these pathways may also be involved in DMV generation for SARS-CoV-2. Recently, a study on SARS-CoV-2 and MHV found pores in the DMVs using cryo-electron microscopy. It is speculated that the pores allow transportation of the transcribed mRNAs from the lumen of the DMVs to the cytosol for translation. The pore for MHV has NSP3 as a key component. However, the characterization of these pores is still an unsolved mystery for SARS-CoV-2 (Wolff *et al.*, 2020).

9.8. Viral mRNA Capping

These DMVs are not sufficient to avoid recognition of the dsRNA — therefore, SARS-CoV-2 mRNA also undergoes capping of the 5' end. This capping occurs to mimic the host mRNA which also has a methylated cap at the 5' end — essentially a N7-methylguanine (m^7G) moiety linked to the first nucleotide via a 5'-5' triphosphate bond. These caps are crucial as they stabilize mRNA, prevent its degradation and initiate translation by recruiting the eukaryotic translation initiation factor 4E (eIF4E). In addition to its helicase domain, NSP13 of SARS-CoV-2 has a triphosphatase domain. This region cleaves the triphosphate at the 5' end of transcribed mRNA following which a host guanylyl transferase (GTase) adds a GTP molecule to the monophosphate. Currently, the identity of the GTase is not known. NSP14 then attaches a methyl group to the N7 position in the guanosine molecule. It has an RNA binding cleft as well as an S-adenosyl methionine (SAM) binding cleft. The methyl group is transferred from SAM to the mRNA by catalytic residues. Next, the NSP10/16 complex attaches a methyl to the 2'-O of the sugar moiety present in the first residue. Here, SAM is also utilized as a substrate for the methyl-transferring reaction. NSP10 is required to stabilize the SAM-binding cleft of NSP16. NSP10 is also known to have RNA-binding properties which may further stabilize the RNA-NSP16 binding. This cap "confuses" the host into sensing that it is a cellular moiety — hence, viral mRNA escapes detection as well as degradation by host factors (Viswanathan *et al.*, 2020).

9.9. Other Strategies for Evading PRR Detection

The nucleocapsid or N protein is another viral protein that helps in evasion from the host immune system. It acts as a protective layer by encapsulating the viral mRNA, thereby preventing mRNA recognition by

PRRs. This is especially needed when mRNA gets exposed during translocation within the cell. The N protein also sequesters dsRNA to prevent its digestion by Dicer molecules. It partially sequesters the siRNA formed at post-Dicer stages, hence inhibiting a common antimicrobial response of the host (Mu *et al.*, 2020). As a last resort to evade identification by PRRs, PKR and OAS, SARS-CoV-2 NSP15 endoribonuclease cleaves its own viral dsRNA at certain points that are needed for detection. It also cleaves the poly-U domain present in negative-strand RNAs that are formed as a result of replication (Amor *et al.*, 2020).

The above mentioned mechanisms enable the evasion of host immune response by avoiding the detection of viral PAMPs by the host PRRs. They may not always be successful, and SARS-CoV-2 thus encodes additional proteins that impede or block subsequent steps in the IFN signaling pathway. These proteins and their functions are further discussed next.

9.10. SARS-CoV-2 Inhibition of IFN Induction

Once PRRs are activated by binding to PAMPs such as dsRNA, they enter different signaling cascades to induce IFN production depending on the PRR. Studies show the involvement of the structural proteins (M and N), non-structural proteins (NSP1, NSP3, NSP6, NSP8, NSP10, NSP13, NSP14, NSP15 and NSP16), and accessory proteins (3a, 3b, 6, 8 and 9b) inhibition of IFN induction (Lei *et al.*, 2020; Xia *et al.*, 2020; Yuen *et al.*, 2020). Much still remains to be uncovered regarding the mechanisms by which these proteins act. In the case of SARS-CoV-2, RIG-I and MDA5 act as PRRs that signal MAVS present in the mitochondria. Activated MAVS forms complexes with different kinases (e.g. TBK, IKK) as well as certain adapter proteins (e.g. TRAF3 and TRAF6) which then send the signal to IRF3/7 and NF-κB. These factors translocate to the nucleus and induce translation of IFNs. These steps are targeted by SARS-CoV-2 in a multitude of ways.

9.11. MAVS, Kinases and Adapter Proteins

In a recent study, the orf3b protein of SARS-CoV-2 was shown to localize to the mitochondria through an unknown mechanism and interfere with RIG-I/MAVS signaling. SARS-CoV-2 ORF3b protein is more than 100 amino acids shorter than its SARS equivalent and yet, it was found to be more potent in IFN inhibition. This new feature suggests a connection between protein length and potency of IFN inhibition. Alarmingly, ORF3b has already mutated in a quasi-species in Ecuador to an optimal length shorter than that of SARS-CoV but longer than that of SARS-CoV-2. This mutated protein is overwhelmingly dominant over IFN production (Konno *et al.*, 2020). Moreover, ORF3b is not the only aspect where SARS-CoV-2 has "outdone" other HCoVs. NSP8 is a part of the replicase in all Coronaviruses, and interacts with the CARD domain of MDA5. This CARD domain is necessary for the K63 ubiquitination of MDA5 which activates it to proceed with signaling (Yang *et al.*, 2020). The M protein also binds with RIG-I and MDA5 individually through an unknown mechanism. This binding interferes with the interactions between RIG-I/MDA5 and MAVS — thus, MAVS does not get activated (Zheng *et al.*, 2020). Yuen *et al.* (2020) also showed that NSP13, NSP14, NSP15 and ORF6 proteins are inhibitors of IRF-mediated IFN production and target RIG-I signaling. ORF6 especially interferes with the RIG-I/MDA5 signaling as well as the activated MAVS signaling cascade to prevent IFN induction. It has additional importance as discussed later in this section (Lei *et al.*, 2020).

The MAVS/TRAF3/TBK1/IKKe complex signals for IRF3/7-mediated translation of IFNs, while the TRAF6/IKKa/IKKb complex signals for NF-κB-mediated translation of IFNs. As mentioned previously, these complexes are targets not only for SARS-CoV-2, but other viruses as well. SARS-CoV-2 M protein is able to bind to each of the factors present in the MAVS/TRAF3/TBK complex. Thus, the M protein acts to inactivate the RIG-I/MDA5/ MAVS/ TRAF3/TBK complex formation, akin to SARS-CoV M protein (Zheng *et al.*, 2020). This shuts down IRF phosphorylation, dimerization, and subsequent translocation to the nucleus. The SARS-CoV-2 ORF9b protein also interacts with RIG-I, MDA5, MAVS, TRIF, STING, and TBK1 individually. This interrupts the complex formations of MDA5/MAVS/RIG-I, TLR/TRIF, and cGAS/STING. Moreover, the ORF9b protein also prevents TBK1 phosphorylation which is another essential step for complex formation with TRAF (Han *et al.*, 2021). Another mechanism of complex formation inhibition by ORF9b protein is attributed to its interaction with the host TOM70 chaperone. TOM70 is important to transmit the signal from MAVS to TRAF since MAVS itself is localized to the mitochondria (Jiang *et al.*, 2020). Using these strategies, ORF9b thus inhibits IRF3/7 activation and IFN production. These strategies orchestrated by ORF9b are quite different from those adopted by SARS-CoV, but they are centered around MAVS. Such observations were made in experiments that mimicked those for SARS and MERS Coronavirus proteins. One such interactome experiment found that TBK1 can interact with NSP13 and NSP15. While NSP13 does so directly, NSP15 interacts with the TBK1 activator ring finger protein 41 or RNF41 (Gordon *et al.*, 2020). Hence, both NSP13 and NSP15 inhibit IFN production via the IRF pathway *in vitro*. NSP13 can bind with TBK1, with the corresponding inactivation of TBK1 phosphorylation — this binding impedes IRF phosphorylation. Although NSP6 can also bind with TBK1, this binding has no effect on TBK1 phosphorylation. Nonetheless, the NSP6-bound TBK1 exhibits reduced efficiency in signaling for IRF phosphorylation (Lei *et al.*, 2020; Xia *et al.*, 2020).

9.12. Targeting Transcription Regulators: IRF3/7 and NF-*κ*B

The last elements to get activated and translocate to the nucleus to promote IFN production are IRF3, IRF7 and NF-*κ*B. IRF3/7 get phosphorylated, dimerize, and enter the nucleus to bind to transcription promoters. NSP3 of SARS-CoV-2 interacts with and inhibits the phosphorylation of IRF3 — it is a strong inhibitor of IFN production. NSP3 also possesses a deubiquitinating domain that cleaves the ISG15 bound to IRF3, since ISG15 is very similar to the ubiquitin or Ub factor. This cleavage immobilizes IRF3 to the cytosol, preventing its movement to the nucleus (Shin *et al.*, 2020). ORF6 impedes phosphorylation as well as translocation of IRF3/7 to the nucleus. The ORF6 C-terminal domain is important for the proper functioning of the protein (Lei *et al.*, 2020). Thus, IRF-mediated translation of IFNs is inhibited. *In vivo*, M protein suppresses translocation of IRF3 into the nucleus (Zheng *et al.*, 2020). In addition, NSP13, NSP14 and NSP15 can also inhibit IRF translocation to the nucleus *in vitro*, but via unknown mechanisms (Yuen *et al.*, 2020). However, the effects of these proteins *in vivo* may be different.

The NF-*κ*B transcription factor also controls IFN production, but utilizes different modulators in its signaling cascade after MAVS activation. To block this signaling as well, SARS-CoV-2 utilizes other strategies. The M protein interferes with the TRAF/IKK complex formation required for NF-*κ*B activation (Zheng *et al.*, 2020). NSP5 also inhibits NF-*κ*B signaling by a unique mechanism. Unlike NSP3, NSP5 utilizes its proteolytic cleavage domain to cleave NLRP12 and TAB1. NLRP12 is a host moiety that helps with the production of cytokines and ISGs induced by NF-κB signaling, while TAB1 downregulates the influx of pro-inflammatory cytokines in the host cell. NSP5 inhibits both of these proteins (NLRP12 and TAB1), thereby targeting the NF-κB pathway (Moustaqil *et al.*, 2021). The NF-κB pathway is also shown to be inhibited by SARS-CoV-2 ORF6, ORF8 and N proteins *in vivo*, albeit by unknown mechanisms (Li *et al.*, 2020).

9.13. Translation Inhibition

While these pathogen–host interactions operate, the SARS-CoV-2 NSP1-induced translational shut-off of host mRNAs affords time for the virus to mount a robust attack on the host's immune system. NSP1 deploys its *C*-terminal domain to bind to the mRNA channel present in the 40S subunit of ribosomes. This blocks the attachment of mRNA to ribosomes and subsequent 80S ribosome formation. Thus, cellular mRNAs, especially those encoding genes of IFNs, remain untranslated. However, viral mRNAs escape this state due to the presence of the leader sequence in their 5′-UTR regions. This sequence is recognized by NSP1 which enables their selective translation. Apart from this, NSP1 selectively marks cellular mRNAs for degradation by host factors which sense that cellular mRNAs lack the leader sequence (Thoms *et al.*, 2020).

Clearly, SARS-CoV-2 expresses an arsenal of proteins that efficiently antagonize the host innate immunity. The IFN production network represents an important target for viruses to enhance their virulence. The IFN signaling cascade is highly influenced by SARS-CoV-2 as well, and this is addressed in the following sections.

9.14. Inhibition of Interferon Signaling and Production of ISGs

Despite SARS-CoV-2 using various strategies to impair IFN production, the cell may still successfully produce some IFN. There is delay in host IFN production that benefits viral replication during early infection, leading to increased viral load in the body and is thus responsible for the symptoms in COVID-19 patients. In general, the virus blocks the activity of IFNs by targeting IFN signaling starting from the IFN receptors on the cell surface (Figure 9.1). SARS-CoV ORF3a and ORF6 proteins down-regulate the surface expression of IFNAR due to enhanced ubiquitination and proteolytic degradation (Kumar *et al.*, 2020) — however, these need validation in the case of SARS-CoV-2 (Figure 9.2). The roles of SARS-CoV-2 proteins in inhibiting IFN signaling have been investigated by studying ISRE activity. Ten viral proteins (i.e. NSP1, NSP6, NSP7, NSP13, NSP14, NSP15, ORF3a, M, ORF6, ORF7a and ORF7b) potentially impede IFN signaling (Lei *et al.*, 2020; Sa Ribero *et al.*, 2020; Xia *et al.*, 2020; Yuen *et al.*, 2020; Zheng *et al.*, 2020). The mechanism of IFN

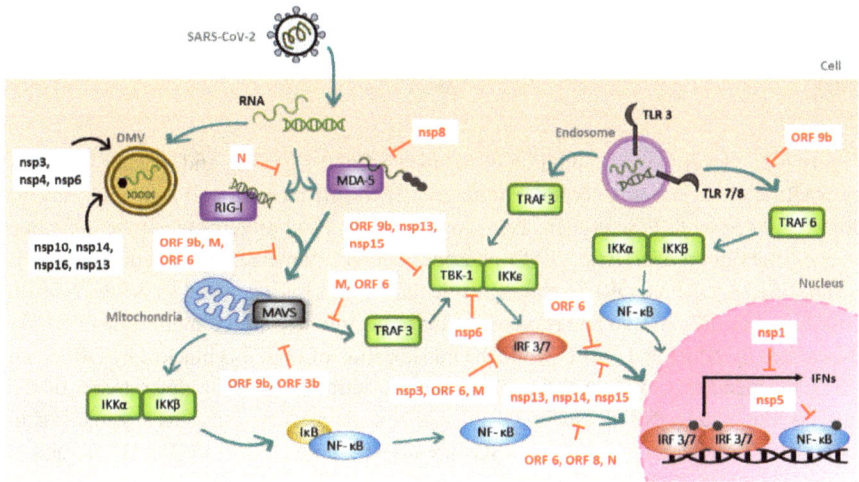

Figure 9.1. Schematic illustration of inhibition of interferon (IFN) induction by SARS-CoV-2 proteins. Upon viral entry, the SARS-CoV-2 genome undergoes translation and the NSP3, NSP4 and NSP6 proteins form DMVs which shield viral PAMPs from PRRs. The synthesized mRNA also has a cap added by NSP10, NSP13, NSP14 and NSP16 which helps evade detection. SARS-CoV-2 N protein also helps "hide" from PRRs such as RIG-I and MDA5. NSP8 binds to MDA5 and inactivates it. Signaling to MAVS is also blocked by ORF9b, M, and ORF6 proteins. ORF9b and ORF3b interact with MAVS to inhibit its functions. ORF6 and M proteins also disrupt subsequent signaling after MAVS activation. ORF9b, NSP13, and NSP15 bind to TBK1, and prevent complex formation with IKKε. NSP6 also does this by inhibiting phosphorylation of TBK1. NSP3, ORF6, and M proteins then block the phosphorylation and translocation of IRF3/7. ORF6, NSP13, NSP14, and NSP15 also inhibit translocation of IRF3/7 into the nucleus. NF-κB signaling is blocked by ORF6, ORF8 and N proteins. ORF9b also blocks the signaling by disrupting TRAF complex formation with other factors. Finally, NSP1 inhibits induction of IFNs by selectively targeting host mRNA for degradation, while NSP 5 cleaves factors that promote inflammatory cytokines produced via the NF-κB pathway.

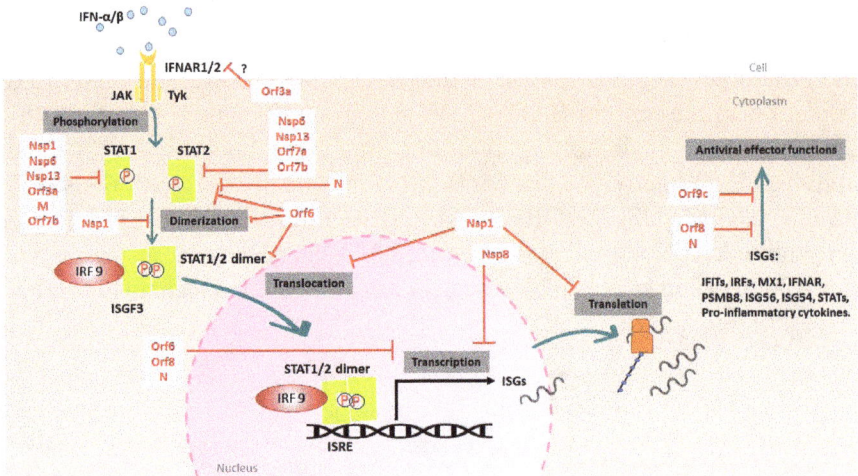

Figure 9.2.   Overview of inhibition of interferon (IFN) signaling and effector functions by SARS-CoV-2 proteins. Type-I interferons (IFN-α/β) receptors (IFNAR1/2) may be downregulated by ORF3a protein. Two sets of SARS-CoV-2 proteins target the inhibition of phosphorylation of STATs. STAT1 phosphorylation is targeted for inhibition by NSP1, NSP6, NSP13, ORF3a, ORF7b and M; while that of STAT2 is targeted by NSP6, NSP13, ORF7a and ORF7b. ORF6 and N proteins also target this step. The dimerization of STATs is inhibited by NSP1 and ORF6; while the translocation of ISGF3 is blocked by ORF6 and NSP1 independently. Within the nucleus, the transcription of ISGs downstream of the ISRE is hindered by NSP8, ORF6, ORF8, and N proteins. Translation as a whole is shut by NSP1. The effector functions of ISGs are directly targeted by ORF9c, ORF8, and N proteins of SARS-CoV-2.

suppression involves two sets of viral proteins groups that interfere with the phosphorylation of STAT1/2, and consequently their nuclear translocation. Overall, NSP1, NSP6, NSP13, ORF3a, M, ORF7b suppress STAT1 phosphorylation, while NSP6, NSP13, ORF7a, ORF7b hinder the STAT2 phosphorylation (Xia *et al.*, 2020). N protein also interacts with STAT1/2 to inhibit their phosphorylation and subsequent translocation to the nucleus (Figure 9.2). ORF6 exerts inhibitory effect on ISRE and ISG56/IFIT1 promoter activity. Since these promoters function downstream of IFN signaling, ORF6 thus affects IFN signaling, and inhibits production of ISGs. The ORF6 protein of SARS-CoV-2 interacts with a nuclear import protein karyopherin $\alpha2$ (KPNA2), which hampers the nuclear translocation of multiple immune-related transcription factors like IRF3 (Bouayad, 2020; Lei *et al.*, 2020; Xia *et al.*, 2020). Upon interaction with karyopherin α2, ORF6 sequesters both karyopherin α2 and karyo-pherin β1. Accordingly, ORF6 affects the nuclear translocation of STAT1, thereby inhibiting the IFN signaling — hence, SARS-CoV-2 blocks the expression of ISGs. SARS-CoV ORF6 is a well-known IFN antagonist with its C-terminus being critical for this antagonistic characteristic. The ORF6 proteins of SARS-CoV and SARS-CoV-2 share 69% sequence identity, where the disparity mainly resides in the C-terminus. Unsurprisingly, the presence of C-terminus (amino acids 53-61) was found to be crucial for its immune modulatory functions. Therefore, ORF6 is a potent IFN antagonist that not only diminishes IFN production, but also impairs downstream IFN signaling (Lei *et al.*, 2020; Xia *et al.*, 2020) (Figure 9.2).

Another efficacious route for immune evasion adopted by SARS-CoV-2 is the inhibition of host protein synthesis. The NSP1 protein of SARS-CoV-2 induces an almost complete shut-down of host mRNA translation and also leads to its degradation, while selectively concealing viral mRNA from degradation by some unknown mechanism (Figure 9.2). In this way, it allows the production of viral proteins, but strongly impairs the host defense that requires the synthesis of antiviral factors involving IFN response, pro-inflammatory cytokines and ISG production (Thoms *et al.*, 2020: Yang *et al.*, 2020). The shut-down of synthesis of many host factors, that can otherwise block viral infection, now renders the cellular environment favorable for effective viral replication. Although SARS-CoV-2 encodes other proteins that manipulate the host immune system, the loss of NSP1 from the viral genome renders the virus more susceptible to clearance by the innate immune response — suggesting that the role of NSP1 is crucial for establishing a successful disease condition. NSP1 is also implicated to bind to STAT1, thereby preventing its phosphorylation and translocation from cytosol to nucleus (Bouayad, 2020; Kikkert, 2020; Thoms *et al.*, 2020) (Figure 9.2). ORF6, ORF8 and nucleocapsid (N) proteins also interfere with IFN signaling. Not only do they inhibit the IFN-β and NF-κB promoters, but also the ISREs present in promoter regions of most ISGs. ORF6 and ORF8 are stronger in antagonizing immune responses as they inhibit the ISRE even after IFN-β treatment (Li *et al.*, 2020) (Figure 9.2).

All the above-mentioned strategies that facilitate IFN inhibition are known to exist in other HCoVs. However, SARS-CoV-2 possesses the ORF9c protein previously unknown in other Coronaviruses, with immune evasion properties (Lu, 2020). ORF9c encodes a 73-amino acid protein containing a transmembrane domain that localizes to any double-membraned organelle in the cell, and interacts with many membrane proteins in diverse cellular compartments to cause IFN inhibition as well as other pathogenic processes. The protein is highly unstable and hinders multiple immune pathways. Some of the biomolecules ORF9c interacts with and downregulates are part of the IFN machinery, including IRF7/IRF1, IFNAR, and IFN-signaling components, including IFI35, multiple IFIT proteins, IRF9, ISG15, MX1, PSMB8, and STAT proteins. ORF9c also modulates the levels of ubiquitin-conjugating enzymes, proteasomal components, and components of antigen processing and presentation (HLA-A/B/C, TAP-1, TAPBP) as well as some proteins of the complement system (Lu, 2020). SARS-CoV-2 ORF3a protein interacts with the inflammasome components (ASC NLRP3), TRAF3 and IC assemblage, leading to the activation of NF-κB and synthesis of pro-inflammatory cytokines via inflammasome-mediated invigoration of IL-1β and IL-18. The PLpro (NSP3) of SARS-CoV-2 has several unique SARS-CoV-2 unique domains (SUD) that are responsible for triggering NLRP3 inflammasome signaling response, resulting in release of excessive amounts of pro-inflammatory cytokines that instigate the infiltration of neutrophils and macrophages to the site of infection (Bouayad, 2020). NSP8 protein of SARS-CoV-2 impairs the transcription of several ISGs (e.g. IFIT1, IFIT2) and certain proinflammatory cytokines, by inhibiting the components upstream in the RIG-I/MDA5 signaling pathway (Yang *et al.*, 2020). Another means exploited by SARS-CoV-2 to suppress IFN signaling is to upregulate the negative regulators of IFN pathway. SOCS proteins (SOCS1 and SOCS3) act at different levels in the JAK/STAT signaling pathway as a "retro-control" mechanism that acts to suppress the response to maintain homeostasis (Sa Ribero *et al.*, 2020).

9.15. Inhibition of ISG Function

ORF6, ORF8 and N proteins of SARS-CoV-2 are implicated in directly inhibiting the functions of certain ISGs (Li *et al.*, 2020). The ORF6 and ORF8 proteins strongly antagonize the expression of antiviral ISGs induced by IFN-β signaling, and they inhibit transcription through ISREs. However, the N protein shows no significant effect. In addition, ORF6, ORF8 and N protein inhibit certain ISGs, including ISG54 and ISG56 (Figure 9.2). Direct suppression of effector functions of ISGs is very well-documented in other HCoVs. Thus, MERS-CoV encodes ORF4b protein that uniquely inhibits the function of the OAS-ribonuclease L (RNase L) machinery. OAS is one of the many ISGs that identifies the free viral RNA in the cytosol, and degrades it (Park and Iwasaki, 2020). The ORF4b of MERS-CoV utilizes its 2′-5′-phosphodiesterase activity that cleaves the product of OAS to prevent activation of RNase L (Park and Iwasaki, 2020). A similar mechanism in SARS-CoV-2 has not yet been documented. These are only some of the numerous ways in which SARS-CoV-2 interacts with the web of host cell pathways. Even minute effects of proteins on different aspects of cell physiology can perturb cellular homeostasis. The multitude of strategies used by SARS-CoV-2 to impair IFN and ISG production may prove detrimental to the host — learning more about them can help to counter COVID-19 and similar threats in future.

9.16. Inhibition of Adaptive Immunity

The secreted IFNs, ISGs, and pro-inflammatory cytokines stimulate the immune system into an active and responsive immune state where large numbers of leukocytes, including activated neutrophils, monocytes, B- and T-lymphocytes, migrate to the site of infection. The alveolar macrophages and B-lymphocytes recognize virus-infected epithelial cells based on the changes in the host cell surface antigens, and phagocytosis occurs. Upon internalization, the viral antigens are processed and presented on the surface of the macrophages with major histocompatibility complex (MHC-II) molecules which prime the adaptive immune responsive. The pathogen-specific immunity targets the virus and virus-infected cells for clearance. The activated B-lymphocytes clonally expand and start secreting large amounts of antibodies against viral determinants. The antibodies help to eliminate the pathogen by enhancing opsonization and phagocytosis, and by neutralizing the viral particles. The antigen presentation by professional antigen-presenting cells or APCs (macrophages, dendritic cells, B-lymphocytes) primes T-lymphocytes that ultimately work to clear the infection (Kumar *et al.*, 2020). SARS-CoV-2 carries proteins that can attenuate certain mechanisms of adaptive immunity. A new feature of SARS-CoV-2 is the presence of the ORF8 protein, which potentially downregulates MHC-I surface presentation and thus antigen presentation. One proposed mechanism is by co-localizing with MHC in lysosomes and re-routing it to autophagosomes. As a result, the surface presentation of viral peptides complexed with MHC-I to T-lymphocytes is impaired — partially disabling the second arm of host immune system. Virus-infected host cells escape detection and clearance, thus benefitting viral replication (Park, 2020; Zhang *et al.*, 2021). Another intriguing protein of SARS-CoV-2 is the 73-amino acid long ORF9c, which downregulates antigen processing (Lu, 2020). The presence of viral ORF9c protein is sufficient to significantly reduce the levels of proteins that mediate various steps of antigen processing, complexing and presentation. These host proteins are involved in antigen loading and display (HLA proteins, β2M, antigen transporters TAP1 and TAP2) to proteins involved in the ubiquitin-proteasome system (ubiquitin-conjugating enzymes UBE2I and UBE2L6; deubiquitinating enzymes USP18 and UPS41; and proteasome components PSMB and PSME).

Studies suggest that mild infection with SARS-CoV-2 successfully develops virus-specific antibodies. The recovered individual not only has specific antibodies, but also memory B-cells and T-cells that confer protective immunity upon antigen re-encounter (Rodda *et al.*, 2021). However, studies on serum samples of recovered COVID-19 patients offer new insights into the body's serologic responses against the virus. The findings suggest that the serological memory decays over a course of 6 months after recovery. The reason behind this short B-cell memory is suspected to be some viral factor that impairs the process of differentiation of the B-cell, which matures from an actively antibody-secreting plasma cell to a stable memory B-cell (Jeffery-Smith *et al.*, 2021). Knowledge of all the viral strategies that target and handicap the host immune system may help to design effective treatment approaches. Evidently, IFNs show protective effects against SARS-CoV, MERS-CoV, and recently SARS-CoV-2 infections. The induction of hundreds of different ISGs can practically target each and every stage of the viral infection cycle, including viral entry, replication, protein synthesis, assembly and exit of new virion particles. Therefore, IFN treatment is a potential therapeutic approach for these diseases, and may mitigate severe disease and even prevent infection. However, the timing of IFN administration is one of the most important determinants of the outcome. IFN treatment is useful only when given prior to infection or early during infection, whereas late administration is generally ineffective and may even be detrimental (Box 9.1). Therefore, combinatorial treatment with other antiviral drugs

Box 9.1.   Setting up a storm: COVID-19 and cytokine imbalance.

Cytokines are key factors that modulate the immune response of the body. When SARS-CoV-2 enters the lungs, IFN production is strongly inhibited, thus facilitating elevated viral proliferation and viral load at the site of infection. This increase in virions induces infected cells to generate pro-inflammatory cytokines which subsequently recruit neutrophils, macrophages, and monocytes. The recruited immune cells produce additional cytokines needed to combat the pathogen. However, in some cases, due to recurrent recruitment of immune cells, an excessive number and/or level of cytokines is produced, leading to a hyper-inflammatory phenomenon known as the "cytokine storm". This storm results from a sudden acute increase in circulating levels of pro-inflammatory cytokines such as IL-6, IL-1, TNF-α. The resultant increased vascular permeability causes arteries and veins to leak blood and plasma, with subsequent decrease in blood pressure. This also gives rise to enhanced extravasation of neutrophils and macrophages from the circulation into the infection site — with destructive effects on tissues such as damage of endothelial cells and capillaries, pulmonary alveolar cells, and obstruction of airways. Especially in the lungs, severe injury can manifest itself as acute respiratory distress syndrome or ARDS (Ragab *et al.*, 2020). Multiple studies reveal significantly higher levels of cytokines and chemokines including IL-6, IL-7, IL-8, IL-9, IL-10, FGF, G-CSF, IP-10, MCP-1, MIP-1A, MIP-1B, TNF-α, CXCL2, and CXCL8 in COVID-19 mortality cases (Chen *et al.*, 2020; Gao *et al.*, 2020; Huang *et al.*, 2020; Ruan *et al.*, 2020). The cytokine-induced ARDS renders other organs of the body susceptible to injury. In fact, ARDS-related multi-organ failure is the leading cause of death in many COVID-19 patients (Ruan *et al.*, 2020). Hyper-inflammation is also promoted by co-morbidities such as aging, smoking, diabetes, and hypertension. Patients with such co-morbidities are at higher risk of severity compared to those without (Jordan *et al.*, 2020). One study demonstrated the effectiveness of blocking IL-1 cytokine signaling to alleviate the hyper-inflammation in sepsis patients (Shakoory *et al.*, 2016). Notably, specific immunosuppression strategies can be effective against the cytokine storm in COVID-19 patients. Tocilizumab, an IL-6 inhibitor, has beneficial effects for the treatment of patients with severe COVID-19 (Xu *et al.*, 2020). Another study reported that immune-suppressants did not increase the risk of COVID-19, while TNF-α inhibitors significantly reduced the chances of severe disease (Veenstra *et al.*, 2020). Hence, it is possible to manage and ameliorate the cytokine storm, by leveraging on the intricacies of the virus–host interactions.

may help to optimize its clinical application to treat SARS-CoV-2 infection. Despite the numerous strategies the virus deploys to dampen the immune system and establish disease, humanity can still have hope in defeating this pandemic.

Acknowledgments

Shashank Tripathi is supported by DBT-IISc partnership funds. Shachee Swaraj is supported by Primer Minister's Research Fellowship. Tanisha Malpani is supported by KVPY Fellowship.

References

Amor S *et al.* Innate immunity during SARS-CoV-2: Evasion strategies and activation trigger hypoxia and vascular damage. *Clin Exp Immunol* 2020; 202:193–209.

Bouayad A. Innate immune evasion by SARS-CoV-2: Comparison with SARS-CoV. *Rev Med Virol* 2020; 30:1–9.

Braciale TJ, Hahn YS. Immunity to viruses. *Immunol Rev* 2013; 255:5–12.

Canton J *et al.* MERS-CoV 4b protein interferes with the NF-κB-dependent innate immune response during infection. *PLoS Pathog* 2018; 14:e1006838.

Chen G *et al.* Clinical and immunologic features in severe and moderate Coronavirus Disease 2019. *J Clin Invest* 2020; 130:2620–2629.

Freundt EC *et al.* Molecular determinants for subcellular localization of the severe acute respiratory syndrome Coronavirus open reading frame 3b protein. *J Virol* 2009; 83:6631–6640.

Frieman M *et al.* SARS-CoV ORF6 antagonizes STAT1 function by sequestering nuclear import factors on the rER/Golgi membrane. *J Virol* 2007; 81: 9812–9824.

Frieman M *et al.* Severe acute respiratory syndrome Coronavirus Papain-like protease Ubiquitin-like domain and catalytic domain regulate antagonism of IRF3 and NF-κB signaling. *J Virol* 2009; 83:6689–6705.

Gao Y *et al.* Diagnostic utility of clinical laboratory data determinations for patients with the severe COVID-19. *J Med Virol* 2020; 92:791–796.

Gordon DE *et al.* A SARS-CoV-2 protein interaction map reveals targets for drug repurposing. *Nature* 2020; 583:459–468.

Han L *et al.* SARS-CoV-2 ORF9b antagonizes type I and III interferons by targeting multiple components of the RIG-I/MDA-5-MAVS, TLR3-TRIF, and cGAS-STING signaling pathways. *J Med Virol* 2021; 93:5376–5389.

Hu Y *et al*. The severe acute respiratory syndrome Coronavirus nucleocapsid inhibits type I interferon production by interfering with TRIM25-mediated RIG-I ubiquitination. *J Virol* 2017; 91:e02143–16.

Huang C *et al*. SARS Coronavirus nsp1 protein induces template-dependent endonucleolytic cleavage of mRNAs: Viral mRNAs are resistant to nsp1-induced RNA cleavage. *PLoS Pathog* 2011; 7:e1002433.

Huang C *et al*. Clinical features of patients infected with 2019 novel Coronavirus in Wuhan, China. *Lancet* 2020; 395:497–506.

Jeffery-Smith A *et al*. SARS-CoV-2-specific memory B cells can persist in the elderly who have lost detectable neutralising antibodies. *J Clin Invest* 2021; e152042.

Jiang H *et al*. SARS-CoV-2 Orf9b suppresses type I interferon responses by targeting TOM70. *Cell Mol Immunol* 2020; 17:998–1000.

Jordan RE *et al*. COVID-19: Risk factors for severe disease and death. *BMJ* 2020; 368:m1198.

Kikkert M. Innate immune evasion by human respiratory RNA viruses. *J Innate Immun* 2020; 12:4–20.

Knoops K *et al*. SARS-Coronavirus replication is supported by a reticulovesicular network of modified endoplasmic reticulum. *PLoS Biol* 2008; 6:e226.

Konno Y *et al*. SARS-CoV-2 ORF3b is a potent interferon antagonist whose activity is increased by a naturally occurring elongation variant. *Cell Rep* 2020; 32:108185.

Kumar S *et al*. Host immune response and immunobiology of human SARS-CoV-2 infection. In: Saxena SK. (Ed.), *Coronavirus Disease 2019 (COVID-19). Medical Virology: From Pathogenesis to Disease Control* (pp. 43–53). Springer, Singapore, 2020.

Lei X *et al*. Activation and evasion of type I interferon responses by SARS-CoV-2. *Nat Commun* 2020; 11:e3810.

Li JY *et al*. The ORF6, ORF8 and nucleocapsid proteins of SARS-CoV-2 inhibit type I interferon signaling pathway. *Virus Res* 2020; 286:198074.

Lim YX *et al*. Human Coronaviruses: A review of virus–host interactions. *Diseases* 2016; 4:26.

Lokugamage KG *et al*. Middle East respiratory syndrome Coronavirus nsp1 inhibits host gene expression by selectively targeting mRNAs transcribed in the nucleus while sparing mRNAs of cytoplasmic origin. *J Virol* 2015; 89:10970–10981.

Lu F. SARS-CoV-2 ORF9c: A mysterious membrane-anchored protein that regulates immune evasion? *Nat Rev Immunol* 2020; 20:648.

Lu X *et al*. SARS-CoV nucleocapsid protein antagonizes IFN-β response by targeting initial step of IFN-β induction pathway, and its C-terminal region is critical for the antagonism. *Virus Genes* 2011; 42:37–45.

Lui PK *et al*. Middle East respiratory syndrome Coronavirus M protein suppresses type I interferon expression through the inhibition of TBK1-dependent phosphorylation of IRF3. *Emerg Microbes Infect* 2016; 5:e39.

Minakshi R *et al*. The SARS Coronavirus 3a protein causes endoplasmic reticulum stress and induces ligand-independent downregulation of the Type 1 interferon receptor. *PLoS One* 2009; 4:e8342.

Moustaqil M *et al*. SARS-CoV-2 proteases cleave IRF3 and critical modulators of inflammatory pathways (NLRP12 and TAB1): Implications for disease presentation across species and the search for reservoir hosts. *Emerg Microbes Infect* 2021; 10:178–195.

Mu J *et al*. SARS-CoV-2-encoded nucleocapsid protein acts as a viral suppressor of RNA interference in cells. *Sci China Life Sci* 2020; 63:1413–1416.

Oudshoorn D *et al*. Expression and cleavage of Middle East respiratory syndrome Coronavirus nsp3-4 polyprotein induce the formation of double-membrane vesicles that mimic those associated with Coronaviral RNA replication. *mBio* 2017; 8:e01658-17.

Park A, Iwasaki A. Type I and Type III interferons — Induction, signaling, evasion, and application to combat COVID-19. *Cell Host Microbe* 2020; 27:870–878.

Park, MD Immune evasion via SARS-CoV-2 ORF8 protein? *Nat Rev Immunol.* 20, 408 (2020).

Ragab D *et al*. The COVID-19 cytokine storm; what we know so far. *Front Immunol* 2020; 11:1446.

Reggiori F *et al*. Coronaviruses Hijack the LC3-I-positive EDEMosomes, ER-derived vesicles exporting short-lived ERAD regulators, for replication. *Cell Host Microbe* 2010; 7:500–508.

Rodda L *et al*. Functional SARS-CoV-2-specific immune memory persists after mild COVID-19. *Cell* 2021; 184:169–183.e17

Ruan Q *et al*. Clinical predictors of mortality due to COVID-19 based on an analysis of data of 150 patients from Wuhan, China. *Intensive Care Med* 2020; 46:846–848.

Sa Ribero M *et al*. Interplay between SARS-CoV-2 and the type I interferon response. *PLoS Pathog* 2020; 16:e1008737.

Santerre M *et al*. Why do SARS-CoV-2 NSPs rush to the ER? *J Neurol* 2020; 268:2013–2022.

Seth R *et al*. Antiviral innate immunity pathways. *Cell Res* 2006; 16:141–147.

Shakoory B *et al*. Interleukin-1 receptor blockade is associated with reduced mortality in sepsis patients with features of macrophage activation syndrome: Reanalysis of a prior phase iii trial. *Crit Care Med* 2016; 44: 275–281.

Shi CS *et al*. SARS-Coronavirus open reading Frame-9b suppresses innate immunity by targeting mitochondria and the MAVS/TRAF3/TRAF6 signalosome. *J Immunol* 2014; 193:3080–3089.

Shin D *et al*. Papain-like protease regulates SARS-CoV-2 viral spread and innate immunity. *Nature* 2020; 587:657–662.

Shokri S *et al*. Modulation of the immune response by Middle East respiratory syndrome Coronavirus. *J Cell Physiol* 2018; 234:2143–2151.

Siu KL *et al*. Severe acute respiratory syndrome Coronavirus M protein inhibits type I interferon production by impeding the formation of TRAF3.TANK. TBK1/IKKepsilon complex. *J Biol Chem* 2009; 284:16202–16209.

Siu KL *et al*. Middle east respiratory syndrome Coronavirus 4a protein is a double-stranded RNA-binding protein that suppresses PACT-induced activation of RIG-I and MDA5 in the innate antiviral response. *J Virol* 2014; 88(9):4866–4876.

Sun L *et al*. Coronavirus papain-like proteases negatively regulate antiviral innate immune response through disruption of STING-mediated signaling. *PloS One* 2012; 7:30802.

Thoms M *et al*. Structural basis for translational shutdown and immune evasion by the Nsp1 protein of SARS-CoV-2. *Science* 2020; 369:1249–1255.

Thornbrough JM *et al*. Middle East respiratory syndrome Coronavirus NS4b protein inhibits host RNase L activation. *mBio* 2016; 7:e00258–16.

Totura AL, Baric RS. SARS Coronavirus pathogenesis: Host innate immune responses and viral antagonism of interferon. *Curr Opin Virol* 2012; 2:264–275.

Veenstra J *et al*. Antecedent immunosuppressive therapy for immune-mediated inflammatory diseases in the setting of a COVID-19 outbreak. *J Am Acad Dermatol* 2020; 83:1696–1703.

Viswanathan T *et al*. Structural basis of RNA cap modification by SARS-CoV-2. *Nat Commun* 2020; 11:e3718.

Wathelet MG *et al*. Severe acute respiratory syndrome Coronavirus evades antiviral signaling: Role of nsp1 and rational design of an attenuated strain. *J Virol* 2007; 81:11620–11633.

Weber F. Antiviral innate immunity: Introduction. *Encyclopedia of Virology* 2021; 1:577–583.

Wolff G *et al*. A molecular pore spans the double membrane of Coronavirus replication organelle. *Science* 2020; 369:1395–1398.

Wong HH *et al*. Accessory proteins 8b and 8ab of severe acute respiratory syndrome Coronavirus suppress the interferon signaling pathway by mediating ubiquitin-dependent rapid degradation of interferon regulatory factor 3. *Virology* 2018; 515:165–175.

Wong LYR *et al*. Middle East respiratory syndrome Coronavirus ORF8b accessory protein suppresses Type I IFN expression by impeding HSP70-dependent activation of IRF3 kinase IKKε. *J Immunol* 2020; 205:1564–1579.

Xia X. Extreme genomic CpG deficiency in SARS-CoV-2 and evasion of host antiviral defense. *Mol Biol Evol* 2020; 37:2699–2705.

Xia H *et al*. Evasion of Type I interferon by SARS-CoV-2. *Cell Rep* 2020; 33:108234.

Xu X *et al*. Effective treatment of severe COVID-19 patients with Tocilizumab. *Proc Natl Acad Sci USA* 2020; 117:11970–11975.

Yang Y *et al*. Middle East respiratory syndrome Coronavirus ORF4b protein inhibits type I interferon production through both cytoplasmic and nuclear targets. *Sci Rep* 2015; 5:e17554.

Yang Z *et al*. Suppression of MDA5-mediated antiviral immune responses by NSP8 of SARS-CoV-2. *bioRxiv* 2020; 2020.08.12.247767.

Yuen CK *et al*. SARS-CoV-2 nsp13, nsp14, nsp15 and orf6 function as potent interferon antagonists. *Emerg Microbes Infect* 2020; 9:1418–1428.

Zhang Y *et al*. The ORF8 protein of SARS-CoV-2 mediates immune evasion through down-regulating MHC-I. *Proc Natl Acad Sci USA* 2021; 118: e2024202118.

Zheng Y *et al*. Severe acute respiratory syndrome Coronavirus 2 (SARS-CoV-2) membrane (M) protein inhibits type I and III interferon production by targeting RIG-I/MDA-5 signaling. *Signal Transduct Target Ther* 2020; 5:299.

Chapter 10

Transcriptomics and Proteomics of SARS-CoV-2 Infection and COVID-19

Kai Sen Tan[*,‡,§,¶]**, Ryan Zhe Zhang Lew**[‡,‖]**,
and De Yun Wang**[‡,**]

**Department of Microbiology and Immunology,
Infectious Diseases Translational Research Program,
Yong Loo Lin School of Medicine,
National University Health System,
National University of Singapore,
Kent Ridge, Singapore*

*‡Department of Otolaryngology,
Infectious Diseases Translational Research Program,
Yong Loo Lin School of Medicine,
National University Health System,
National University of Singapore, Kent Ridge, Singapore*

*§NUSMed BSL-3 Core Facility,
Yong Loo Lin School of Medicine,
National University Health System,
National University of Singapore,
Kent Ridge, Singapore*

¶kaistan@nus.edu.sg
‖entlzzr@nus.edu.sg
**entwdy@nus.edu.sg

Abstract

The emergence of the novel severe acute respiratory syndrome Coronavirus-2 (SARS-CoV-2) Coronavirus resulted in a global pandemic due to its nature of rapid transmission and variable severities that facilitated its spread worldwide. Correspondingly, owing to advances in molecular technologies, information on this virus is generated at an unprecedented pace. Since the onset of the pandemic, multiple high-throughput "omics" analyses — including transcriptomics and proteomics of different viral infection models — have been made readily available to the research and wider community. The availability and ability to rapidly generate these data facilitate the deciphering of virus–host interactions during SARS-CoV-2 infection — thus enhancing understanding of the viral transmission, host susceptibility, pathogenesis, viral evolution, and disease complications. Such information is vital for eventual applications towards biomarker and treatment discovery against Coronavirus disease 2019 (COVID-19), and can serve as useful models for future pandemic responses.

Keywords: Coronavirus; SARS-CoV-2; COVID-19; respiratory viral infection; high-throughput analysis; transcriptomics; proteomics; host–pathogen interactions; infection models; inflammation; immune responses; host responses; marker discovery; target discovery; therapeutics

10.1. Overview

Severe acute respiratory syndrome Coronavirus-2 SARS-CoV-2 is a novel Coronavirus and the causative agent of Coronavirus disease 2019 (COVID-19) that first emerged in China in late 2019, and spread rapidly across the globe within the span of months, resulting in a pandemic (Guan *et al.*, 2020; Li *et al.*, 2020b). The high transmissibility of the virus and the propensity to cause severe complications, including pneumonia and acute respiratory distress syndrome (ARDS), has wreaked a heavy healthcare and economic toll on a global scale (Fu *et al.*, 2020; Hu *et al.*, 2020). Like any newly emerging virus, there are still a great number of gaps in understanding and unpredictability of SARS-CoV-2 pathogenesis and its course of infection. While severe cases of COVID-19 have been attributed to the cytokine storm, the exact mechanisms and determinants triggering the event remain unknown and are likely heterogeneous (Guo *et al.*, 2020). In addition, the virus is also mutating and adapting to its new human host, thus contributing further to the variability in severity (Gamage *et al.*, 2020). Hence, comprehensive analyses that take into account the virus and host interactions, along with the host responses during the infection, are required to provide new management strategies against SARS-CoV-2 infection (Pizzorno *et al.*, 2020).

When a virus infects its host, it interacts with the host to facilitate its replication; while the host elicits a wide array of responses against the virus in order to clear the virus as well as to cope with the damage from the infection (Gamage *et al.*, 2020; Pizzorno *et al.*, 2020). The responses exerted by the host can be either beneficial or detrimental to the virus and host alike. Hence, accurately classifying and understanding these interactions are vital in uncovering the viral transmission and pathogenesis mechanisms associated with the development of the disease and pathology in the host. In the case of SARS-CoV-2, there is a high degree of variability in the symptoms following infection, mirroring other infections such as influenza A (Gamage *et al.*, 2020). Therefore, to be able to interrogate determinants of COVID-19 disease severity caused by SARS-CoV-2, studies of gene and protein expression changes following infection via transcriptomics and proteomics are currently a subject of intense research.

10.2. Transcriptomics and Proteomics Studies as High-Throughput Analysis Tools to Understand the Science of SARS-CoV-2 and COVID-19

With the advent of high-throughput assays, the field of "omics" has witnessed a boom of interest and activity. The ability to quickly uncover the wide array of responses from cells and tissues using *in vitro* and *in vivo* models could rapidly advance the field of viral-host interactions. By investigating the gene and protein expression profiles following infection and comparing them to uninfected controls, the changes in expression can be associated with specific infection outcomes. These studies thus provide an important first step to identify important biomarkers and targets for diagnostic, prognostic and therapeutic purposes.

Since its conception and application, "omics" studies have been harnessed to study and analyze many different disease conditions including cancer, metabolic diseases, genetic diseases, chronic diseases as well as infectious diseases. The ability to uncover and correlate gene expression alterations in disease conditions facilitated the advancement of clinical guidelines and public health policies that aid in the effective diagnosis and treatment of diseases. In the field of infectious diseases, this tool is highly valuable as the "omics" platform can capture acute changes following infection, given that acute inflammation following pathogen infection generally induces rapid changes in genome transcription. Therefore, transcriptomics and proteomics in the field of viral infectious diseases are vital in understanding the transmission and pathology of novel infectious diseases such as COVID-19 (Grenga and Armengaud, 2020).

During acute infection caused by an RNA virus like SARS-CoV-2, many of the responses by the host are rapid, and hence mostly clustered as mRNA and protein changes. To investigate these signatures, technologies like microarray and RNA sequencing (including single cell RNA sequencing) are employed to investigate transcriptomic changes at the mRNA or microRNA level; while mass spectrometry is utilized for proteomic analysis to unravel post-translational changes following infection. In addition, secretomics studies using conventional and multiplex ELISA are able to detect proteins (e.g. cytokines and chemokines) in the blood and serum of patients, which also constitute another aspect of proteomics. Given that the changes during an acute infection are temporal and complex, the benefits of "omics" analysis is that it can offer a snapshot of "global" alterations occurring during the infection at a specific point in time. The data and information gleaned from these experiments would then allow researchers to infer the specific events occurring only in infected samples that are significant to the course of the infection. Such inferences can be made by comparing the changes in infected samples with reference to matched controls without the infection. Upon obtaining "omics" information of infected samples, the signatures can then be correlated to molecular pathway databases to uncover the critical pathway alterations contributing to pathogenesis of COVID-19; or in clinical settings, be correlated to specific clinical events to serve as diagnostic biomarkers for the disease. In the longer term, such identified markers may also serve as treatment targets to be explored for better management strategies against SARS-CoV-2 infection and COVID-19 (Gordon *et al.*, 2020).

10.3. Deciphering the Wealth of Transcriptomics and Proteomics Data

Since the first discovery and isolation of SARS-CoV-2 virus, "omics" data, particularly transcriptomics data, were generated at an unprecedented pace. Because of this, there is a wealth of complex "omics" data available which requires deciphering for their differential importance and clinical significance (Fagone *et al.*, 2020). The "omics" data are usually generated from different sources, including *in vitro* cell lines and primary cell models, and *in vivo* animal models (mice, ferrets, non-human primates), as well as human samples. Each model has its own merits and the data obtained may be interpreted differently, contributing a piece to the whole picture towards understanding the host responses against SARS-CoV-2 infection and the pathogenesis of COVID-19.

As the basic building blocks of the host organism, the epithelial cells in the airway represent the primary target of SARS-CoV-2 infection. Hence, the usage of homogenous epithelial cell lines offers a relevant glimpse of primary responses when infected with the SARS-CoV-2 virus. Transcriptomic data derived from cell lines are often the easiest to be generated, and they provide the initial knowledge of cellular responses against SARS-CoV-2 infection. In addition, immune cell lines are also exploited to interrogate the immune responses elicited upon contact with the virus or viral components. Although simple, these cell line models form the initial baseline of "omics" studies and can highlight key pathways to focus on during subsequent analyses in more complex models. However, the simplicity of cell lines also contributed to their shortcomings. These simple, homogenous models are often derived from the immortalization of cell samples or cancerous cells — in which the information that they will provide may sometimes be an over- or under-estimation of what occurs physiologically when compared to a systemic model. This is due to the lack of interactions with other cell types that may also influence the responses during infection. In addition, "omics" data from immune cell lines are usually generated by direct interaction with the virus, which is usually not the case in systemic immune responses. Hence, findings based on these simple models may be further confounded by their inherent simplicity.

Therefore, to compensate for the simplicity of cell line models, "omics" studies involving transcriptomics and proteomics have expanded in recent years towards heterogeneous models of 3D cultures using primary cells or progenitor cells (Tan *et al.*, 2018b, 2019; Zhao *et al.*, 2012). These 3D models consist of air-liquid interface (ALI) cultures, *ex vivo* organ explants and organoids. Unlike cell lines, these cell models are established by isolating stem or progenitor cells from biopsies of human donors. When grown *in vitro* to maturity, these models closely mimic the physiological morphology of the respiratory airway, the actual source of the cells. The model consists of the different cell types that are present in the respiratory airway with a similar pseudo-stratified structure. Conducting transcriptomics or proteomics analyses using these *in vitro* models would be able to provide insights into the early cellular events of SARS-CoV-2 infection in the airway that are driving its pathogenesis and severity. In addition, interactions between the different cell types will also be reflected in these models, and hence exhibit more physiological responses against the infection when performing "omics" analyses. While these models provide physiologically relevant "omics" responses against SARS-CoV-2 infection, they are usually limited to the early events within the epithelium. This is because the model lacks the immune components of the host that can clear the virus infection, and the model is unable to capture downstream activation of the immune system following infection (Gamage *et al.*, 2020; Tan *et al.*, 2018a; Yan *et al.*, 2016). Although immune responses can be inferred to a certain extent by "omics" responses of the epithelium based on the associated pathways of the "omics" changes, the prediction may not be completely accurate due to the absence of immune cells to drive the full responses. Recently however, there are attempts to rectify this shortcoming by inclusion of immune cells in co-cultures of 3D models or respiratory organoids (Luukkainen *et al.*, 2018); but such strategies are still in their infancy and have to surmount multiple limitations to be able to accurately recapitulate the physiological cross-talk between epithelial and immune cells.

On the other hand, in order to elucidate the responses against SARS-CoV-2 infection at a systemic level, animal models are used to represent systemic models that are able to recapitulate events of an infection at an organismal level. Given that model organisms can respond to viral infections in similar fashion as humans (including transmission, pathology and recovery), the "omics" analyses performed on these models can provide information about the complete temporal changes in the responses following infection, all the way to viral clearance and recovery from infection. Since its discovery, there have been studies on the pathology of SARS-CoV-2 infection in different animal models in attempts to investigate the pathogenesis of COVID-19. Animal models include rodent models such as mice, hamsters, ferrets (which is a key model organism for respiratory viral infections), and non-human primate models that potentially behave the closest to humans in terms of their responses towards SARS-CoV-2 infection (Blanco-Melo *et al.*, 2020; Cleary *et al.*, 2020). The "omics" analyses performed on animal models will be able to comprehensively reveal the disease progression of COVID-19, and to elucidate the changes at each point of the disease process. However, while being able to provide comprehensive temporal "omics" responses against SARS-CoV-2 infection, several fundamental differences between animals and humans remain — hence, not all findings from animal models may be generalizable to humans. Therefore, findings from animal models will usually be correlated with findings from *in vitro* human models to acquire a more accurate prediction of transcriptomics and proteomics signatures that may serve as diagnostic biomarkers or therapeutic targets.

Finally, "omics" studies in humans represent the most physiologically relevant investigations in the case of SARS-CoV-2 infection and COVID-19. However, due to ethical concerns, controlled infection experiments would usually not be allowed for severe infections such as SARS-CoV-2. Therefore, most human studies focus on collecting samples from infected patients, and then matching the samples for analysis according to various criteria such as age, time of infection, and underlying diseases. The "omics" analyses in humans will then facilitate the identification of potential diagnostic biomarkers in severely infected patients, or further testing their utility as treatment targets. However, as there are significant variations between individuals, proper sampling and matching are imperative to ensure the accuracy of the studies. Hence, the challenge in human-based transcriptomics and proteomics lies in the ability to control for inter-individual variation to make meaningful comparisons. In addition, sample integrity also presents another layer of difficulty since patient sample degradation is harder to control compared to studies using cell and animal models. Nevertheless, valuable "omics" data can be forthcoming if these issues are properly addressed, and they may serve as the "raw" data to design further studies that contribute to immediate impact and improved clinical practice in the management of COVID-19 patients.

When analyzing transcriptomics and proteomics data of infections with viruses such as SARS-CoV-2, there are several pathways of interest that can potentially lead to differential severity of the infection. Firstly, differences in innate and adaptive immune pathways (including cytokine and chemokine expression) which form the bulk of the pathology, are usually compared between different degrees of severity, as well as between different virus strains. Next, changes in epithelial cell functions and their metabolic alterations may also offer clues on the pathogenesis of COVID-19, since the epithelial cells act as the physical barrier against incoming pathogens and may compromise the airway when damaged (Tan *et al.*, 2017, 2020). Cell death pathways such as apoptosis, necroptosis and pyroptosis may also influence barrier function, viral replication and inflammation, potentially altering the course and severity of the disease (Robinson *et al.*, 2020; Tan *et al.*, 2018b). Changes in cell cycle, gene expression and transcription factors may also determine the course of SARS-CoV-2 infection. Finally, microRNA transcriptomics may also contribute to the acute inflammatory process during infection as well as recovery following infection, thus warranting detailed investigation and analysis. By considering mRNA, microRNA and protein expression changes in these pathways, as well as the model where the changes are observed, and the overlaps that exist across different models, vital information contributing towards deciphering SARS-CoV-2 pathogenesis can be acquired.

10.4. Transcriptomic and Proteomic Analyses of ACE2, the Entry Receptor of SARS-CoV-2

During its infection, SARS-CoV-2 enters the susceptible host cell via the angiotensin-converting enzyme 2 (ACE2). Given that SARS-CoV-2 is highly related to SARS-CoV (which also uses ACE2 as its entry receptor), the entry receptor of SARS-CoV-2 was predicted to bind ACE2 as well, and this has been experimentally verified (Ziegler *et al.*, 2020). Since its confirmation as the SARS-CoV-2 entry receptor, transcriptomics and proteomics data on the tissue expression of ACE2 have been generated rapidly. These sets of data revealed that the ACE2 receptor is ubiquitous across multiple tissues including the kidney, nervous system and endothelial system (Ahmetaj-Shala *et al.*, 2020; Wang *et al.*, 2020b; Wu *et al.*, 2020a). Surprisingly, the airway tissue expression of ACE2 is not as strong as expected, which raised the hypothesis of co-factor(s) for SARS-CoV-2 infection. Further transcriptomic profiling revealed TMPRSS2 as a co-factor of viral entry that aids SARS-CoV-2 infection in the airway, and it is expressed at higher abundance in the airway (Liu *et al.*, 2020b).

In addition, transcriptomic and proteomic analyses further identified other SARS-CoV-2-associated proteases, cathepsins B and L, which can also function as co-factors of viral entry and are generally more highly expressed in severe COVID-19 patients (Wu *et al.*, 2020b). Therefore, the transcriptomic and proteomic profiling performed during the early phases of the pandemic helped to explain the potential complications that SARS-CoV-2 may cause, due to the presence of its entry receptor(s) in multiple tissues, and laid the foundation for many clinical studies that further investigated the mechanisms of such complications.

10.5. Transcriptomic and Proteomic Alterations During SARS-CoV-2 Infection

10.5.1. *Changes in immune responses*

The immune responses are crucial for the host in combating foreign pathogens such as SARS-CoV-2. Since SARS-CoV-2 is an RNA virus, the response against such viruses by the host is initiated by generically detecting foreign biological components unique to the virus and its life-cycle, such as double-stranded RNAs, which occur with replication of the viral genomes. Such components, called pathogen-associated molecular patterns (PAMPs), are detected by the host via toll-like receptors (TLRs) and their associated pathways in the innate immunity arm of the host responses (Guo *et al.*, 2020). The activation of the TLR pathways initiated by the detection of viral PAMPs of SARS-CoV-2 will then trigger the interferon (IFN) pathways that prime the cells for antiviral responses in an attempt to restrict viral spread. Following the priming of the host epithelial cells, these cells will further secrete immune-signaling molecules (cytokines and chemokines) to recruit professional immune cells to initiate the adaptive immune responses. The adaptive immune responses against viral pathogens are generally dominant for type 1 inflammation, in which the main activation of adaptive immune cells is skewed towards CD8+ T-cells. The latter cells are the primary cells that remove infected cells by triggering cell death pathways in these cells. While type 1 inflammation is dominant, type 2 inflammation by the CD4+ T-cells remains important in order to clear free viral particles and to ensure immunologic memory against SARS-CoV-2 virus. The CD4+ T-cells cooperate with the other professional immune cells like macrophages and monocytes to process viral components and generate specific immunity, including antibody-producing B-cells against the virus. This will ensure that free viruses are removed from the host system, and that the persistence of immune memory will prevent re-infection of SARS-CoV-2 in the same host (Guo *et al.*, 2020).

Antiviral responses are important for the clearance of all respiratory viruses, including SARS-CoV-2. Therefore, transcriptomic and proteomic analyses focusing on the immune responses against SARS-CoV-2 will allow us to understand if SARS-CoV-2 infection will cause the host to mount the required responses against the virus. Through "omics" analyses, deviation from the "normal" pathways against viral infection can be detected, and hence identified as factors that may contribute to SARS-CoV-2 transmission, pathogenesis, and COVID-19 severity compared to other respiratory viruses.

10.5.1.1. *Innate response changes in COVID-19*

The innate immune responses against SARS-CoV-2, like other respiratory viruses, center along the activation of IFNs through the TLR pathways. However, as shown by early transcriptomics studies, the IFN activation of SARS-CoV-2-infected epithelial cells is highly subdued (Blanco-Melo *et al.*, 2020). Furthermore, as the initial IFN induction is suppressed, many interferon-stimulated genes (ISGs) are similarly weakly expressed or delayed in airway ALI culture model of infection (Gamage *et al.*, 2020; Pizzorno *et al.*, 2020). Using influenza virus infection as comparison, a robust IFN induction can be detected in ALI models as early as 8 hours post-infection, as opposed to 72 hours post-infection by SARS-CoV-2 (Gamage *et al.*, 2020). This finding was also confirmed by transcriptomics analysis of human swab samples of the upper airway, where innate immune responses against SARS-CoV-2 infection are dampened (Mick *et al.*, 2020). However, the initial suppression of innate immune responses does not reflect the overall pathogenesis of SARS-CoV-2. The pathology of SARS-CoV-2 infection is often linked to the cytokine storm, a state of uncontrolled activation of immune cells that accompanies certain viral infections such as influenza (Ryabkova *et al.*, 2020). Therefore, it is hypothesized that the suppression of upper airway innate immune responses upon initial contact with the virus may drive the strong activation of immune responses later in the infection. Indeed, the transcriptomics analysis of broncho-alveolar lavage fluid from the lower airway of COVID-19 patients revealed that the innate immune responses are strongly activated (Zhou *et al.*, 2020). These innate immune responses include IFN and ISGs that perpetuate the immune responses in the lower airway, likely contributing to the cytokine storm, lower airway and lung injury, and pneumonia that culminate in severe COVID-19 and death in SARS-CoV-2-infected patients.

Further transcriptomic and proteomic profiling was also performed on severe COVID-19 patients. It was observed that in severe COVID-19, IFN and ISGs, as well as leukocytic signatures were often highly expressed and represented (Gill *et al.*, 2020). This led to further downstream studies that implicated granulocytes, particularly neutrophils, in the pathogenesis of COVID-19 (Park and Lee, 2020; Shaath *et al.*, 2020; Vitte *et al.*, 2020; Wang *et al.*, 2020a). On the other hand, innate T-cells, particularly mucosal-associated invariant T-cells (MAIT), their activation and cytokine secretion were found to be reduced (Parrot *et al.*, 2020). MAIT cells have been strongly implicated in favorable responses against viral infections, and hence their reduction may contribute to COVID-19 pathology (Parrot *et al.*, 2020; van Wilgenburg *et al.*, 2018). Following this, transcriptomic analyses of leukocytes and immune cells then further revealed cytokine and chemokine profiles that may contribute to the pathogenesis and severity of SARS-CoV-2 infection and COVID-19, which will be elaborated in the subsequent section.

In addition to the aberrant innate immune responses likely caused by the viral suppression mechanisms of SARS-CoV-2, the differences in innate immune responses may directly contribute to the infection site of SARS-CoV-2. The viral entry receptor ACE2 is initially found to be induced by IFN, and to function as an ISG (Sajuthi *et al.*, 2020; Ziegler *et al.*, 2020). This is currently a point of contention as it was later found that the ACE2 increase detected by the transcriptomics analysis was attributed to a shorter transcript, dACE2, which does not bind SARS-CoV-2 (Saffern, 2020). Therefore, this finding highlighted the importance of further experimental verification of "omics" experiments, since there may exist limitations of the current "omics" technology in discerning the functional isoforms of specific genes. Nevertheless, the "omics" finding spurred further experimental validation and clinical studies that contributed to the utility of recombinant IFNs in the treatment of SARS-CoV-2 (Busnadiego *et al.*, 2020).

10.5.1.2. *Cytokines and chemokines in COVID-19*

The innate immune responses triggered by viral infections such as SARS-CoV-2 function to keep viral replication in check so that the adaptive immune responses can effectively clear the viral infection without inflicting excessive damage on the host. To achieve this, the initial site of infection and the initially recruited immune cells (including macrophages, granulocytes and innate T-cells) further secrete cytokines and chemokines to mediate crosstalk with the adaptive immune cells to mount appropriate responses against the SARS-CoV-2 infection. As stated previously, SARS-CoV-2 infections that lead to severe COVID-19 manifestations are often the result of cytokine storm. Hence, the transcriptomic and proteomic analyses of the initial infection site, and the recruited innate cells can offer further clues on the cytokines and chemokines that exacerbate the disease progression of SARS-CoV-2 infection.

Many studies have investigated the cytokine profiles following SARS-CoV-2 infection. Some studies indicate that expression of key cytokines during SARS-CoV-2 infection may not arise from the upper airway epithelial cells, where their antiviral responses are muted (Gamage *et al.*, 2020). Instead, most of the cytokines and chemokines produced in response to SARS-CoV-2 may arise from the initially recruited innate immune cells, in which their overexpression may then contribute to a potential cytokine storm that culminates in the pathology of COVID-19. At the epithelial cell level in the upper airway, the release of cytokines is similarly muted with only CXCL10 (IP-10) being actively secreted by infected nasal epithelial cells (Gamage *et al.*, 2020). In contrast, the lower airway is observed to elicit stronger but similarly delayed responses of IFIT1, MX1, CXCL10 and CXCL11 during infection of alveolar epithelial cells (Huang *et al.*, 2020b). These findings by transcriptomics and proteomics show that the epithelial airways may not be the major producer of cytokines and chemokines, which is unlike many other respiratory infections where the epithelial cells elicit good cytokine and chemokine production (Tan *et al.*, 2019). However, samples of broncho-alveolar lavage fluid, serum, and peripheral blood mononuclear cells (PBMCs) from COVID-19 patients exhibited strong and almost excessive production of cytokines and chemokines — thus signifying the imbalance of cytokine production by the epithelial and immune cells which likely contributes to the cytokine storm in the pathology of COVID-19. These studies reveal that in immune cells, cytokines and chemokines including CCL2, CXCL9, CXCL10, CCL3, CCL4 are elevated and their increased levels are often associated with more severe disease and mortality (Abers *et al.*, 2020; Xiong *et al.*, 2020).

10.5.1.3. *Inflammation and adaptive response*

Inflammation and the adaptive response represent the late and vital response to ensure viral clearance and long-term immune memory against viral infection in the host. A well-timed and appropriate inflammation supported by the relevant cell types ensure that free viruses and infected cells are cleared from the system with minimal damage (Qiao *et al.*, 2018).

However, SARS-CoV-2 infection is observed to mostly cause aberrant inflammation and adaptive responses, likely due to the imbalance in innate and cytokine responses from the epithelial and immune cells. The enhanced and prolonged inflammation, despite viral clearance in some patients, may lead to damage of the respiratory system and even multi-organ injury (Chen *et al.*, 2020b; Sadanandam *et al.*, 2020). Indeed, characterization of the inflammatory and adaptive immune responses in mice and humans alike revealed excessive and prolonged expression of inflammatory factors such as NF-κB, TNF, IL-6, IL-8, IL-15, IL-2 and IL-10, which are usually associated with severity and cytokine storm-like pathology in COVID-19 patients (Abers *et al.*, 2020; Chen *et al.*, 2020b; Li *et al.*, 2020a; Winkler *et al.*, 2020; Xiong *et al.*, 2020). In addition to the aberrant inflammation, transcriptomics and proteomics of SARS-CoV-2 infection elucidated skewing towards Th2 inflammation and adaptive immune responses, a diversion from the normal Th1 inflammation" and Th17 inflammation that is required for viral clearance (Liao *et al.*, 2020; Meckiff *et al.*, 2020; Vaz de Paula *et al.*, 2020). In addition, the Th2 inflammatory factor IL-13 was found to be strongly expressed following SARS-CoV-2 infection, and may promote ACE2 and TMPRSS2 expression which may then contribute to virus replication, thus aggravating COVID-19 severity and duration (Sajuthi *et al.*, 2020; Vaz de Paula *et al.*, 2020). The diversion from the norm of the adaptive immune response in SARS-CoV-2 infection may explain the clinically severe and prolonged COVID-19 in some patients, as the virus is not properly cleared from the system and continually activates inflammatory pathways that may result in host injury. The mechanisms and interactions that lead to these shunts warrant further investigation and verification in order to better understand SARS-CoV-2 pathogenesis.

10.5.2. *Changes in epithelial barrier functions and metabolism*

The airway epithelia (including both the upper and lower airways) form the mechanical barrier against invading pathogens — their tight formation, mechanical movement and mucus secretion constitute the first line of defense against preventing infection, on top of their immune functions (Tan *et al.*, 2017, 2020). Their tight formation via the tight junctions prevent easy access of the pathogens to other parts of the tissue (Huang *et al.*, 2020c; Tian *et al.*, 2018). Mechanical beating of the cilia then removes pathogens bound to the mucus layer of the epithelium to facilitate their expulsion from the system (Guan *et al.*, 2018; Tan *et al.*, 2020). Hence, it is important that the airway epithelium remains intact during an infection to keep viral replication in check during the early stages of the infection. In view of this, metabolism in the epithelium is also an important topic for further studies given that any alteration of metabolism may compromise epithelial function (Tan *et al.*, 2017, 2020). In addition, the metabolic pathways in the immune cells during SARS-CoV-2 infection bear similar importance since metabolic compounds may contribute to normal immune signaling in immune cells (Andonegui-Elguera *et al.*, 2020).

Upon infection by SARS-CoV-2, the epithelial cells also undergo changes that may alter their barrier function on top of their immune responses. Most notably, ciliated cell markers undergo rapid and strong down-regulation in expression, negatively correlating with immune responses (Nunnari *et al.*, 2020). This is coupled with the increased expression of mucus-related genes and proteins such as MUC5AC and TMPRSS2 (Sajuthi *et al.*, 2020).The finding is further corroborated by clinical assessment of mucus production in COVID-19 patients (Huang *et al.*, 2020a; Liu *et al.*, 2020a; Lu *et al.*, 2020). The increased expression of mucus-related genes and decreased expression of ciliary genes may be attributed to the expression of IL-13 following SARS-CoV-2 infection, given that IL-13 is a strong inducer of goblet cell differentiation and mucus production (Liu *et al.*, 2018; Sajuthi *et al.*, 2020). In addition to the barrier function, lipid synthesis, MMP2, MMP9 and keratin sulfate synthesis pathways are also altered in the infected epithelial cells which may further compromise signaling processes and epithelial integrity (Karakurt and Pir, 2020; Shaath and Alajez, 2020). These transcriptomic findings indicate that the induction of immune responses against

SARS-CoV-2 infection may lead to the epithelial barrier being compromised — such findings may significantly contribute to COVID-19 severity as well as the risk of secondary bacterial infection.

On top of the changes to the epithelial barrier, transcriptome and proteome profiling of immune cells also reveal changes to their metabolism. One transcriptomic profile of PBMCs from COVID-19 patients showed increase in the oxidative phosphorylation pathway, likely implicating altered mitochondrial functions following SARS-CoV-2 infection (Gardinassi *et al.*, 2020). This change may be indicative of respiratory burst from immune cells to generate heightened levels of reactive oxygen species (ROS) to counter the infection (White *et al.*, 2005). However, overproduction of ROS may also damage the host and result in the pathology of COVID-19. Therefore, subsequent analyses should also focus on host metabolic changes to identify biomarkers that can discern COVID-19 severity.

10.5.3. *Modifications in cell death pathways*

Programmed cell death is an early physiological attempt at removing viral-infected cells (Fujikura and Miyazaki, 2018). However, viruses may also be leverage on cell death processes as a means of spreading to healthy cells in the infection site (Arora *et al.*, 2016). So far, three types of programmed cell death are identified, namely apoptosis, necroptosis and pyroptosis, each serving different purposes and playing different roles during viral infections (Fujikura and Miyazaki, 2018). While apoptosis serves to remove infected cells without releasing its cellular contents; necroptosis and pyroptosis burst and bloat the cells, respectively, triggering inflammatory responses that alert the immune system towards the infection site (Fujikura and Miyazaki, 2018; Robinson *et al.*, 2020; Silke *et al.*, 2015). Similar to inflammation, these processes are beneficial when induced at appropriate levels, but may be detrimental if prolonged or unchecked, culminating in tissue damage that contributes to the severity of infection.

Like any viral infection, SARS-CoV-2 infection triggers cell death of infected cells at the advanced stages of the infection. However, the levels of cell death appear to differ across the different regions of the airways. Studies using *in vitro* 3D cultures suggest that upper airway infection leads to minimal cell death events compared to lower and alveolar infection (Gamage *et al.*, 2020; Katsura *et al.*, 2020). Additionally, inflammatory cell death factors such as NLRP3 that trigger pyroptosis and the inflammasome, appear to be also subdued in the upper airway, consistent with findings of the low inflammation in the upper airway (Mick *et al.*, 2020). However, systemic profiling of COVID-19 patient blood and plasma samples showed sustained expression of apoptotic proteins (CASP8, TNFSF14, HGF, TGFB1) especially in severe COVID-19 patients, indicating potential tissue damage triggered by the infection events (Haljasmagi *et al.*, 2020). Hence, the study of cell death remains an important area of focus to define the pathogenic and tissue injury mechanisms of SARS-CoV-2 infection, particularly in severe COVID-19.

10.5.4. *Changes in cell cycle factors and transcription factors*

Along with cell death, levels of cell cycle and general transcription factors can also be altered in response to cellular stress such as during viral infection (Tan *et al.*, 2018b). These transcription factors constitute general stress factors that may modulate multiple physiologic processes in response to a stressor like SARS-CoV-2 infection. While not specific to infection, the changes in the levels of these factors regulate cell division, differentiation and physiologic processes in reaction to SARS-CoV-2 infection, but may also contribute to the clinical manifestations and pathology of COVID-19 if not properly regulated.

A key transcription pathway with many genes upregulated following SARS-CoV-2 infection is the Akt/mTOR/HIF-1a pathway (Appelberg *et al.*, 2020). This pathway activation may result in the activation of immune responses and immune environment to aid antiviral processes. In addition, the involvement of HIF-1a pathway is usually a response to hypoxic conditions likely to occur with SARS-CoV-2 infection, which may also trigger inflammatory responses as a consequence (Zhong *et al.*, 2020). In addition, FGF1, a growth factor involved in the cell cycle and inflammatory responses is also elevated in response to SARS-CoV-2 infection *in vitro* (Alsamman and Zayed, 2020). With the many transcriptomic and proteomic studies focusing on deciphering the immune responses against COVID-19, not much attention is paid to these general transcription factors since it is challenging to harness these factors as markers or treatment targets. Nevertheless, their roles during SARS-CoV-2 infection remain crucial for understanding the pathogenesis and pathologic mechanisms of COVID-19.

10.5.5. *Transcriptomics of microRNAs and non-coding RNAs*

Non-coding RNAs (ncRNAs) are RNAs that are not translated into proteins. A key group of ncRNAs, microRNAs (or miRNAs) are small RNAs of ~23 nucleotides that play vital roles in post-transcriptional regulation of physiologic processes (Tan *et al.*, 2014). In terms of a viral infection, miRNAs can be involved in all the processes elaborated in the previous sections, which will likely be similar in the context of SARS-CoV-2 infection. Profiling of miRNA via transcriptomics is important in the "omics" studies of COVID-19 since identification of the critical miRNAs and their targets may create avenues for diagnosing and/or preventing SARS-CoV-2 replication and COVID-19 pathology. It is also established that miRNAs are involved in the regeneration of the airway following viral infection (Tan *et al.*, 2014). Therefore, understanding the temporal miRNA expression during and after SARS-CoV-2 infection can facilitate the discovery of diagnostic and treatment targets across the various stages of COVID-19.

Following SARS-CoV-2 infection, pathways related to miRNA processing are increased, indicating miRNA activities as a response against the infection (Alsamman and Zayed, 2020). In a study of blood markers predicting the severity and prognosis of COVID-19 patients, the miRNAs of the let-7 family were delineated as extracellular miRNA predictors of severity and immune suppression (Chen *et al.*, 2020b). Another study identified long ncRNAs that may be involved in upstream regulation of SARS-CoV-2 responses (Vishnubalaji *et al.*, 2020). Currently, ncRNAs studies on SARS-CoV-2 infection and COVID-19 are still in their infancy — further investigations are warranted in future to complement the wealth of transcriptomic and proteomic studies, which will aid in target discovery for SARS-CoV-2 treatment.

10.6. Common Themes from "Omics" Analyses and their Links to Pathogenesis

With the myriad of "omics" data generated within the relatively short span following the discovery of SARS-CoV-2 in the year 2020, much of the information obtained sheds light on the potential pathways and mechanisms of the infection and COVID-19 pathology. In general, the current consensus from the transcriptomics and proteomics studies points to a suppressed immune response at the upper airway epithelium, with a delayed but enhanced response in the lower airway and lung epithelium. In contrast, there is an enhanced, uncontrolled expression of immune mediators and modulators at the level of professional immune cells. Moreover, there is a tendency of shunting the immune mediators towards the less efficient Th2 inflammation against viral infection, which may contribute to augmented mucus production and diminished ciliary markers likely through the modulation by IL-13. Furthermore, the expression of IL-13 may also be involved in enhancing the expression of the cell entry receptor ACE2 and TMPRSS2 for SARS-CoV-2 infection. These are coupled with the destruction and compromised function of the epithelial barrier and metabolism, which further contribute to the pathology of COVID-19. Finally, induction of stress-related transcription factors and miRNAs may also serve as modulators of COVID-19 pathology. With further verifications, findings from these studies will contribute to the discovery of diagnostic markers and treatment targets against SARS-CoV-2 infection, especially for patients with severe manifestations of COVID-19.

10.7. Application of "Omics" Findings to Clinical Settings

Transcriptomics and proteomics data have been exploited to reveal specific markers in various models following SARS-CoV-2 infection. The next steps are to leverage on these discovered markers, to verify them experimentally and clinically before they can be applied to benefit patients. In addition, the expression levels of these markers can also be evaluated for their modifications in patients with risk factors or conditions that increase susceptibility to SARS-CoV-2 infection and severe COVID-19. Some established predisposing factors include age, cardiovascular diseases, and metabolic disorders like diabetes mellitus (Guan *et al.*, 2020; Zhu *et al.*, 2020). Other conditions under investigation include chronic airway inflammatory diseases such as asthma and chronic obstructive pulmonary disease or COPD (Jacobs *et al.*, 2020; Murphy *et al.*, 2020), and smoking (Jacobs *et al.*, 2020; Rossato *et al.*, 2020). Information gained from these follow-up studies will have public health and clinical implications to improve the management of SARS-CoV-2 infection and COVID-19.

Moreover, a number of proteomic studies have analyzed the potential of specific proteins as treatment targets against SARS-CoV-2 infection

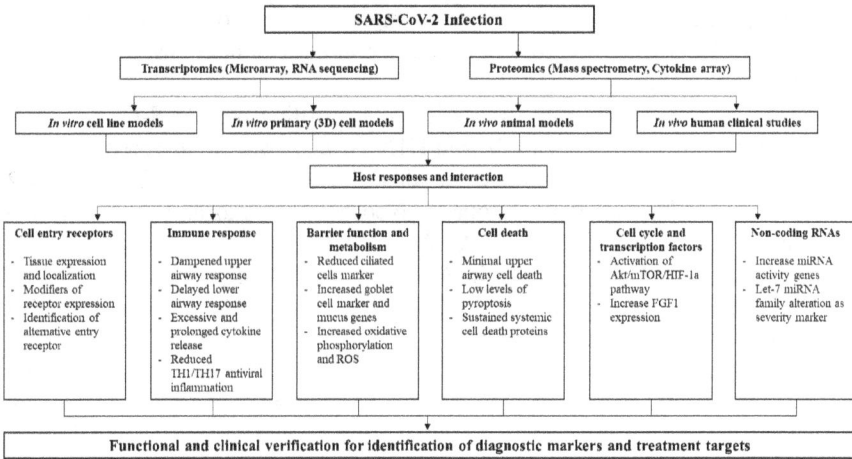

Figure 10.1. Applications of "omics" platforms to study host responses and interactions during SARS-CoV-2 infections.

(Chen *et al.*, 2020a; Gordon *et al.*, 2020; Li *et al.*, 2021). These targets can then be further tested experimentally in pre-clinical models, followed by lead optimization for the development of potential novel treatments especially for severe COVID-19, to complement the implementation of vaccine strategies.

10.8. Conclusion

As summarized in Figure 10.1, the application of "omics" platforms is vital for emerging viral infectious diseases such as COVID-19 to rapidly obtain a large amount of information that aids in the investigation of host–viral interactions which contribute to the transmission, pathogenesis, and severity of COVID-19. By critically analyzing the "omics" data in fine detail, the narrative on the pathology of SARS-CoV-2 infection and COVID-19 will accelerate future studies pertaining to the discovery and development of diagnostic biomarkers and treatment targets.

References

Abers MS *et al.* An immune-based biomarker signature is associated with mortality in COVID-19 patients. *JCI Insight* 2020; 6:e144455.

Ahmetaj-Shala B *et al.* Cardiorenal tissues express SARS-CoV-2 entry genes and Basigin (BSG/CD147) increases with age in endothelial cells. *JACC Basic Transl Sci* 2020; 5:1111–1123.

Alsamman AM, Zayed H. The transcriptomic profiling of SARS-CoV-2 compared to SARS, MERS, EBOV, and H1N1. *PLoS One* 2020; 15:e0243270.

Andonegui-Elguera S *et al.* Molecular alterations prompted by SARS-CoV-2 infection: Induction of hyaluronan, glycosaminoglycan and mucopolysaccharide metabolism. *Arch Med Res* 2020; 51:645–653.

Appelberg S *et al.* Dysregulation in Akt/mTOR/HIF-1 signaling identified by proteo-transcriptomics of SARS-CoV-2 infected cells. *Emerg Microbes Infect* 2020; 9:1748–1760.

Arora S *et al.* Influenza A virus enhances its propagation through the modulation of Annexin-A1 dependent endosomal trafficking and apoptosis. *Cell Death Differ* 2016; 23:1243–1256.

Blanco-Melo D *et al.* Imbalanced host response to SARS-CoV-2 drives development of COVID-19. *Cell* 2020; 181:1036–1045.e9.

Busnadiego I *et al.* Antiviral activity of Type I, II, and III interferons counterbalances ACE2 inducibility and restricts SARS-CoV-2. *mBio* 2020; 11: e01928–20.

Chen X *et al.* Immunomodulatory and antiviral activity of metformin and its potential implications in treating Coronavirus disease 2019 and lung injury. *Front Immunol* 2020a; 11:2056.

Chen YM *et al.* Blood molecular markers associated with COVID-19 immunopathology and multi-organ damage. *EMBO J* 2020b; 39:e105896.

Cleary SJ *et al.* Animal models of mechanisms of SARS-CoV-2 infection and COVID-19 pathology. *Br J Pharmacol* 2020; 177:4851–4865.

Fagone P *et al.* Transcriptional landscape of SARS-CoV-2 infection dismantles pathogenic pathways activated by the virus, proposes unique sex-specific differences and predicts tailored therapeutic strategies. *Autoimmun Rev* 2020; 19:102571.

Fu L *et al.* Clinical characteristics of Coronavirus disease 2019 (COVID-19) in China: A systematic review and meta-analysis. *J Infect* 2020; 80:656–665.

Fujikura D, Miyazaki T. Programmed cell death in the pathogenesis of influenza. *Int J Mol Sci* 2018; 19:2065.

Gamage AM *et al.* Infection of human Nasal Epithelial Cells with SARS-CoV-2 and a 382-nt deletion isolate lacking ORF8 reveals similar viral kinetics and host transcriptional profiles. *PLoS Pathog* 2020; 16:e1009130.

Gardinassi LG *et al.* Immune and metabolic signatures of COVID-19 revealed by transcriptomics data reuse. *Front Immunol* 2020; 11:1636.

Gill SE *et al.* Transcriptional profiling of leukocytes in critically ill COVID19 patients: Implications for interferon response and coagulation. *Intensive Care Med Exp* 2020; 8:75.

Gordon DE *et al*. A SARS-CoV-2 protein interaction map reveals targets for drug repurposing. *Nature* 2020; 583:459–468.

Grenga L, Armengaud J. Proteomics in the COVID-19 battlefield: First semester check-up. *Proteomics* 2020; 21:e2000198.

Guan WJ *et al*. Motile ciliary disorders in chronic airway inflammatory diseases: Critical target for interventions. *Curr Allergy Asthma Rep* 2018; 18:48.

Guan WJ *et al*. Clinical characteristics of Coronavirus disease 2019 in China. *N Engl J Med* 2020; 382:1708–1720.

Guo YR *et al*. The origin, transmission and clinical therapies on Coronavirus disease 2019 (COVID-19) outbreak — An update on the status. *Mil Med Res* 2020; 7:11.

Haljasmagi L *et al*. Longitudinal proteomic profiling reveals increased early inflammation and sustained apoptosis proteins in severe COVID-19. *Sci Rep* 2020; 10:20533.

Hu Y *et al*. Prevalence and severity of corona virus disease 2019 (COVID-19): A systematic review and meta-analysis. *J Clin Virol* 2020; 127:104371.

Huang C *et al*. Clinical features of patients infected with 2019 novel Coronavirus in Wuhan, China. *Lancet* 2020a; 395:497–506.

Huang J *et al*. SARS-CoV-2 infection of pluripotent stem cell-derived human lung alveolar Type 2 cells elicits a rapid epithelial-intrinsic inflammatory response. *Cell Stem Cell* 2020b; 27:962–973.

Huang ZQ *et al*. Interleukin-13 alters tight junction proteins expression thereby compromising barrier function and dampens rhinovirus induced immune responses in nasal epithelium. *Front Cell Dev Biol* 2020c; 8:572749.

Jacobs M *et al*. Increased expression of ACE2, the SARS-CoV-2 entry receptor, in alveolar and bronchial epithelium of smokers and COPD subjects. *Eur Respir* J 2020; 56:2002378.

Karakurt HU, Pir P. Integration of transcriptomic profile of SARS-CoV-2 infected normal human bronchial epithelial cells with metabolic and protein-protein interaction networks. *Turk J Biol* 2020; 44:168–177.

Katsura H *et al*. Human lung stem cell-based alveolospheres provide insights into SARS-CoV-2-mediated interferon responses and pneumocyte dysfunction. *Cell Stem Cell* 2020; 27:890–904.

Li J *et al*. Virus-host interactome and proteomic survey reveal potential virulence factors influencing SARS-CoV-2 pathogenesis. *Med (NY)* 2020a; 2:99–112.

Li Q *et al*. Early transmission dynamics in Wuhan, China, of novel Coronavirus–infected pneumonia. *N Engl J Med* 2020b; 382:1199–1207.

Li G *et al*. Transcriptomic signatures and repurposing drugs for COVID-19 patients: Findings of bioinformatics analyses. *Comput Struct Biotechnol J* 2021; 19:1–15.

Liao M *et al*. Single-cell landscape of bronchoalveolar immune cells in patients with COVID-19. *Nat Med* 2020; 26, 842–844.

Liu J *et al*. Role of IL-13Ralpha2 in modulating IL-13-induced MUC5AC and ciliary changes in healthy and CRSwNP mucosa. *Allergy* 2018; 73: 1673–1685.

Liu Y *et al*. Mucus production stimulated by IFN-AhR signaling triggers hypoxia of COVID-19. *Cell Res* 2020a; 30:1078–1087.

Liu Y *et al*. Expression pattern of the SARS-CoV-2 entry genes ACE2 and TMPRSS2 in the respiratory tract. *Viruses* 2020b; 12:1174.

Lu W *et al*. Elevated MUC1 and MUC5AC mucin protein levels in airway mucus of critical ill COVID-19 patients. *J Med Virol* 2020; 93:582–584.

Luukkainen A *et al*. A co-culture model of PBMC and stem cell derived human nasal epithelium reveals rapid activation of NK and innate T cells upon Influenza A virus infection of the nasal epithelium. *Front Immunol* 2018; 9:2514.

Meckiff BJ *et al*. Imbalance of regulatory and cytotoxic SARS-CoV-2-reactive CD4(+) T cells in COVID-19. *Cell* 2020; 183:1340–1353.

Mick E *et al*. Upper airway gene expression reveals suppressed immune responses to SARS-CoV-2 compared with other respiratory viruses. *Nat Commun* 2020; 11:5854.

Murphy RC *et al*. Effects of asthma and human rhinovirus A16 on the expression of SARS-CoV-2 entry factors in human airway epithelium. *Am J Respir Cell Mol Biol* 2020; 63:859–863.

Nunnari G *et al*. Network perturbation analysis in human bronchial epithelial cells following SARS-CoV2 infection. *Exp Cell Res* 2020; 395:112204.

Park JH, Lee HK. Re-analysis of single cell transcriptome reveals that the NR3C1-CXCL8-neutrophil axis determines the severity of COVID-19. *Front Immunol* 2020; 11:2145.

Parrot T *et al*. MAIT cell activation and dynamics associated with COVID-19 disease severity. *Sci Immunol* 2020; 5:eabe1670.

Pizzorno A *et al*. Characterization and treatment of SARS-CoV-2 in nasal and bronchial human airway epithelia. *Cell Rep Med* 2020; 1:100059.

Qiao Y *et al*. CD151, a novel host factor of nuclear export signaling in influenza virus infection. *J Allergy Clin Immunol* 2018; 141:1799–1817.

Robinson KS *et al*. Enteroviral 3C protease activates the human NLRP1 inflammasome in airway epithelia. *Science* 2020; 370:eaay2002.

Rossato M *et al*. Current smoking is not associated with COVID-19. *Eur Respir J* 2020; 55:2001290.

Ryabkova VA *et al*. Influenza infection, SARS, MERS and COVID-19: Cytokine storm — The common denominator and the lessons to be learned. *Clin Immunol* 2020; 223:108652.

Sadanandam A *et al*. A blood transcriptome-based analysis of disease progression, immune regulation, and symptoms in Coronavirus-infected patients. *Cell Death Discov* 2020; 6:141.

Saffern M. ACE2 is not induced by interferon. *Nat Rev Immunol* 2020; 20:521.

Sajuthi SP *et al*. Type 2 and interferon inflammation regulate SARS-CoV-2 entry factor expression in the airway epithelium. *Nat Commun* 2020; 11:5139.

Shaath H, Alajez NM. Computational and transcriptome analyses revealed preferential induction of chemotaxis and lipid synthesis by SARS-CoV-2. *Biology* (Basel) 2020; 9:260.

Shaath H *et al*. Single-cell transcriptome analysis highlights a role for neutrophils and inflammatory macrophages in the pathogenesis of severe COVID-19. *Cells* 2020; 9:2374.

Silke J *et al*. The diverse role of RIP kinases in necroptosis and inflammation. *Nat Immunol* 2015; 16:689–697.

Tan KS *et al*. Micro-RNAs in regenerating lungs: An integrative systems biology analysis of murine influenza pneumonia. *BMC Genomics* 2014; 15:587.

Tan KS *et al*. Impact of respiratory virus infections in exacerbation of acute and chronic rhinosinusitis. *Curr Allergy Asthma Rep* 2017; 17:24.

Tan KS *et al*. In vitro model of fully differentiated human nasal epithelial cells infected with rhinovirus reveals epithelium-initiated immune responses. *J Infect Dis* 2018a; 217:906–915.

Tan KS *et al*. Comparative transcriptomic and metagenomic analyses of influenza virus-infected nasal epithelial cells from multiple individuals reveal specific nasal-initiated signatures. *Front Microbiol* 2018b; 9:2685.

Tan KS *et al*. RNA sequencing of H3N2 influenza virus-infected human nasal epithelial cells from multiple subjects reveals molecular pathways associated with tissue injury and complications. *Cells* 2019; 8:986.

Tan KS *et al*. Respiratory viral infections in exacerbation of chronic airway inflammatory diseases: Novel mechanisms and insights from the upper airway epithelium. *Front Cell Dev Biol* 2020; 8:99.

Tian T *et al*. H3N2 influenza virus infection enhances oncostatin M expression in human nasal epithelium. *Exp Cell Res* 2018; 371:322–329.

van Wilgenburg B *et al*. MAIT cells contribute to protection against lethal influenza infection in vivo. *Nat Commun* 2018; 9:4706.

Vaz de Paula CB *et al*. IL-4/IL-13 remodeling pathway of COVID-19 lung injury. *Sci Rep* 2020; 10:18689.

Vishnubalaji R *et al*. Protein coding and long noncoding RNA (lncRNA) transcriptional landscape in SARS-CoV-2 infected bronchial epithelial cells highlight a role for interferon and inflammatory response. *Genes (Basel)* 2020; 11:760.

Vitte J *et al*. A granulocytic signature identifies COVID-19 and its severity. *J Infect Dis* 2020; 222:1985–1996.

Wang J *et al*. Excessive neutrophils and neutrophil extracellular traps in COVID-19. *Front Immunol* 2020a; 11:2063.

Wang P *et al*. A cross-talk between epithelium and endothelium mediates human alveolar-capillary injury during SARS-CoV-2 infection. *Cell Death Dis* 2020b; 11:1042.

White MR *et al*. Respiratory innate immune proteins differentially modulate the neutrophil respiratory burst response to influenza A virus. *Am J Physiol Lung Cell Mol Physiol* 2005; 289:L606–L616.

Winkler ES *et al*. SARS-CoV-2 infection of human ACE2-transgenic mice causes severe lung inflammation and impaired function. *Nat Immunol* 2020; 21:1327–1335.

Wu B *et al*. Single-cell sequencing of glioblastoma reveals central nervous system susceptibility to SARS-CoV-2. *Front Oncol* 2020a; 10:566599.

Wu M *et al*. Transcriptional and proteomic insights into the host response in fatal COVID-19 cases. *Proc Natl Acad Sci USA* 2020b; 117:28336–28343.

Xiong Y *et al*. Transcriptomic characteristics of bronchoalveolar lavage fluid and peripheral blood mononuclear cells in COVID-19 patients. *Emerg Microbes Infect* 2020; 9:761–770.

Yan Y *et al*. Human nasal epithelial cells derived from multiple individuals exhibit differential responses to H3N2 influenza virus infection in vitro. *J Allergy Clin Immunol* 2016; 138:276–281.

Zhao XN *et al*. The use of nasal epithelial stem/progenitor cells to produce functioning ciliated cells in vitro. *Am J Rhinol Allergy* 2012; 26:345–350.

Zhong B *et al*. Hypoxia-induced factor-1alpha induces NLRP3 expression by M1 macrophages in noneosinophilic chronic rhinosinusitis with nasal polyps. *Allergy* 2020; 76:582–586.

Zhou Z *et al*. Heightened innate immune responses in the respiratory tract of COVID-19 patients. *Cell Host Microbe* 2020; 27:883–890.

Zhu N *et al*. A novel Coronavirus from patients with pneumonia in China, 2019. *N Engl J Med* 2020; 382:727–733.

Ziegler *et al*. SARS-CoV-2 receptor ACE2 is an interferon-stimulated gene in human airway epithelial cells and is detected in specific cell subsets across tissues. *Cell* 2020; 181:1016–1035.

Index